Nitric Oxide and Endothelin in the Pathogenesis of Glaucoma

Editor

Ivan O. Haefliger, M.D.
Head, Laboratory of Ocular Pharmacology and Physiology
Department of Ophthalmology
School of Medicine
University of Basel
Basel, Switzerland

Co-Editor

Josef Flammer, M.D.
Head, Department of Ophthalmology
School of Medicine
University of Basel
Basel, Switzerland

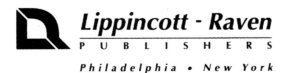

Lippincott - Raven
P U B L I S H E R S
Philadelphia • New York

Printed in Belgium

9 8 7 6 5 4 3 2 1

Library of Congress Cataloging-in-Publication Data

Nitric oxide and endothelin in the pathogenesis of glaucoma/editor,
 Ivan O. Haefliger, co-editor, Josef Flammer.
  p. cm.
 Includes bibliographical references and index.
 ISBN 0-781-71600-4
  1. Glaucoma—Pathogenesis. 2. Nitric oxide—Pathophysiology.
 3. Endothelins—Pathophysiology. I. Haefliger, Ivan O.
 II. Flammer, J. (Josef)
  [DNLM: 1. Glaucoma—physiopathology. 2. Glaucoma—therapy.
 3. Nitric Oxide—physiology. 4. Endothelins—physiology.   WW 290
 N731 1998]
 RE871.N54   1998
 617.7′4107—dc21
 DNLM/DLC
 for Library of Congress   98-34799
                                                                                              CIP

Contents

Glaucoma Therapy

Contributors

Albert Alm, M.D.   *Department of Ophthalmology, University Hospital, Uppsala University, S-751 85 Uppsala, Sweden*

Douglas R. Anderson, M.D.   *Department of Ophthalmology, Bascom Palmer Eye Institute, University of Miami School of Medicine, Miami, Florida 33101-6880*

David R. Bacon, M.D.   *Ocular Microcirculation Unit, Devers Eye Institute; R.S. Dow Neurological Science Institute, Legacy Portland Hospital, Portland, Oregon 97210*

Claude Bonne, Ph.D.   *Laboratoire de Physiologie Cellulaire. Université de Montpellier, F-34 060 Montpellier, France*

Evrydiki A. Bouzas, M.D.   *Neuro-ophthalmology Unit, Neurology Department, Athens University, Athens, Greece*

George A. Cioffi, M.D.   *Ocular Microcirculation Unit, Devers Eye Institute; R.S. Dow Neurological Science Institute, Legacy Portland Hospital, Portland, Oregon 97210*

Eike S. Dettmann, Ph.D. (cand.)   *Laboratory for Ocular Pharmacology and Physiology, Department of Ophthalmology, School of Medicine, University of Basel, 4012 Basel, Switzerland*

Guy Donati, M.D.   *Department of Clinical Neurosciences, University Eye Department, Geneva University Hospital, 1211 Geneva 14, Switzerland*

H. Ferdinand A. Duijm, M.D.   *Glaucoma Center of the University of Amsterdam, Academic Medical Center, 1100 DE Amsterdam, The Netherlands*

Dorette Ellis, Ph.D.   *Department of Neurology, Harvard Medical School; Neuropharmacology Research Laboratory, Massachusetts General Hospital, Charlestown, Massachusetts 02129*

Erich F. Elstner, Ph.D.   *Lehrstuhl für Phytopathologie, Technische Universität München, 85350 Freising, Weihenstephan, Germany*

Josef Flammer, M.D.   *Department of Ophthalmology, School of Medicine, University of Basel, 4012 Basel, Switzerland*

Andreas Gass, M.D.   *Department of Ophthalmology, School of Medicine, University of Basel, 4012 Basel, Switzerland*

Paul Gasser, M.D. *Department of Ophthalmology, School of Medicine, University of Basel, 4012 Basel, Switzerland*

H. Caroline Geijssen, M.D. *Glaucoma Center of the University of Amsterdam, Academic Medical Center, 1100 DE Amsterdam, The Netherlands*

Erik L. Greve, M.D. *Glaucoma Center of the University of Amsterdam, Academic Medical Center, 1100 DE Amsterdam, The Netherlands*

Walter E. Haefeli, M.D. *Division of Clinical Pharmacology, Departments of Internal Medicine and Pharmacy, University Hospital, CH-4031 Basel, Switzerland*

Ivan O. Haefliger, M.D. *Laboratory for Ocular Pharmacology and Physiology, Department of Medicine, School of Medicine, University of Basel, 4012 Basel, Switzerland*

Roger A. Hitchings, M.D. *Glaucoma Service, Moorfields Eye Hospital, London EC1 2PD, England*

Satoshi Kashii, M.D., Ph.D. *Department of Ophthalmology and Visual Sciences, Graduate School of Medicine, Kyoto University, Kyoto 606, Japan*

Günter K. Krieglstein, M.D. *Universitäts-Augenklinik, D-50924 Köln, Germany*

Lilly Linder, M.D. *Division of Clinical Pharmacology, Department of Internal Medicine, University Hospital, CH-4031 Basel, Switzerland*

Elke Lütjen-Drecoll, M.D. *Department of Anatomy, University of Erlangen-Nürnberg, D-91054 Erlangen, Germany*

Denis Monard, Ph.D. *Friedrich Miescher Institut, CH-4002 Basel, Switzerland*

Agnes Muller, Ph.D. *Laboratoire de Physiologie Cellulaire, Université de Montpellier, F-34 060 Montpellier, France*

James Nathanson, M.D. *Department of Neurology, Harvard Medical School; Neuropharmacology Research Laboratory, Massachusetts General Hospital, Charlestown, Massachusetts 02129*

Selim Orgül, M.D. *Department of Medicine, School of Medicine, University of Basel, 4012 Basel, Switzerland*

Lutz E. Pillunat, M.D. *Universitäts Augenklinik und Poliklinik, D-20246 Hamburg, Germany*

Constantin J. Pournaras, M.D. *Department of Clinical Neurosciences, University Eye Department, Geneva University Hospital, 1211 Geneva 14, Switzerland*

Charles E. Riva, D.Sc. *Institut de Recherche en Ophtalmologie, 1950 Sion, Switzerland*

Silvana C. Romerio, M.D. *Division of Clinical Pharmacology, Department of Internal Medicine, University Hospital, CH-4031 Basel, Switzerland; Department of Ophthalmology, School of Medicine, University of Basel, 4012 Basel, Switzerland*

Harold Schempp, Ph.D. *Lehrstuhl für Phytopathologie, Technische Universität München 85350 Freising, Weihenstephan, Germany*

Ernst R. Tamm, M.D. *Laboratory of Molecular and Developmental Biology, National Eye Institute, National Institutes of Health, Bethesda, Maryland 20892*

E. Michael Van Buskirk, M.D. *Ocular Microcirculation Unit, Devers Eye Institute; R.S. Dow Neurological Science Institute, Legacy Portland Hospital, Portland, Oregon 97210*

Michael Wiederholt, M.D. *Institut für Klinische Physiologie, Universitätsklinikum Benjamin Franklin, Freie Universität Berlin, 12200 Berlin, Germany*

Preface

Recently, major progress has been made in the pathophysiology, clinical approach, and treatment of glaucoma. In this regard, nitric oxide (NO) and endothelin appear to play a major role in the regulation of the intraocular pressure, the control of ocular blood flow, and, in the case of NO, the loss of retinal ganglion cells by apoptosis. These three fundamental aspects are generally considered to be involved in the pathogenesis of glaucoma.

This book is intended primarily for glaucomatologists and general ophthalmologists who do not necessarily have a strong background in basic science but would like to stay in touch with the latest developments in research influencing clinical care of glaucoma patients. Basic researchers as well as pharmacologists also will find essential relationships between fundamental aspects of research on NO and endothelin implemented in a clinical context.

Therefore, this book should fulfill the expectations of both clinicians and scientists interested in NO, endothelin, and the care of glaucoma patients.

Ivan O. Haefliger, M.D.
Josef Flammer, M.D.

Acknowledgments

The editors thank the Association for Continuing Education in Ophthalmology, who made possible the publication of this book and the organization of the Glaucoma Meeting in Basel (Switzerland), on March 21 and 22, 1997, under the main theme ''Role of NO and Endothelin in the Pathogenesis of Glaucoma.'' In particular, the editors acknowledge Daniela Stümpfig, Elisabeth Meier, Birgitta Henzi, Phillip Hendrickson, Hedwig Kaiser, Selim Orgül, Christian Prünte, and Carl Erb for their valuable help.

Nitric Oxide and Endothelin in the Pathogenesis of Glaucoma, edited by I. O. Haefliger and J. Flammer. Lippincott–Raven Publishers, Philadelphia © 1998.

1

Risk Factors in Glaucoma

Erik L. Greve, H. Ferdinand A. Duijm, and H. Caroline Geijssen

Glaucoma Center of the University of Amsterdam, Academic Medical Center, Amsterdam, The Netherlands

To discuss risk factors in glaucoma, we first must define the disease. The common feature in all glaucomas is optic neuropathy. This is usually a typical optic neuropathy, characterized by excavation and visual field defect of the nerve fiber bundle type. Here we arrive immediately at the limitations of the definition. There is no such thing as *the* glaucomatous excavation. There are different types of excavations in different types of glaucoma patients. There are also different types of visual field defects. There is the entire spectrum of glaucomatous disease ranging from acute angle-closure glaucoma and the secondary open-angle glaucomas to primary open-angle and normal pressure glaucoma.

This chapter is limited to primary open-angle glaucoma, including normal pressure glaucoma. Even with this limitation there is a wide variety of presentations among glaucoma patients. They may be young or old, healthy or sick, and they may have high intraocular pressures or normal intraocular pressures. At one end of the spectrum is the young, healthy patient with high intraocular pressures, sometimes called late congenital glaucoma. At the other end of the spectrum are the patients with normal-pressure glaucoma, usually old and with systemic vascular disease e.g., in so-called senile sclerotic glaucoma (16).

The best definition of glaucoma probably is a typical optic neuropathy leading ultimately to blindness. However, the causes of this optic neuropathy may be quite variable. Glaucoma is usually considered a multifactorial disease. The factors that increase the chance for development of glaucomatous optic neuropathy are the risk factors.

RELEVANCE OF INTRAOCULAR PRESSURE MEASUREMENT

It should be emphasized that the applanation intraocular pressure (IOP) measurement is not as reliable a part of risk factor management as many believe it is. The fact that it is a simple method that provides a simple number does not give it the magic quantitative value that is so often attached to it. The problem with IOP measurements is the value of a pressure measurement in the individual patient. There is a wide range of IOP in the normal population. Within this normal range, the upper end of the IOP spectrum (20 mm Hg) may be twice as high as the lower end of the spectrum (10 mm Hg). Both represent statistically normal pressures. This means, for example, that an IOP of 20 mm Hg, within the normal range, can represent either completely normal IOP for a given patient or a pressure that is 10 mm Hg higher than the patient's original IOP of 10 mm Hg, i.e., double the original pressure. Therefore, although an individual IOP measurement can be obtained in each patient, there is no way to determine how far this IOP level has changed from the patient's original normal pressure. Although statistics indicate that pressures above 24 mm Hg are rare in the normal population, an IOP of 26 mm Hg could be either slightly elevated or extremely high, depending on the individual patient. This wide range of normal IOP makes it difficult to assess from a pressure measurement alone the impact of IOP on the pathogenesis of glaucomatous disease in the individual patient. There are many patients who have run pressures of 25 mm Hg or higher for periods of 10 or more years without any change in the optic disc. There are also normal-pressure glaucoma patients with IOP in the range of 15 mm Hg who have developed severe glaucomatous damage. It is obvious that more than IOP measurements is needed to classify the open-angle glaucomas according to pathogenesis.

OTHER RISK FACTORS

The IOP is the best-known risk factor. However, it is clear that the IOP cannot in itself explain quite a number of glaucomatous optic neuropathies. There must be other factors as well. Well-known risk factors include age (possibly due to the reduced number of nerve fibers or to age-related changes in the supporting structures of the optic disc or blood supply), family history, genetic disposition, race, and myopia. A person from a family with glaucoma has a higher chance of developing glaucoma. Primary open-angle glaucomas and normal-pressure glaucomas may run in the same family. Among the black population, glaucoma appears at an earlier age and with greater severity. Myopia is a serious risk factor for progression of glaucoma. Patients with the combination of glaucoma and myopia have more vision-threatening visual field defects and a higher progression rate.

The second major risk factor after IOP is the vascular risk factor. There is abundant evidence that vascular risk factors play a role in the pathogenesis of glaucoma, particularly in normal pressure glaucoma. Furthermore, the only risk factors that can be measured are IOP and blood flow-related factors. It is not possible to measure the impact of myopia, anatomic, structural, and chemical changes and differences in the individual optic nerve. Vascular risk factors can be subdivided into systemic and local vascular risk factors.

Systemic Vascular Risk Factors

It has been demonstrated that in up to 70% of normal pressure glaucomas cardiovascular or cerebrovascular systemic risk factors are present (15).

Systemic Blood Pressure

Both high and low systemic blood pressure have been incriminated as risk factors in glaucoma. There is a borderline relationship between high systemic blood pressure and glaucomatous disease. A clearer relationship exists between perfusion pressure and glaucomatous disease (40). Low blood pressure has also been linked to glaucoma. In particular, episodes of nocturnal hypotension have been shown to be involved in the progression of at least some glaucoma patients. Glaucoma patients have more episodes of nocturnal hypotension than healthy control subjects. In glaucoma patients treated for systemic hypertension, progression is related to nocturnal episodes of hypotension (3,4,19,20,22).

Migraine and the Vasospastic Syndrome

Research groups in Basel and Vancouver have paid particular attention to the vasospastic syndrome (8,12,14,17). They have proposed that the vasospasms in the eye are part of a syndrome that is active in the whole body and that can, for example, be demonstrated in the small fingernail vessels. Migraine was frequently found in patients with normal-pressure glaucoma.

Silent myocardial ischemia and cerebral ischemia are more common in patients with normal-pressure glaucoma than in control groups (43). Normal-pressure glaucoma patients with headaches have lower IOP than those without headaches (31).

These findings suggest that for at least some patients with glaucoma and particularly for those with normal-pressure glaucoma, vasospasm may play a role in the pathogenesis. The important lesson from these studies is that some normal-pressure glaucoma patients have vasospasms and that these vasospasms may respond favorably to treatment. However, the patients with vasospasm must be identified. It is also of interest that reversible vasospasm can be demonstrated after inhalation of carbon dioxide (see below).

From all these data on systemic vascular risk factors, it appears that many glaucoma patients do not have a healthy vascular system. It has been suggested that glaucoma in these patients may represent part of a general vascular disease. This may be true for at least a certain group of patients with glaucoma, whereas different factors, or a combination of factors, may play a role in other groups.

Local Vascular Risk Factors

The history of local vascular risk factors is a long one. Bjerrum, in the beginning of this century, demonstrated the presence of disc hemorrhages and their relationship with glaucoma. A hemorrhage is an important local vascular risk factor that can be seen by any ophthalmologist with an ophthalmoscope.

Over the years, several other ophthalmoscopically visible risk factors have been added: peripapillary atrophy, choroidal sclerosis, and local peripapillary vasoconstrictions (35). A relationship between hemorrhages (21), peripapillary atrophy (1), and choroidal sclerosis (15) and progression of glaucomatous disease has been established. Therefore, it is clear that the presence of such a *local* vascular risk factor, easily diagnosed by the ophthalmologist, has an impact on management of the glaucoma patient. The only *systemic* vascular risk factor for which a relationship with progression has been established is an episode of nocturnal hypotension.

TYPES OF NORMAL PRESSURE GLAUCOMA

The concept of vascular risk factors is also demonstrated in the different types of normal pressure glaucoma patients. The differentiation of these types is based on the aspect of the excavation. We have suggested that the concentric enlargement type of disc is mostly present in pressure-related glaucomas (Fig. 1). The

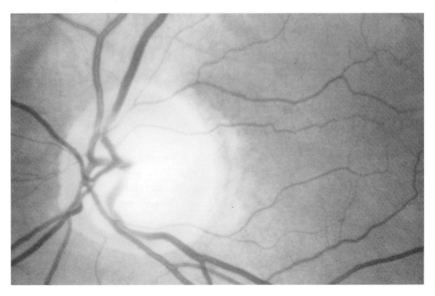

FIG. 1. Concentric enlargement of the excavation in "pressure-related" miscellaneous glaucoma types.

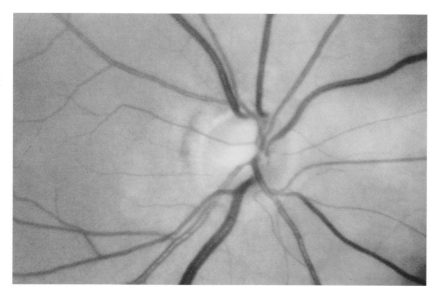

FIG. 2. Excavation in focal "ischemic" normal pressure glaucoma. Typical focal notch with corresponding nerve fiber layer defect and visual field defect.

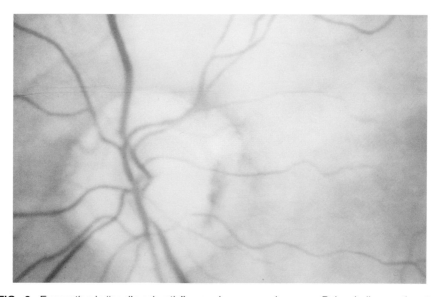

FIG. 3. Excavation in "senile sclerotic" normal pressure glaucoma. Pale, shallow moth-eaten excavation, peripapillary atrophy, and choroidal sclerosis.

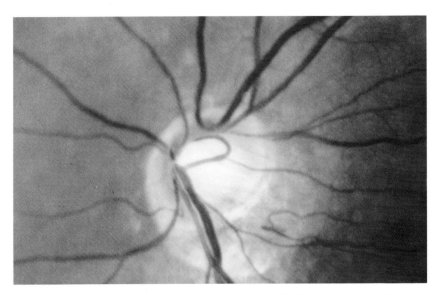

FIG. 4. Excavation in myopic normal pressure glaucoma. Shallow excavation with nasal su-pertraction and peripapillary atrophy.

vascular types of glaucomas include the focal ischemic type (Fig. 2) and the senile sclerotic type (Fig. 3). Vascular factors probably also play a role in myopic glaucoma (Fig. 4). Decreased blood flow has been demonstrated in senile sclerotic glaucoma (27). A relationship between focal ischemic glaucoma and vasospasm has been demonstrated (2). Reduced blood flow–related factors have also been demonstrated in myopia (13). Therefore, it is possible that focal ischemic normal-pressure glaucoma is related to the vasospastic syndrome and that that senile sclerotic glaucoma is the expression of a more generalized vascular sclerosis, whereas myopic normal pressure glaucoma is particularly the result of a locally compromised blood supply in the posterior part of the eye. In myopia, other non-blood flow–related structural factors may also play a role. Findings in these subgroups demonstrate not only that vascular risk factors play an important role in normal-pressure glaucoma but that different types of vascular risk factors may act in the different subgroups of normal pressure glaucoma, requiring different diagnostic and therapeutic approaches.

QUANTITATIVE BLOOD FLOW MEASUREMENTS

The above-mentioned local vascular risk factors are qualitative risk factors. In recent years, many investigations have been devoted to the development of methods that can quantitatively measure the blood flow–related factors in or around the optic nerve. These methods are listed in Table 1 (5,6,9–11,18,24–

TABLE 1. *Selected methods for quantitative assessment of ocular blood flow*

(Scanning laser) angiography
Laser Doppler velocimetry/flowmetry
Scanning laser Doppler flowmetry
Blue field entoptic simulation
Pulsatile ocular blood flow measurements
Oculo-oscillo dynamography
Color Doppler imaging

26,34,36,37,39,42,44,45). These methods differ regarding the aspect of blood flow (if at all) that is measured and the location and area in the eye at which the measurement is performed. Methods range from measurement of pulsations and dye dilution curves to laser Doppler measurements. None of these techniques can achieve a true blood flow measurement. Some methods measure the retinal vasculature, others the choroidal vasculature. Some methods claim to measure the entire choroid, some part of the choroid, and others the retrobulbar vessels. Thus far there are few data on the relationships among the different methods for the measurement of blood flow–related factors. To our knowledge, there are also no measurements on the importance of these vascular risk factors for progression of the disease in a long-term follow-up study. Although each of these methods measures different aspects of ocular blood flow–related factors, they have one common finding: there is a reduced blood flow in many glaucoma patients and in up to 50% of normal pressure glaucoma patients.

Because there is more disturbed blood flow in normal-pressure glaucoma compared to high-pressure glaucoma it is unlikely that this is secondary to elevated IOP. It is more likely that it is caused by a general or local primary vascular disease. In asymmetric glaucoma, reduction of blood flow–related factors is usually more pronounced in the more damaged eye (7,29).

SCANNING LASER ANGIOGRAPHY OF THE RETINAL VESSELS AND PERIPAPILLARY CHOROID

Using the scanning laser ophthalmoscope, image analysis, and sophisticated software, we have developed a method for the quantitative measurement of arteriovenous passage time (AVPT) and choroidal blood refreshment time (BRT). The method is based on the well-known pinciples of fluorescein angiography. It allows simultaneous quantitative evaluation of retinal and choroidal blood flow–related factors. In animal experiments, a satisfactory correlation between blood flow measurements obtained from scanning laser angiography of the peripapillary choroid and labeled microspheres was demonstrated (9). The area of measurement is indicated in Fig. 5. Retinal AVPT and choroidal BRT are illustrated in Fig. 6. We have shown that a reduced choroidal BRT is present in about 30% of our primary open-angle glaucoma patients and in 50% of our patients with normal pressure glaucoma (10). In contrast, the retinal AVPT was prolonged, particularly in the primary open-angle glaucoma patients and more so than in the normal-pressure glaucoma patients (11). This indicates that the choroidal and retinal vascular systems behave differently in these types of glaucoma patients. It may be that the retinal measurements are more pressure-related, whereas the choroidal measurements have a better relationship to primary vascular disease.

The findings on retinal AVPT and choroidal BRT can be divided into three clusters (Fig. 7): cluster 1 with a normal retinal AVPT and a normal choroidal BRT, cluster 2 with a normal retinal AVPT and a slow choroidal BRT, and cluster 3 with a normal retinal AVPT and a slow choroidal BRT. Cluster 2

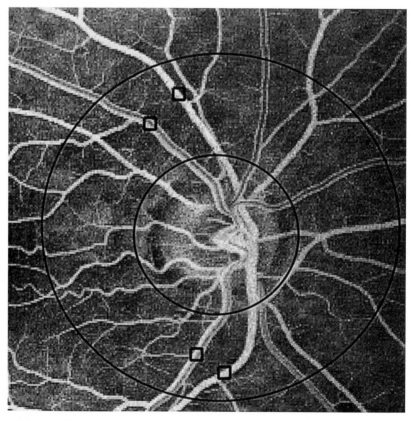

FIG. 5. Peripapillary choroid between two circles and pairs of locations on arteries and veins for the measurement of choroidal blood refreshment time and retinal arteriovenous passage time.

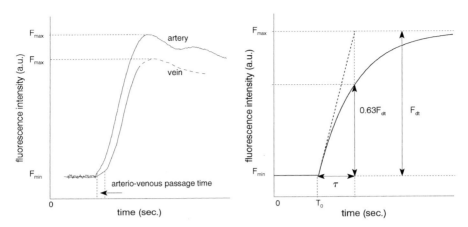

FIG. 6. Measurement principle of retinal (*left*) arteriovenous passage time and (*right*) choroidal blood refreshment time (τ).

includes the majority of NPG patients, whereas in cluster 3 mostly POAG patients are represented.

It was found that the well-known local risk factors; peripapillary atrophy and myopic discs, are correlated with cluster 2, i.e., with prolonged choroidal BRT, and not with cluster 3, i.e., the prolonged retinal findings. Not only is choroidal BRT particularly affected in NPG but it also is related to PPA and myopia. PPA

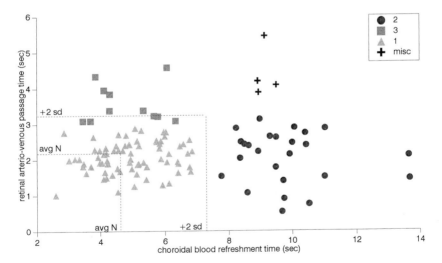

FIG. 7. Retinal arteriovenous passage time vs. choroidal blood refreshment time. Three clusters can be identified: △ with normal RAVP time and normal CBR time; ● with normal RAVP time and slow CBR time (almost all NPG); and ■ with slow RAVP time and normal CBR time (almost all POAG).

is a local vascular risk factor more evident in NPG than in POAG, more related to vascular disease than to IOP, and also correlated with progression, and so is myopia.

PRESSURE VERSUS VASCULAR RISK FACTORS

It is clear that pressure factors play a major role in some patients with glaucoma, whereas in others it appears that vascular factors are the major culprit. Between these two extremes there is an entire range of possible ratios between pressure and vascular involvement. It will be extremely interesting to know the extent of pressure involvement and of vascular involvement in the individual patient. We need more experience with the relative significance of IOP measurements on the one hand and blood flow-related measurements on the other hand. Once we know more about this pressure/blood flow ratio we could base our management of individual patients on these data. We have suggested that the choroidal measurements (and possibly also measurements in the posterior cilliary arteries) have a more direct relationship to primary vascular disease than measurements in the retinal system. This concept, of course, requires validation. If it is true, this might be another approach to establishment of a pressure/vascular ratio.

CAN BLOOD FLOW BE IMPROVED?

Improvement of blood flow–related factors has been demonstrated by two approaches. Several studies with different techniques have shown that blood flow–related factors may improve after successful surgical reduction of IOP (41). This shows the impact of perfusion pressure.

It has been demonstrated in two studies that inhalation of carbon dioxide may improve bloodflow in suitable patients (18,33). One group of investigators has also suggested that this improvement in blood flow is accompanied by an improvement in the visual field (32,33). Again, the importance of these findings is that evidently there is the possibility of improvement of blood flow, even irrespective of IOP lowering, and thus of improving the prognosis of our patients. It has been proposed to use the method of carbon dioxide inhalation for selection of those patients who may have a postive response to vasodilatation.

BLOOD FLOW AND MANAGEMENT
OF THE GLAUCOMA PATIENT

This brings us to the practical question of whether the concept of vascular risk factors is useful for daily management of the glaucoma patient. This potential usefulness can be divided into the usefulness in terms of the risk factor score and usefulness in terms of treatment. We incorporate in our decision-making process the presence or absence of vascular risk factors. For example, the presence of a disc hemorrhage or peripapillary atrophy may lead to earlier or more vigorous treatment. The presence of a reduced choroidal blood refreshment rate, as measured with the SLO technique, may lead us to search for low IOP. Particularly in normal-pressure glaucoma patients, these low pressures can usually be obtained by filtering surgery. The presence of myopia in combination with other risk factors may lead us to opt for earlier surgery. Therefore, the search for and the quantitative measurements of vascular risk factors are of primary importance for the decision-making process in management of the glaucoma patient. As already indicated, the relative importance of pressure and vascular risk factors may be decisive for the therapeutic approach. In that case, we should have more than one option for treatment, i.e., more than merely reduction of IOP.

BLOOD FLOW AND TREATMENT

Long-term improvement of blood flow other than reduction of IOP has been the object of several studies (23,28,32). The results are still controversial. It appears that the major reason for the difference in results lies in the selection process. Patients entering a study on blood flow improvement should clearly have a reduced blood flow, i.e., quantitative blood flow measurement should be included in the study. As indicated earlier, the majority of POAG patients and half of the NPG patients do not have reduced local hemodynamics. Effects of blood flow-improving medication are not to be expected in these patients. Proper selection of the patients is therefore vital. Such selection procedures might include a demonstration of short-term reversibility after CO_2 inhalation. Positive results have been described for calcium-channel blockers and magnesium. No doubt the near future will tell us which patients will react positively to which type of medication. Medical blood flow improvement will undoubtedly be part of the therapeutic armamentarium in the fight against progression of glaucomatous damage.

REFERENCES

1. Araie M, Sekine M, Suzuki Y, Koseki N. Factors contributing to the progression of visual field damage in eyes with normal tension glaucoma. *Ophthalmology* 1994;101:1440–4.
2. Bresson-Dumont H, Béchetoille A. Syndrome vasospastic et glaucome focal ischemic. *Ophtalmologie* 1995;9:56–9.
3. Bresson-Dumont H, Béchetoille A. Hypotension artérielle dans le glaucome à pression normale ou modérément élevée. *J Fr Ophtalmol* 1995;18:128–34.
4. Bresson-Dumont H, Béchetoille A. Rôle de la tension artérielle dans l'évolutivité des lésions glaucomateuses. *J Fr Ophtalmol* 1996;19:435–42.
5. Butt Z, McKillop G, O'Brien C, Allan P, Aspinall P. Measurement of ocular blood flow velocity using color Doppler imaging in low tension glaucoma. *Eye* 1995;9:29–33.

6. Butt Z, O'Brien C, McKillop G, Aspinall P, Allan P. Color Doppler imaging in untreated high-and normal-pressure glaucoma. *Invest Ophthalmol Vis Sci* 1997;38:690–6.
7. Costa VP, Sergott RC, Smith M, et al. Color Doppler imaging in glaucoma patients with asymmetric optic cups. *J Glaucoma* 1994;3:91–7.
8. Drance SM, Douglas GR, Wijsman K, Schulzer M, Britton RJ. Response of bloodflow to warm and cold in normal and low-tension glaucoma patients. *Am J Ophthalmol* 1988;105:35–9.
9. Duijm HFA, Rulo AHF, Astin M, Mäepea O, van den Berg TJTP, Greve EL. Study of choroidal bloodflow by comparison of SLO fluorescein angiography and microspheres. *Exp Eye Res* 1996;63:693–704.
10. Duijm HFA, van den Berg TJTP, Greve EL. Choroidal haemodynamics in glaucoma. *Br J Ophthalmol* 1997;81:735–42.
11. Duijm HFA, van den Berg TJTP, Greve EL. A comparison of retinal and choroidal haemodynamics in patients with primary open-angle glaucoma and normal-pressure glaucoma. *Am J Ophthalmol* 1997;123:644–56.
12. Flammer J, Guthauser U, Mahler M. Do ocular vasospasms help cause low-tension glaucoma. *Doc Ophthalmol Proc Ser* 1987;49:397–9.
13. Galassi F, Sodi A, Vielmo A, Saint Prere Fd, Rossi MG, Ciardullo P. Glaucoma and myopia. A study by means of color Doppler imaging. Third European Professor Workshop on the Quantification of Ocular Blood Flow in Glaucoma. Edinburgh, October 7, 1995.
14. Gasser P. Ocular vasospasm: a risk factor in the pathogenesis of low-tension glaucoma. *Int Ophthalmol* 1989;13:281–90.
15. Geijssen HC. Studies on normal pressure glaucoma. Thesis. Amstelveen: Kugler Publications, 1991.
16. Greve EL, Geijssen HC. The relation between excavation and visual field in glaucoma patients with high and with low intraocular pressures. *Doc Ophthalmol Proc Ser* 1983;35:35–42.
17. Guthauser U, Flammer J, Mahler F. The relationship between digital and ocular vasospasm. *Graefes Arch Clin Exp Ophthalmol* 1988;226:224–6.
18. Harris A, Sergott RC, Spaeth GL, Katz JL, Shoemaker JA, Martin BJ. Color Doppler analysis of ocular vessel blood velocity in normal tension glaucoma. *Am J Ophthalmol* 1994;118:642–9.
19. Hayreh SS, Zimmerman MB, Podhajsky P, Alward WLM. Nocturnal arterial hypotension and its role in optic nerve head and ocular ischemic disorders. *Am J Ophthalmol* 1994;117:603–24.
20. Hayreh SS, Zimmerman MB, Podhajski P, Alward WLM. The role of nocturnal hypotension in ocular and optic nerve ischemic disorders. *Invest Ophthalmol Vis Sci* 1993;34:994.
21. Hendryckx KH, Van Den Enden A, Rasker MT, Hoyng PFJ. Cumulative incidence of patients with disc hemorrhages in glaucoma and the effect of therapy. *Ophthalmology* 1994;101:1165–72.
22. Kaiser HJ, Flammer J, Graf T, Stuempfig D. Systemic blood pressure in glaucoma patients. *Graefes Arch Clin Exp Ophthalmol* 1993;231:677–80.
23. Kitazawa Y, Shirai H, Go FJ. The effect of Ca^{2+}-antagonist on visual field in low-tension glaucoma. *Graefes Arch Clin Exp Ophthalmol* 1989;227:408–12.
24. Michelson G, Schmauss B, Langhans MJ, Harazny J, Groh MJM. Principle, validity, and reliability of scanning laser Doppler flowmetry. *J Glaucoma* 1996;5:99–105.
25. Michelson G, Langhans MJ, Groh MJ. Perfusion of the juxtapapillary retina and the neuroretinal rim area in primary open angle glaucoma. *J Glaucoma* 1996;5:91–8.
26. Nicolela MT, Walman BE, Buckley AR, Drance SM. Various glaucomatous optic nerve appearances. A color Doppler imaging study of retrobulbar circulation. *Ophthalmology* 1996;103:1670–9.
27. Nicolela MT, Drance SM, Rankin SJA, Buckley AR, Walman BE. Color Doppler imaging in patients with asymmetric glaucoma and unilateral visual field loss. *Am J Ophthalmol* 1996;121:502–10.
28. Netland PA, Chaturvedi N, Dreyer EB. Calcium channel blockers in the management of low-tension glaucoma and open-angle glaucoma. *Am J Ophthalmol* 1993;115:608–13.
29. O'Brien C, Saxton V, Crick RP, Meire H. Doppler carotid artery studies in asymmetric glaucoma. *Eye* 1992;6:273–6.
30. Ong K, Farinelli A, Houang M, Stern M. Comparative study of brain magnetic resonance

imaging findings in patients with low tension glaucoma and control subjects. *Ophthalmol* 1995;102:1632–8.

31. Orgül S, Flammer J. Headache in normal tension glaucoma patients. *J Glaucoma* 1994;3: 292–5.

32. Pillunat LE, Lang GK: Nimodipine and carbon dioxide reactivity in normal pressure glaucoma [Abstract]. *Invest Ophthalmol Vis Sci* 1993(Suppl 4):1287.

33. Pillunat LE, Lang GK, Harris A: The visual response to increased ocular blood flow in normal pressure glaucoma. *Surv Ophthalmol* 1994;38S:139–147; discussion S:147–8.

34. Quaranta L, Manni G, Donato F, Bucci MG: The effect of increased intraocular pressure on pulsatile ocular blood flow in low tension glaucoma. *Surv Ophthalmol* 1994;38:177–82.

35. Rader J, Feuer WJ, Anderson DR. Peripapillary vasoconstriction in the glaucomas and the anterior ischemic optic neuropathies. *Am J Ophthalmol* 1994;117:72–80.

36. Riva CE, Harino S, Petrig BL, Shonat RD. Laser Doppler flowmetry in the optic nerve. *Exp Eye Res* 1992;55:499–506.

37. Rojanapongpun P, Drance SM, Morrison BJ. Ophthalmic artery flow velocity in glaucomatous and normal subjects. *Br J Ophthalmol* 1993;77:25–9.

38. Schmidt KG, Mittag TW, Pavlovic S, Hessemer V. Influence of physical exercise and nifedipine on ocular pulse amplitude. *Graefes Arch Clin Exp Ophthalmol* 1996;234:527–32.

39. Tamaki Y, Araie M, Kawamoto E, Egadri S, Fujii H. Noncontact, two-dimensional measurement of retinal microcirculation using laser speckle phenomenon. *Invest Ophthalmol Vis Sci* 1994;35:3825–34.

40. Tielsch JM, Katz J, Sommer A, Quigley HA, Javitt JC. Hypertension, perfusion pressure, and primary open angle glaucoma. A population-based assessment. *Arch Ophthalmol* 1995;113:216–21.

41. Trible JR, Sergott RC, Spaeth GL, et al. Trabeculectomy is associated with retrobulbar hemodynamic changes. A color Doppler analysis. *Ophthalmology* 1994;101:340–51.

42. Ulrich Ch, Helm W, Ulrich A, Barth A, Ulrich W-D. Störung der peripapillären Mikrozirkulation bei Glaukom-patienten. *Ophthalmologe* 1993;90:45–50.

43. Waldmann E, Gasser P, Dubler B, Huber C, Flammer J. Silent myocardial ischemia in glaucoma and cataract patients. *Graefes Arch Exp Ophthalmol* 1996;234:595–8.

44. Wolf S, Arend O, Sponsel WE, Schulte K, Cantor LB, Reim M. Retinal hemodynamics using scanning laser ophthalmoscopy and hemorrheology in chronic open-angle glaucoma. *Ophthalmology* 1993;100:1561–6.

45. Yamazaki Y, Miyamoto S, Hayamizu F. Color Doppler velocimetry of the ophthalmic artery in glaucomatous and normal subjects. *Jpn J Ophthalmol* 1994;38:317–21.

Nitric Oxide and Endothelin in the Pathogenesis of Glaucoma, edited by I. O. Haefliger and J. Flammer. Lippincott–Raven Publishers, Philadelphia © 1998.

2

The Concept of Vascular Dysregulation in Glaucoma

Josef Flammer

Department of Ophthalmology, University of Basel, Basel, Switzerland

Glaucoma is a progressive optic neuropathy characterized by optic nerve head excavation with consecutive defects in retinal sensitivity. The pathogenesis is still not yet well understood. The intraocular pressure (IOP) is often elevated and is a major risk factor for many individuals (9). There is little doubt, however, that there are other risk factors as well. Such risk factors may be damaging by themselves or in concert with other risk factors, especially when combined with an increased IOP. A number of risk factors have been described (5). This review is confined to the role of vascular factors (15). It should be emphasized, however, that this concentration on vascular factors by no means implies a denial of the importance of other risk factors, including the high clinical relevance of IOP (10).

Traditionally, chronic glaucoma has been divided into different groups, especially in primary open-angle glaucoma and in normal-tension glaucoma. Such separations are helpful for epidemiologic studies (57). In terms of pathophysiology, however, there is a continuum. As a general rule, the lower the IOP at which damage occurs or progresses, the higher the chance of finding additional risk factors. This discussion therefore does not distinguish between high-tension and normal-tension glaucoma. However, vascular changes clearly are more often found on the normal-tension side of the spectrum than on the high-tension side.

IS OCULAR BLOOD FLOW ABNORMAL IN GLAUCOMA?

Although ocular vessels can relatively easily be seen, methods to quantify ocular blood flow have only recently been available (19). To summarize many recently published studies applying different methods, it can be stated that the blood flow velocity in the eye is, on the average, reduced in glaucoma patients. There is obviously overlap between normal subjects and glaucoma patients, indicating that not all glaucoma patients have compromised blood flow. The

14

present methods basically allow the quantification of blood flow velocity. Although the velocity is, on the average, clearly decreased, we can only assume that the blood flow is also decreased. In different parts of the eye the reduction might be different. There are indications that normal-tension glaucoma patients may have more reduction in choroidal blood flow, whereas high-tension glaucoma patients might have more reduction in retinal circulation (15).

Changes in the conjunctival vessels (48), disc hemorrhages (7), narrowing of the retinal arteries at the optic nerve head (55), preservation of nerve fiber layers in the vicinity of retinal vessels inside the scleral ring, (2) and the occurrence of gliosis-like retinal alterations (27) further support the assumption that ocular blood flow is disturbed in glaucoma.

ARE THE VASCULAR CHANGES IN GLAUCOMA OF A GENERAL NATURE?

A basic and important question is whether we are dealing with a vascular problem confined to the eye or with a systemic disease in which the eye is especially involved. In some glaucoma patients, vascular changes can also be found in other parts of the body. Extensive studies of the retro-ocular vessels clearly indicate decreased blood flow velocity (34) and increased resistance to blood flow (1). Even in the systemic circulation, the blood flow velocity appears to be decreased (43), especially in the capillaries (25). Furthermore, ischemic brain lesions have been detected with MRI (46,58). Impaired hearing (59) and silent myocardial ischemia (60) have been observed. Taking this information together, we can state that in some patients the vascular changes are of a general nature or, at least, multifocal.

ARE OCULAR VASCULAR CHANGES PRIMARY OR SECONDARY?

There is little doubt that a markedly mechanically damaged optic nerve head may lead to secondary vascular changes (10). However, the fact that hemodynamic changes can precede the glaucomatous damage (45) and that changes can also be observed in other parts of the body, especially in the retrobulbar vessels, together with the observation that a non-ischemic optic atrophy does not lead to changes in orbital hemodynamics (26) indicates that the ocular vascular changes are at least partially primary. In other words, the changes are not necessarily only secondary.

WHAT IS THE GENESIS OF THE HEMODYNAMIC ALTERATIONS?

In general, arteriosclerosis is the most important cause of vascular insufficiency. The risk factors for arteriosclerosis, such as systemic hypertension, hypercholesterolemia, smoking, and diabetes mellitus, are well known. However, it is quite surprising that glaucomatous damage is strongly related neither to arteriosclerosis nor to one of its major risk factors. Although experimental studies indicate that arteriosclerosis may make the eyes slightly more sensitive to increased IOP (30), arteriosclerosis does not appear to play a major role in human glaucomatous disease. Therefore, we have to search for other causes of vascular insufficiency. One is the blood pressure or, more exactly, the perfusion pressure. A large number of studies have found a relationship between glaucomatous damage and systemic hypotension (13,31). Low perfusion pressure in the eye may result, both through increased IOP and decreased systemic blood pressure. If a drop in the perfusion pressure exceeds the autoregulatory capacity, local ischemia results. However, the fact that reduced perfusion pressure caused by carotid stenosis (52) or by diseases of the autonomic nervous system (12) may not (or at least not consistently) lead to glaucomatous damage indicates that the pathogenesis might be more complex. Indeed, an association between systemic hypotension and vasospasm has been clinically observed (23). The sensitivity to endothelin-1, the most potent vasoconstrictor known (29), also depends on the level of blood pressure (22). This indicates that patients with systemic hypotension also have a higher resistance to flow in some vascular beds. This brings us to another important cause of vascular insufficiency, i.e., local vasospasm or a vascular dysregulation.

WHAT IS THE OCULAR VASOSPASTIC SYNDROME?

We introduced this term at a time when it was not yet possible to quantify ocular blood flow. In a number of patients with unexplained visual field defects, peripheral vasospasms were observed. Visual field defects worsened in some of these patients after cold provocation and often improved after treatment with a calcium-channel blocker (28). Therefore, we assumed an involvement of the visual system in the vasospastic disorder. The topography of the presumed vasospasm remained unclear. However, the fact that the visual field defects observed were not homonymous suggested that the location was prechiasmal. Considering this, together with the fact that we had not (or only very rarely) seen changes in the retinal vessels, we assumed that the spasms occur mainly in the choroid or ciliary vessels (16). In other words, we hypothesized that the choroid circulation or possibly even the optic nerve head circulation might participate in the generalized vasospastic syndrome (23). This assumption was later supported by studies with the help of choroidal angiography (53). Such ocular vasospasms appear to be risk factors for anterior ischemic neuropathy in young patients (32), for retinal vein occlusions in young individuals (42), and for central serous chorioretinopathy (54).

The similarity between the visual field defects of patients with a presumed ocular vasospastic syndrome and those of glaucoma patients led to the hypothesis that the vasospastic syndrome might also be a risk factor for glaucoma (17). This hypothesis was later confirmed by control studies (6,25).

THE CONCEPT OF VASCULAR DYSREGULATION IN GLAUCOMA

The fact that vascular insufficiency is present in at least some glaucoma patients and that this insufficiency is not (or only rarely) related to arteriosclerosis but relatively strongly related to low systemic blood pressure and to vasospastic diathesis indicates that vascular dysregulation is indeed involved in the pathogenesis of the damage in at least some glaucoma patients. This hypothesis is further supported by the observation that normal-tension glaucoma occurs much more often in females than in males (49) and in patients under psychological stress (8,18). Whereas low blood pressure may induce arterial vasospasm (22), a basic underlying vascular dysregulation may also explain low blood pressure. This could be due partly to a venous dysregulation. A disturbance on the venous side may also explain the optic disc splinter hemorrhages. The fact that these hemorrhages usually precede functional damage indicates that they might be the cause rather than the consequence of local ischemia (47).

RELATIONSHIP BETWEEN VASCULAR DYSREGULATION AND GLAUCOMATOUS DAMAGE

The fact that vascular dysregulation is related to glaucomatous damage does not automatically imply that this is always due to ischemia. Vascular dysregulation can obviously lead to local ischemia. Such an ischemia, however, may rarely be so pronounced that it leads to irreversible structural damage. It may also be that some type of reperfusion damage might lead to free radicals, thus finally leading to apoptosis of some cells. However, it is also possible that vascular dysregulation may lead to damage other than ischemia. It is known that the glial cells are in contact with both the endothelial cells of the blood vessels and the neural tissue. A basic underlying disorder of vascular endothelial cells therefore may lead to a change in cell-to-cell interactions and finally to apoptosis of some cells, including glial cells. Such an assumption is also supported by the interesting observation that anterior ischemic neuropathy caused by arteriosclerosis does not lead to optic nerve head excavation, whereas ischemia caused by giant-cell arteritis often does so (50). This could imply not only that a sufficient supply of oxygen and other nutrition is prerequisite to the survival of the tissue but that a normal vessel wall is also necessary, allowing normal cell-to-cell interactions, especially with the glial cells.

WHAT IS THE CAUSE OF VASCULAR DYSREGULATION?

The regulation of ocular blood flow, and even more so that of the optic nerve head, is quite complex. A detailed review has appeared elsewhere (19). Both metabolic and myogenic autoregulation occur, and there is both neurogenic and humoral control of blood flow. The endothelial cells play a major role in this regulation by releasing vasoactive factors (29). In such a complex regulatory system it is not surprising that dysregulation might occur. However, which factors are involved in which stages remains to be clarified. It is also possible that in different patients there are different causes. Clinical observations, however, indicate that there might be a genetic predisposition. Because such dysregulation occurs more often in females indicates that estrogen may be involved. The concentration of endothelin-1 in the peripheral blood is increased in some of these patients (33). The real cause, however, is not yet known, and further research in this direction is needed.

RELATIONSHIP BETWEEN REGULATION OF IOP AND REGULATION OF VASCULAR TONE

The IOP and the vascular dysregulation might act together, because both can reduce ocular perfusion. On the other hand, it is conceivable that dysregulation of IOP and dysregulation of vessels might often occur together, because both are regulated by endothelin and nitric oxide (NO) (61). A basic underlying disorder might involve aqueous humor production, outflow resistance, blood pressure, and local vascular resistance.

THERAPEUTIC CONSEQUENCES

The fact that at least some patients suffer from progressive damage despite normal IOP or despite a normalization of an increased IOP substantiates the need for additional treatment. The strong association between glaucomatous damage and its progression to low systemic blood pressure leads to the logic consequence that low blood pressure should be avoided or, when necessary, that a very low blood pressure should be increased, if possible, to the normal range. However, to the best of our knowledge no control studies have been done with blood pressure–increasing therapy. On the other hand it is our clinical experience that the avoidance of blood pressure decreases by simple means, such as increased intake of salt and increased physical activity and, if necessary, a blood pressure-increasing treatment with a low dosage of fludrocortisone, are helpful. Treatment of systemic hypotension often improves the general condition of a patient as well. More information is available about treatment of spasms. In patients with ocular vasospastic syndrome, a quick improvement of the visual fields can often be observed after treatment with a calcium-channel blocker

(11,16,28). This improvement is especially impressive in young patients and when the optic nerve head is not (or not yet markedly) damaged (21). It has been questioned whether this visual effect might be due to a changes in the circulation or a direct effect on the neural tissue. However, the fact that a similar improvement can be observed with CO_2 breathing (51) and that the improvement of visual function is correlated with the improvement in peripheral blood flow (28) indicates that such visual improvement might indeed be due to an improvement of blood flow. Because endothelin is involved in the pathogenesis of the vascular dysregulation (14,33,39), calcium antagonists may indeed be helpful because of their ability to modulate the vascular response to endothelin-1 (37,41). Although a positive short-term response is of major diagnostic interest and improves our understanding of the pathophysiology, it does not automatically indicate that patients would profit from long-term treatment. There are, however, placebo-controlled studies (36,56) and non-controlled studies (16,24,44) suggesting beneficial effects in selected patients. In clinical routine, in selected glaucoma patients we have routinely used low dosages of nifedipine for more than a decade. The clinical impression is very promising.

In addition to calcium-channel blockers, other therapeutic modalities may influence vascular dysregulation. Dipyridamole dilatates ocular vessels in vitro (40) and increases the retro-ocular blood flow velocity in vivo (35). Magnesium can release endothelin-induced spasms in vitro (3,4) and appears to be of some benefit in vivo (20), and endothelin receptor antagonists exert a major influence in vitro (39) and might therefore be of future help for glaucoma patients (14). Finally, other useful drugs, such as phytogenic compounds, might be found (38) in the future.

REFERENCES

1. Butt Z, O'Brien C, McKillop G, Aspinall P, Allan P. Color Doppler imaging in untreated high- and normal-pressure open-angle glaucoma. *Invest Ophthalmol Vis Sci* 1997;38:690–6.
2. Chihara E, Honda Y. Preservation of nerve fiber layer by retinal vessels in glaucoma. *Ophthalmology* 1992;99:208–14.
3. Dettmann ES, Flammer J, Haefliger I. Magnesium and vascular tone modulation. In: Drance SM, ed. *Glaucoma ocular blood flow and drug treatment.* Amsterdam, New York: Kugler Publications, 1997:79–86.
4. Dettmann ES, Lüscher TF, Flammer J, Haefliger I. Modulation of endothelin-1–induced contractions by magnesium/calcium in porcine ciliary arteries. *Graefes Arch Clin Exp Ophthalmol* (in press).
5. Drance SM. The concept of chronic open-angle glaucoma: a personal view. *Ophthalmologica* 1996;210:251–6.
6. Drance SM, Douglas GR, Wijsman K, Schulzer M, Britton RJ. Response of blood flow to warm and cold in normal and low-tension glaucoma patients. *Am J Ophthalmol* 1988;105:35–9.
7. Drance SM, Fairclough M, Butler DM, Kottler MS. The importance of disc hemorrhage in the prognosis of chronic open-angle glaucoma. *Arch Ophthalmol* 1977;95:226–8.
8. Erb C, Batra A, Lietz A, Bayer AU, Flammer J, Thiel H-J. Psychological characteristics of patients with normal-tension glaucoma (Submitted).
9. Fechtner RD, Weinreb RN. Mechanisms of optic nerve damage in primary open-angle glaucoma. *Surv Ophthalmol* 1994;39:23–42.

10. Flammer J. Psychophysics in glaucoma. A modified concept of the disease. In: Greve EL, Leydhecker W, Raitta C, eds. *Proc Eur Glaucoma Soc.* Dordrecht: Dr. W. Junk, 1985:11–17.
11. Flammer J. Therapeutic aspects of normal-tension glaucoma. *Curr Opin Ophthalmol* 1993;4:58–64.
12. Flammer J. The vascular concept of glaucoma. *Surv Ophthalmol* 1994;38:3–6.
13. Flammer J. To what extent are vascular factors involved in the pathogenesis of glaucoma? In: Kaiser HJ, Flammer J, Hendrickson Ph, eds. *Ocular blood flow.* Basel: Karger, 1996:12–39.
14. Flammer J. Endothelin in the pathogenesis of glaucoma. In: Drance SM, ed. *Glaucoma ocular blood flow and drug treatment.* Amsterdam: Kugler Publications, 1997:97–103.
15. Flammer J, Gasser P, Prünte Ch, Yao K. The probable involvement of factors other than ocular pressure in the pathogenesis of glaucoma. In: Drance SM, Van Buskirk EM, Neufeld AH, eds. *Pharmacology of glaucoma.* Baltimore: Williams & Wilkins, 1992:273–83.
16. Flammer J, Guthauser U. Behandlung chorioidaler Vasospasmen mit Kalzium-antagonisten. *Klin Mbl Augenheilk* 1987;190:299–300.
17. Flammer J, Guthauser U, Mahler M. Do ocular vasospasms help cause low-tension glaucoma? *Doc Ophthalmol Proc Ser* 1987;49:397–9.
18. Flammer J, Messerli J, Haefliger I. Sehstörungen durch vaskuläre Dysregulationen. *Therapeutische Umschau* 1996;53:37–42.
19. Flammer J, Orgül S. Optic nerve blood-flow abnormalities in glaucoma. *Prog Retinal Eye Res* (in press)
20. Gaspar AZ, Gasser P, Flammer J. The influence of magnesium on visual field and peripheral vasospasm in glaucoma. *Ophthalmologica* 1995;209:11–3.
21. Gaspar AZ, Flammer J, Hendrickson Ph. Influence of nifedipine on the visual fields of patients with optic nerve head disease. *Eur J Ophthalmol* 1994;1:24–8.
22. Gass A, Flammer J, Linder L, Romerio SC, Gasser P, Haefeli WE. Inverse correlation between endothelin-1-induced peripheral microvascular vasoconstriction and blood pressure in glaucoma patients. *Graefes Arch Clin Exp Ophthalmol* (in press).
23. Gasser P, Flammer J. Influence of vasospasm on visual function. *Doc Ophthalmol* 1987;66:3–18.
24. Gasser P, Flammer J. Short- and long-term effect of nifedipine on the visual field in patients with presumed vasospasm. *J Int Med Res* 1990;18:334–9.
25. Gasser P, Flammer J. Blood-cell velocity in the nailfold capillaries of patients with normal-tension or high-tension glaucoma and of healthy controls. *Am J Ophthalmol* 1991;111:585–8.
26. Goh KY, Kay MD, Hughes JR. Orbital color Doppler imaging in nonischemic optic atrophy. *Ophthalmology* 1997;104:330–3.
27. Graf Th, Flammer J, Prünte CH, Hendrickson Ph. Gliosis-like retinal alterations in glaucoma patients. *J Glaucoma* 1993;2:257–9.
28. Guthauser U, Flammer J, Mahler F. The relationship between digital and ocular vasospasm. *Graefes Arch Clin Exp Ophthalmol* 1988;226:224–6.
29. Haefliger IO, Meyer P, Flammer J, Lüscher Th. The vascular endothelium as a regulator of the ocular circulation: a new concept in ophthalmology? *Surv Ophthalmol* 1994;39:123–32.
30. Hayreh SS, Bill A, Sperber GO. Effects of high intraocular pressure on the glucose metabolism in the retina and optic nerve in old atherosclerotic monkeys. *Graefes Arch Clin Exp Ophthalmol* 1994;232:745–52.
31. Kaiser HJ, Flammer J, Graf Th, Stümpfig D. Systemic blood pressure in glaucoma patients. *Graefes Arch Clin Exp Ophthalmol* 1993;231:677–80.
32. Kaiser HJ, Flammer J, Messerli J. Vasospasm—a risk factor for nonarteric anterior ischemic optic neuropathy? *Neuro-ophthalmology* 1996;16:5–10.
33. Kaiser HJ, Flammer J, Wenk M, Lüscher Th. Endothelin-I plasma levels in normal-tension glaucoma: abnormal response to postural changes. *Graefes Arch Clin Exp Ophthalmol* 1995;233:484–8.
34. Kaiser HJ, Schötzau A, Stümpfig D, Flammer J. Blood-flow velocities of the extraocular vessels in patients with high-tension and normal-tension primary open-angle glaucoma. *Am J Ophthalmol* 1997;123:320–7.
35. Kaiser HJ, Stümpfig D, Flammer J. Short-term effect of dipyridamole on blood-flow velocities in the extraocular vessels. *Int Ophthalmol* 1996;19:355–8.
36. Kitazawa J, Shirai H, Go FJ. The effect of calcium antagonists on visual field in low-tension glaucoma. *Graefes Arch Clin Exp Ophthalmol* 1989;277:408–12.

37. Lang MG, Zuh P, Meyer P, et al. Amlodipine and benazeprilat differently affect the responses to endothelin-1 and bradykinin in porcine ciliary arteries: effects of a low and high dose combination. *Curr Eye Res* 1997;16:208–13.
38. Liu SXL, Chiang CH, Yao QS, Chiou GCY. Increase of ocular blood flow by some phytogenic compounds. *J Ocul Pharmacol* 1996;12:95–101.
39. Meyer P, Flammer J, Lüscher Th. Endothelin-dependent regulation of the ophthalmic microcirculation in perfused porcine eye: role of nitric oxide and endothelins. *Invest Ophthalmol Vis Sci* 1993;34:3614–21.
40. Meyer P, Flammer J, Lüscher Th. Effect of dipyridamole on vascular responses of porcine ciliary arteries. *Curr Eye Res* 1996;15:387–93.
41. Meyer P, Lang MG, Flammer J, Lüscher Th. Effects of calcium-channel-blockers on the response to endothelin-1 bradykinin and sodium nitroprusside in porcine ciliary arteries. *Exp Eye Res* 1995;60:505–10.
42. Messerli J, Flammer J. Zentralvenenthrombosen bei jüngeren Patienten. *Klin Mbl Augenheilk* 1996;208:303–5.
43. Nasemann JE, Carl Th, Spiegel D. Measurement of systemic and ocular blood flow velocities in normal-tension glaucoma. In: Kaiser HJ, Flammer J, Hendrickson Ph, eds. *Ocular blood flow.* Basel: Karger, 1996:207–16.
44. Netland PA, Chaturvedi N, Dreyer EB. Calcium-channel blockers in the management of low-tension and open-angle glaucoma. *Am J Ophthalmol* 1993;115:608–13.
45. Nicolela MT, Drance SM, Rankin SJA, Buckley AR, Walman BE. Color Doppler imaging in patients with asymmetric glaucoma and unilateral visual field loss. *Am J Ophthalmol* 1996;121:502–10.
46. Ong K, Farinelli A, Billson F, Houang M, Stern M. Comparative study of brain magnetic resonance imaging findings in patients with low-tension glaucoma and control subjects. *Ophthalmology* 1995;102:1632–8.
47. Orgül S, Flammer J. Optic disc hemorrhages. *Neuro-ophthalmology* 1994;14:97–101.
48. Orgül S, Flammer J. Perilimbal aneurysms of conjunctival vessels in glaucoma patients. *Ger J Ophthalmol* 1995;4:94–6.
49. Orgül S, Flammer J, Gasser P. Female preponderance in normal-tension glaucoma. *Ann Ophthalmol* 1995;27:355–9.
50. Orgül S, Gass A, Flammer J. Optic disc cupping in arteric anterior ischemic optic neuropathy. *Ophthalmologica* 1994;208:336–8.
51. Pillunat LE, Lang GK, Harris A. The visual response to increased ocular blood flow in normal pressure glaucoma. *Surv Ophthalmol* 1994;38(suppl):S139–48.
52. Pillunat LE, Stodtmeister R. Inzidenz des Niederdruckglaukoms bei hämodynamisch relevanter Karotisstenose. *Spektrum Augenheilk* 1988;2:24–7.
53. Prünte Ch, Flammer J. Choroidal angiography findings in patients with glaucoma-like visual field defects. In: Heijl A, ed. *Perimetry update 88/89.* Amstelveen: Kugler & Ghedini, 1989:325–7.
54. Prünte Ch, Flammer J. Choroidal capillary and venous congestion in central serous chorioretinopathy. *Am J Ophthalmol* 1996;121:26–34.
55. Rader J, Feuer WJ, Anderson DR. Peripapillary vasoconstriction in the glaucomas and the anterior ischemic optic neuropathies. *Am J Ophthalmol* 1994;117:72–80.
56. Sawada A, Kitazawa Y, Yamamoto T, Okabe I, Ichien K. Prevention of visual field defect progression with brovincamine in eyes with normal-tension glaucoma. *Ophthalmology* 1996;103:283–8.
57. Sommer A. Doyne Lecture: Glaucoma: facts and fancies. *Eye* 1996;10:295–301.
58. Stroman GA, Stewart WC, Golmik KC, Cure JK, Olinger RE. Magnetic resonance imaging in patients with low-tension glaucoma. *Arch Ophthalmol* 1995;113:168–72.
59. Susanna R, Basseto FL. Hemorrhage of the optic disc and neurosensorial dysacousia. *J Glaucoma* 1992;1:248–53.
60. Waldmann E, Gasser P, Dubler B, Huber Ch, Flammer J. Silent myocardial ischemia in glaucoma and cataract patients. *Graefes Arch Clin Exp Ophthalmol* 1996;234:595–8.
61. Wiederholt M, Sturm A, Lepple-Wienhues A. Relaxation of trabecular meshwork and ciliary muscle by release of nitric oxide. *Invest Ophthalmol Vis Sci* 1994;35:2515–20.

Nitric Oxide and Endothelin in the Pathogenesis of Glaucoma, edited by I. O. Haefliger and J. Flammer. Lippincott–Raven Publishers, Philadelphia © 1998.

3

Nitric Oxide and Endothelin in the Pathogenesis of Glaucoma: An Overview

Ivan O. Haefliger and *Eike S. Dettmann

*Laboratory of Ocular Pharmacology and Physiology, Departments of Medicine and *Ophthalmology, University of Basel, Basel, Switzerland*

To coordinate inter- and intracellular activity, living organisms have developed complex chemical signaling systems. Intercellular signals are generally mediated by chemical messengers known as hormones or neurotransmitters, whereas intracellular signals are usually mediated by second messengers (1). In the context of biochemical communication, nitric oxide (NO) and endothelin are two cellular mediators that have recently been identified and that act primarily as hormones or neurotransmitters (2,3).

In the eye, NO and endothelin are involved in regulation of the intraocular pressure (IOP) (4–7), local modulation of ocular blood flow (8,9), and control of retinal ganglion cell death by apoptosis (10–12), three fundamental aspects generally considered to be involved in the pathogenesis of glaucoma (13).

This review article provides a short and simplified overview of some fundamental biochemical aspects of NO and endothelin that are described in detail in other chapters of this book dealing with their respective roles in the pathogenesis of glaucoma. The basic biochemical mechanisms of NO and endothelin are described here as they occur in a blood vessel.

NITRIC OXIDE

Although for more than a century the relaxing effect of NO released from drugs such as nitroglycerin has been used to treat coronary artery diseases (14), it has only been recently recognized that vascular endothelial cells can themselves produce NO and thus induce local relaxation of the underlying smooth-muscle cells (15,16). The stimulation of a membrane receptor on the surface of endothelial cells by an agonist (i.e., acetylcholine) leads to an increase in intracellular calcium, which in turn activates the enzyme nitric oxide synthase (NOS) to produce NO (Fig. 1) (16).

The NOS enzyme has the amino acid L-arginine as substrate and by oxidation leads to the formation of NO and the amino acid L-citrulline (16). The NO formation can be inhibited by analogues of L-arginine, such as N^ω-nitro-L-arginine methyl ester (L-NAME) or N^ω-monomethyl-L-arginine (L-NMMA), which are competitive inhibitors of NOS and thus inhibit the production of NO (Fig. 1) (17).

In contrast to other hormones and neurotransmitters, which are usually polypeptides, amino acid derivatives, or steroids, NO is an inorganic free radical gas ($^\cdot N{=}O$). Like O_2 and CO_2, which are lipophylic molecules, NO rapidly diffuses across cell membranes, cannot be stored in vesicles, and does not act on specific membrane receptors. Therefore, the NO produced in a single endothelial cell rapidly diffuses and penetrates surrounding cells (18).

Because NO is very unstable, it is often considered to have a half-life of a few seconds and therefore to have an area of activity limited to a region near its site of production. In particular, NO can react with oxygen to form nitrites or nitrates ($O_2 + NO \rightarrow NO_3^-/NO_2^-$) or with hemoglobin, which acts as a scaven-

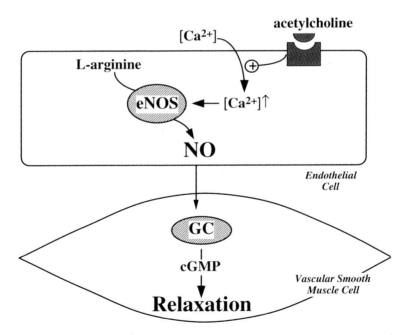

FIG. 1. Simplified scheme of the nitric oxide pathway in a blood vessel. In endothelial cells, the stimulation of a membrane receptor leads to an influx of calcium [Ca^{2+}]. The increase in calcium activates the enzyme nitric oxide synthase (NOS), responsible for the production of nitric oxide (NO) from the amino acid L-arginine. After diffusion of NO to the underlying smooth-muscle cells, NO activates the enzyme guanylate cyclase (GC), responsible for the production of the second messenger cGMP, leading ultimately to relaxation of these muscle cells.

ger of NO. In the presence of the free radical superoxide anion it forms toxic products, such as peroxynitrite and the hydroxy radical (18,19).

When NO reaches its target cell (e.g., smooth-muscle cells) it activates the enzyme guanylate cyclase, responsible for the production of 3'5'-cyclic guanosine monophosphate (cGMP), a second messenger. This increase in cGMP ultimately leads to smooth-muscle cell relaxation by reducing the intracellular calcium content (Fig. 1) (20).

It therefore appears that in endothelial cells of a blood vessel, after stimulation of a membrane receptor (which increases intracellular calcium), NOS is activated and the NO then produced causes relaxation of the underlying vascular smooth-muscle cells through increased production of cGMP (Fig. 1).

NO SYNTHASE ISOFORMS

In addition to the NOS found in endothelial cells (eNOS), there exist two additional major NOS isoforms (Table 1) (18,21). One of them is the neuronal NOS (nNOS), which can be found in nonadrenergic–noncholinergic (NANC) neurons, nerves responsible for the relaxation of smooth-muscle cells and thus vasodilatation (e.g., GUT, cerebral and ocular circulation). Both eNOS and nNOS are constitutive, which means that they are normally expressed in endothelial cells or in some neurons. These eNOS and nNOS isoforms are very similar, in the sense that they both are calcium-dependent (and calmodulin-dependent) and therefore are activated by an increase in intracellular calcium. As mentioned above, in vascular endothelial cells the intracellular calcium increase is triggered by the activation of a membrane receptor (e.g., acetylcholine, bradykinin, histamine), whereas in neurons the increase

TABLE 1. *NOS isoforms*

Isoenzyme	Tissue	Regulation	Physiologic function
Isoenzyme I: neuronal, nNOS	Brain	Calmodulin and calcium	Long-term regulation of synaptic transmission in the central nervous system; central blood pressure regulation; smooth muscle relaxation and vasodilatation via peripheral NANC nitrergic nerves
Isoenzyme II: inducible, iNOS	Macrophage	Cytokine and LPS	Major cytotoxic effector function of macrophages
Isoenzyme III: endothelial, eNOS	Endothelium	Calmodulin and calcium	Blood vessel dilatation; prevention of platelet adhesion; inhibition of VSMC proliferation

in calcium can result either from nerve impulses or from postsynaptic activation of a glutamate (Glu) receptor (Fig. 2).

In contrast to the eNOS and nNOS, the third major NOS isoform, called inducible NOS (iNOS), is not expressed under normal conditions but is only transcriptionally induced after exposure to cytokines or bacterial products, such as endotoxins. This means that first the gene responsible for the iNOS enzyme has to be activated in the nucleus and then the information has to be transcribed into mRNA before being translated to its enzymatic active form. iNOS is primarily involved in inflammatory processes. In macrophages and neutrophils several hours after exposure to cytokines or endotoxins, these cells begin to produce large quantities of NO and continue to do so for many hours. The same cells also produce superoxide anion ($O_2^{-\cdot}$), which chemically combines with NO to form the toxic peroxynitrite anion ($OONO^-$), which is unstable and rapidly decomposes to form the even more toxic hydroxide radical ($OH^\cdot$), used to kill ingested bacteria (Fig. 3). The cytotoxic action of macrophages can be blocked by NOS inhibitors, and NO has been implicated in the vasodilatation observed in endotoxic shock.

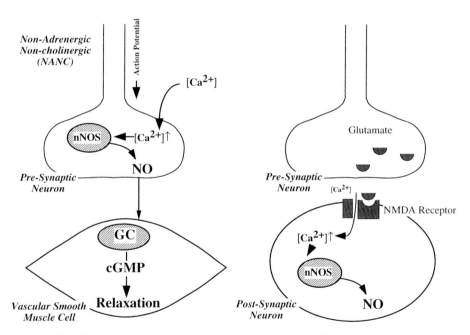

FIG. 2. Simplified scheme of neuronal nitric oxide synthase (nNOS) that can be found in pre- or postsynaptic neurons. In some presynaptic nonadrenergic–noncholinergic (NANC) neurons, action potential propagation leads to an extracellular influx of calcium with the activation of nNOS and production of nitric oxide (NO). The NO produced by NANC neurons surrounding some vessels diffuses to the underlying vascular smooth-muscle cells to activate a guanylate cyclase (GC) that increases cGMP production, inducing vasorelaxation. In some other neurons, postsynaptic activation of an *N*-methyl-D-aspartate (NMDA) membrane receptor by glutamate increases intracellular calcium [Ca^{2+}] concentration and activates of nNOS to produce NO.

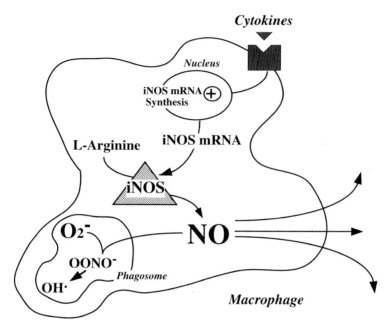

FIG. 3. Schematic and simplified scheme of the inducible nitric oxide synthase (iNOS) in a macrophage. After stimulation by cytokines, de novo production of the enzyme iNOS is induced after activation of the iNOS gene in the nucleus and its transcription into mRNA. Once activated, iNOS produces large quantities of nitric oxide (NO), which leads in phagosomes, after interaction with the superoxide anion (O_2^-), to formation of the peroxynitrite anion ($OONO^-$) and the very toxic hydroxide radical ($OH^·$), used to kill ingested bacteria.

ENDOTHELIN

In contrast to NO, which is a relaxing agent, endothelin-1 is the most potent physiologic vasoconstrictor presently known (22–24). Endothelin-1 is part of a family of small 21–amino-acid peptides with close structural analogies to bee and snake venom, suggesting an early phylogenetic origin of this molecule. Endothelin-1 is essentially produced in endothelial cells. It is formed from a precursor peptide of approximately 200 amino acids called preproendothelin. This precursor is itself cleaved by an endopeptidase into a smaller 38–amino-acid peptide called big endothelin. Then, in a final step, the endothelin-converting enzyme (ECE) cleaves again the big endothelin to the biologically active 21–amino-acid peptide endothelin (Fig. 4). Inhibitors of the ECE enzyme are currently under development. Most of the endothelin produced by endothelial cells is released abluminally and only a small proportion into the lumen of the vessel, suggesting that endothelin mainly acts locally.

Two main endothelin receptors exist, ET_A and ET_B. On vascular smooth-muscle cells, it is mainly the stimulation of ET_A receptors that evokes marked and sustained vasoconstriction. Indeed, ET_A receptors have been shown to be

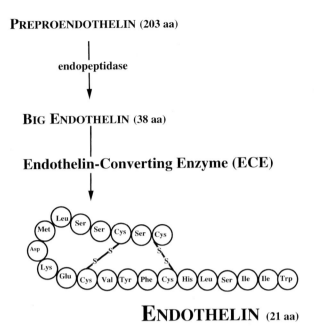

FIG. 4. Schematic representation of the formation (after cleavage from a precursor) of the 21−amino-acid (aa) endothelin peptide.

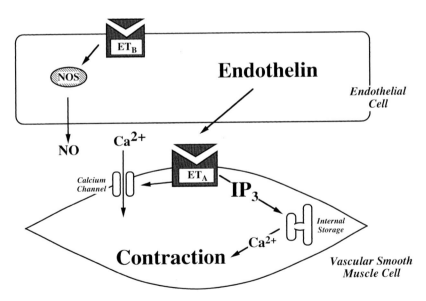

FIG. 5. Simplified scheme of ET_A and ET_B endothelin receptors in a blood vessel. On vascular smooth-muscle cells, stimulation of an ET_A receptor leads to an increase in intracellular calcium (Ca^{2+}) and to potent vasoconstriction. On endothelial cells of some vessels, stimulation of ET_B receptors can activate nitric oxide synthase (NOS), leading to nitric oxide (NO) production and transient vasodilatation. IP_3, inositol triphosphate.

linked to phospholipase C, known to induce the formation of the second messengers inositoltriphosphate (IP_3) and diacylglycerol. Activation of these messengers can lead to an increase in intracellular calcium (usually from internal storage, but in certain vessels from external sources through voltage-operated calcium channels). It is this increase in intracellular calcium that ultimately leads to sustained contractions. On endothelial cells, ET_B receptors are expressed. By stimulation of these receptors NO and/or prostacyclin can be released, evoking transient vasodilatation (Fig. 5).

NO AND ENDOTHELIN IN GLAUCOMA

NO and Endothelin in Vasospastic Reaction

Glaucoma is an optic nerve head neuropathy associated with different risk factors, such as high levels of intraocular pressure (IOP), or blood flow dysregulation, such as vasospastic reactions (24–26). There are conditions in which a lack

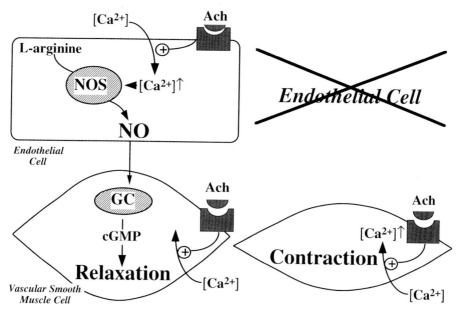

FIG. 6. Simplified scheme illustrating how a lack of NO production from endothelial cells in a vessel can lead to a vasospastic reaction. On the surface of endothelial and smooth-muscle cells, activation of the membrane receptor by an agonist, such as acetylcholine, increases intracellular concentration of calcium [Ca^{2+}]. In endothelial cells this increase stimulates the production of nitric oxide (NO) by the enzyme nitric oxide synthase (NOS), whereas in smooth-muscle cells it induces contraction. Under normal conditions the relaxing effect of NO overcomes the direct contracting effect of acetylcholine on smooth-muscle cells. In the case of endothelial damage, absence of NO production can lead to a localized vasospastic reaction. GC, guanylate cyclase; cGMP, cyclic GMP.

of NO production from endothelial cells can lead to a vasospastic reaction. As mentioned earlier, the endothelial activation of a membrane receptor (acetylcholine) can lead to an increase in the concentration of intracellular calcium, which in turn activates NOS and the production of NO, leading to relaxation of the underlying smooth-muscle cells and thus to vasodilatation (Fig. 1). It should be noted that, on the surface of smooth-muscle cells, the same agonist (acetylcholine) can also interact with a receptor and, in a similar manner, increase the intracellular concentration of calcium, which can potentially lead to contraction of these muscle cells. Under normal conditions this vasoconstrictive effect is counterbalanced by the strong relaxing effect of NO. However, in some pathologic conditions, e.g., in the case of an endothelial dysfunction and a decrease in NO production, it is possible to observe that such an agonist can provoke local vasoconstriction instead of relaxation (Fig. 6) (15).

On the other hand, local production of ET can also lead to a vasospastic reaction. For example, in endothelial cells the production of ET can be stimulated by Ox-LDL, a substance associated with hypercholesterolemia. For example, in isolated ciliary arteries after exposure to Ox-LDL sustained contractions could be observed. Contractions were abolished either by the removal of endothelial cells or by pretreatment with an ET_A receptor antagonist (Fig. 7) (27).

NO and Endothelin in Intraocular Pressure Regulation

There is evidence that the trabecular meshwork has intrinsic contractile elements that can be relaxed by NO or contracted endothelin (5,6). Owing to these

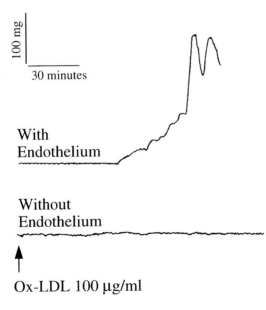

100 mg

30 minutes

With
Endothelium

Without
Endothelium

↑

Ox-LDL 100 µg/ml

FIG. 7. Effect of Ox-LDL on an isolated porcine ciliary artery. Exposure to Ox-LDL evokes spontaneous contractions that can be abolished by removal of the endothelium.

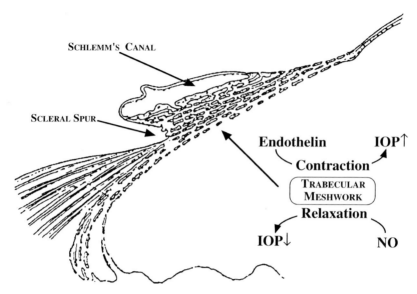

FIG. 8. Scheme of iridocorneal angle and the potential role of nitric oxide (NO) and endothelin on intraocular pressure (IOP) regulation. Because of its intrinsic contractile properties the trabecular meshwork is believed to influence aqueous humor outflow resistance and thus to participate in regulation of IOP.

contractile properties, it has been suggested that the trabecular meshwork could participate in the regulation of aqueous humor outflow and that NO could increase aqueous humor outflow and, thus, lower IOP, whereas endothelin could decrease outflow, resulting in an increase in IOP (Fig. 8) (4–7).

It could also be shown that in the aqueous humor of glaucoma patients, levels of endothelin were significantly higher than those in matched control subjects (28), however on the other hand it could be demonstrated histologically that in the eyes of glaucoma patients there was a marked decrease in NOS, the enzyme responsible for production of NO (29).

Therefore, it appears that NO and endothelin not only are important physiologic modulators of IOP but might be directly involved in the increase in IOP observed in glaucoma, either because of a decrease in NO production or an excess of ET secretion.

NO AND RETINAL GANGLION CELL APOPTOSIS

The irreversible functional visual loss observed in glaucoma is a manifestation of retinal ganglion cell death possibly through a process called apoptosis (10,30). Under the influence of different factors, a genetically programmed mechanism can be activated within the retinal ganglion cells, leading cells to commit a kind of "suicide" and to rapidly die without evoking any sign of inflammation (12). Apoptosis can be induced by glutamate activation of the *N*-methyl-D-aspartate (NMDA) membrane receptor, which stimulates the production of large quantities of NO, as well as by the production of the free radical superoxide anion in mitochondria (Fig. 9). In macrophages, NO reacts with the superoxide anion to form the very toxic peroxynitrite, which triggers cell death by apoptosis (Fig. 3).

In the vitreous body of glaucoma patients, increased levels of glutamate have been measured (31). It has also been shown that the large retinal ganglion cells are much more susceptible to NMDA-mediated neurotoxicity (32). Because typical glaucomatous visual field defects reflect loss of large retinal ganglion cells, the increased sensitivity of these ganglion cells to glutamate may explain the geographic distribution of these glaucomatous defects (13).

In conclusion, it appears that NO and endothelin are two mediators that play a key role in the regulation of several ocular functions which are of major importance in glaucoma, particularly the regulation of IOP (4–7), ocular blood flow (8,9), and retinal ganglion cell death by apoptosis (10–12). This offers new perspectives in the understanding of the pathogenesis of glaucoma and, as a consequence, opens new potential therapeutic approaches for an affliction that is still a leading cause of blindness.

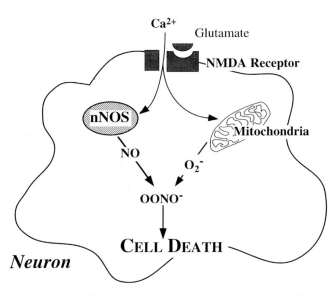

FIG. 9. Schematic and simplified scheme of neuronal apoptosis induced by activation of an *N*-methyl-D-aspartate (NMDA) membrane receptor by glutamate. Activation of NMDA receptor stimulates production of large quantities of nitric oxide (NO) by neuronal nitric oxide synthase (nNOS) and production of the free radical superoxide anion in mitochondria. By reacting with the superoxide anion (O_2^-), NO forms the very toxic compound peroxynitrite (OONO⁻), which triggers cell death by apoptosis.

REFERENCES

1. Voet D, Voet JG. Biochemical communications: hormones and neurotransmitters. In: Voet D, Voet JG, eds. *Biochemistry*. 2nd ed. New York: John Wiley & Sons, 1995:1261–301.
2. Bredt DS, Snyder SH. Nitric oxide, a novel neuronal messenger. *Neuron* 1992;8:3–11.
3. Lowenstein CJ, Dinerman JL, Snyder SH. Nitric oxide: a physiologic messenger. *Ann Intern Med* 1994;120:227–37.
4. Behar-Cohen FF, Goureau O, D'Hermies F, Courtois Y. Decreased intraocular pressure induced by nitric oxide donors is correlated to nitrite production in the rabbit eye. *Invest Ophthalmol Vis Sci* 1996;37:1711–5.
5. Tamm ER, Lütjen-Drecoll E. Nitric oxide in the outflow pathways of the aqueous humor. In: Haefliger IO, Flammer J, eds. *Nitric oxide and endothelin in the pathogenesis of glaucoma*. New York: Lippincott-Raven, 1997:158–67.
6. Wiederholt M. Nitric oxide and endothelin in aqueous humor outflow regulation. In: Haefliger IO, Flammer J, eds. *Nitric oxide and endothelin in the pathogenesis of glaucoma*. New York: Lippincott-Raven, 1997:168–77.
7. Ellis D, Nathanson J. Nitric oxide in the human eye: sites of synthesis and physiological actions on intraocular pressure, blood flow, sodium transport and neuronal viability. In: Haefliger IO, Flammer J, eds. *Nitric oxide and endothelin in the pathogenesis of glaucoma*. New York: Lippincott-Raven, 1997:178–204.
8. Haefliger IO, Meyer P, Flammer J, Lüscher TF. The vascular endothelium as a regulator of the ocular circulation: a new concept in ophthalmology. *Surv Ophthalmol* 1994;39:123–32.
9. Riva CE. Nitric oxide and endothelin in optic nerve head blood flow regulation. In: Haefliger IO, Flammer J, eds. *Nitric oxide and endothelin in the pathogenesis of glaucoma*. New York: Lippincott-Raven, 1997:44–58.
10. Bonne C, Muller A. The glaucoma excitotoxicity theory. In: Haefliger IO, Flammer J, eds. *Nitric oxide and endothelin in the pathogenesis of glaucoma*. New York: Lippincott-Raven, 1997:205–12.
11. Kashii S. Delayed retinal neuronal death in glaucoma. In: Haefliger IO, Flammer J, eds. *Nitric oxide and endothelin in the pathogenesis of glaucoma*. New York: Lippincott-Raven, 1997:221–9.
12. Monard D. Mechanisms of neuronal apoptosis. In: Haefliger IO, Flammer J, eds. *Nitric oxide and endothelin in the pathogenesis of glaucoma*. New York: Lippincott-Raven, 1997:213–20.
13. Shields MB. Primary open-angle glaucoma. In: Shields MD, ed. *Textbook of glaucoma*. 3rd ed. Baltimore: Willams & Wilkins, 1992:172–97.
14. Feelisch M, Stamler JS. Donors of nitrogen oxides. In: Feelisch M, Stamler JS, eds. *Methods in nitric oxide research*. New York: John Wiley & Sons, 1996:71–115.
15. Furchgott RF, Zawadzki JV. The obligatory role of endothelial cells in the relaxation of arterial smooth muscle by acetylcholine. *Nature* 1980;288:373–6.
16. Palmer RMJ, Ashton DS, Moncada S. Vascular endothelial cells synthesize nitric oxide from L-arginine. *Nature* 1988;333:664–6.
17. Griffith OW, Gross SS. Inhibitors of nitric oxide synthases. In: Feelisch M, Stamler JS, eds. *Methods in nitric oxide research*. New York: John Wiley & Sons, 1996:187–208.
18. Stamler JS, Feelisch M. Biochemistry of nitric oxide and redox-related species. In: Feelisch M, Stamler JS, eds. *Methods in nitric oxide research*. New York: John Wiley & Sons, 1996:19–27.
19. Wink DA, Beckman JS, Ford PC. Kinetics of nitric oxide reaction in liquid and gas phases. In: Feelisch M, Stamler JS, eds. *Methods in nitric oxide research*. New York: John Wiley & Sons, 1996:27–37.
20. Moncada S, Higgs EA. The L-arginine–nitric oxide pathway. *N Engl J Med* 1993;329:2002–12.
21. Michel T, Xie Q-W, Nathan C. Molecular biological analysis of nitric oxide synthases. In: Feelisch M, Stamler JS, eds. *Methods in nitric oxide research*. New York: John Wiley & Sons, 1996:161–75.
22. Yanagisawa M, Kurihara H, Kimura S, et al. A novel potent vasoconstrictor peptide produced by vascular endothelial cells. *Nature* 1988;332:411–5.
23. Nayler WG. *The endothelins*. Berlin: Springer-Verlag, 1990.
24. Flammer J. To what extent are vascular risk factors involved in the pathogenesis of glaucoma?

In: Kaiser HJ, Flammer J, Hendrickson Ph, eds. *Ocular blood flow. New insights into the pathogenesis of ocular diseases.* Basel: Karger, 1996:12–39.

25. Greve EL, Duijm HFA, Geijssen HC. Risk factors in glaucoma. In: Haefliger IO, Flammer J, eds. *Nitric oxide and endothelin in the pathogenesis of glaucoma.* New York: Lippincott-Raven, 1997:1–13.

26. Flammer J. The concept of vascular dysregulation in glaucoma. In: Haefliger IO, Flammer J, eds. *Nitric oxide and endothelin in the pathogenesis of glaucoma.* New York: Lippincott-Raven, 1997:14–21.

27. Zhu P, Resink TJ, Flammer J, Lüscher TF, Haefliger IO. ET_A-antagonist inhibits endothelium-dependent contraction to Ox-LDL in porcine ciliary artery. *Invest Ophthalmol Vis Sci* 1997;38:S1136.

28. Noske W, Hensen J, Wiederholt M. Endothelin-like immunoreactivity in aqueous humor of primary open angle glaucoma and cataract patients. *Graefes Arch Clin Exp Ophthalmol* 1997;235:551–2.

29. Nathanson JA, McKee M. Alteration of ocular nitric oxide synthase in human glaucoma. *Invest Ophthalmol Vis Sci* 1995;36:1774–84.

30. Quigley HA, Nickells RW, Kerrigan LA, Pease ME, Thibaut DJ, Zack DJ. Retinal ganglion cell death in experimental glaucoma and after axotomy occurs by apoptosis. *Invest Ophthalmol Vis Sci* 1995;36:774–86.

31. Dreyer EB, Zurakowski D, Schumer RA, Podos SM, Lipton SA. Elevated levels in the vitreous body of human and monkeys with glaucoma. *Arch Ophthalmol* 1996;114:299–305.

32. Dreyer EB, Pan ZH, Storm S, Lipton SA. Greater sensitivity of larger retinal ganglion cells to NMDA-mediated cell death. *Neuroreport* 1994;5:629–31.

Nitric Oxide and Endothelin in the Pathogenesis of Glaucoma, edited by I. O. Haefliger and J. Flammer. Lippincott–Raven Publishers, Philadelphia © 1998.

4

Optic Nerve and Choroidal Circulation: Physiology

Albert Alm

Department of Ophthalmology, University Hospital, Uppsala University, Uppsala Sweden

It is generally assumed that the damage in glaucoma starts in the optic nerve head. The fact that glaucomatous damage occurs in eyes at normal intraocular pressure (IOP) indicates that factors in addition to the IOP contribute to the damage. One such factor may be disturbed ocular blood flow. Whether or not disturbed blood flow is a primary effect responsible for glaucomatous damage has not been clarified, but one can also expect secondary effects on blood flow through the retina and the optic nerve. For a better understanding of these possibilities, an understanding of the normal regulation of blood flow through the eye is important. Both systemic and local factors are involved in the regulation of blood flow. This review of the physiology of optic nerve and choroidal blood flow focuses on aspects relevant to glaucoma and to the nitric oxide (NO) and endothelins (ET).

ANATOMY

The vessels of the optic nerve and the choroid derive from the ophthalmic artery. In the orbit, it branches into the central retinal artery, two or three posterior ciliary arteries, and several anterior ciliary arteries (1). The main part of the choroid is supplied by the short posterior ciliary arteries, and anterior ciliary arteries supply part of the peripheral choroid and the anterior uvea. The retrobulbar portion of the optic nerve is supplied with small branches from the central retinal artery and from pial vessels. As the nerve enters the eye, no more vessels are delivered from the central retinal artery, with the exception of the superficial capillaries on the nerve head. The remaining part of the optic nerve head (ONH), including the lamina cribrosa, is supplied mainly by branches from the short posterior ciliary arteries. Apart from this common origin the two vascular beds have little in common. The choriocapillaris has a thin wall with fenestrations covered by a porous membrane that permits even large molecules, such as albumin, to pass. The capillaries of the ONH have the same structure as those of the brain and the retina, with tight junctions between endothelial cells constituting part of the blood–retinal barrier.

NORMAL FLOW RATES, GLUCOSE, AND OXYGEN EXTRACTION

Blood flow through the various ocular tissues of anesthetized cats and monkeys is presented in Table 1 (2,3). In both species, choroidal blood flow corresponds to 75–85% of total ocular blood flow. The perfusion through the choroid is one of the largest in the body, three to four times that through the kidney cortex. For choroidal blood flow there is an interesting difference between the two species. In monkeys there is a distinct regional distribution of blood flow with flow levels in the submacular area that are about 10 times those in the periphery (3). In the cat, which does not have a well-developed fovea, this regional distribution is much less pronounced (2).

Blood flow through the optic nerve is on the same order as in the brain, 120–200 ml/min per 100 g tissue in the ONH and 50–60 ml/min per 100 g in the retrobulbar part (4). The higher rate in the ONH compared to the remaining part of the optic nerve is explained by the lack of myelin in the ONH.

The reason for the high rate of flow through the choroid is probably twofold. One reason could be regulation of the temperature at the level of the photoreceptors (5–8). This is particularly important for the fovea, where light is focused, and the high rate of submacular blood flow helps to dissipate the heat and keep the temperature at the stable level required for most biologic processes. Another reason is to meet the metabolic needs of the retina. The energy consumption in the photoreceptor layer is high, and the choroid delivers a large fraction of the total amount of glucose and oxygen consumed by the retina. Thus, in anesthetized pigs about 60% of the oxygen and 80% of the glucose consumed by the retina

TABLE 1. *Blood flow through the ocular tissues in anesthetized cats and monkeys; blood flow was determined with labeled microspheres and values are given as mg/min for the entire tissue (mean ± SEM)*

Tissue	Cats (n = 12–13)	Monkeys (n = 15)
Retina	15 ± 2	34 ± 2
Iris	60 ± 11	8 ± 1
Ciliary body	262 ± 30	81 ± 6
Choroid	734 ± 94	677 ± 67

Data from refs. 2 and 3.

TABLE 2. *Choroidal and retinal contribution to retinal metabolism; figures are calculated from blood flow values and arteriovenous differences for choroidal and retinal blood flow in anesthetized pigs (nmol/min)*

	Glucose	Oxygen
Choroid	121	191
Retina	28	138
Total	149	329

Data from ref. 9.

are delivered by the choroid (Table 2) (9). Nevertheless, because of the large choroidal blood flow the normal choroidal arteriovenous differences are quite small; only a few percent of the arterial oxygen and glucose are extracted from the choroid.

The peculiar arrangement with such a distant source of supply as the choroid is obviously necessary for good visual acuity but is nevertheless a risky arrangement. In addition, it is interesting to note that the retina appears to be prepared for a certain level of hypoxia. The oxygen tension is low in the layers between the two vascular beds, the retinal capillary bed and the choriocapillaris (10), and is reduced during increased IOP (11). However, the glucose metabolism in the retina differs from that of the brain, with a substantial portion of the glucose being metabolized anaerobically (9). This is only marginally changed in animals breathing pure oxygen (12), suggesting that anaerobic glycolysis is a normal and important source of energy for the retina.

PERFUSION PRESSURE AND AUTOREGULATION

The driving force of ocular blood flow is the perfusion pressure (PP), which is the difference between the pressure in the arteries entering the eye and the pressure in the veins leaving it. The pressure in the arteries entering the eye cannot be determined, and as a rule the mean arterial pressure (MAP) in the brachial artery is used as a substitute. MAP is defined as the diastolic pressure plus one-third of the pulse pressure (systolic less diastolic pressure). Consequently, at a blood pressure of 140/80 mm Hg the MAP is 100 mm Hg. There is a loss of pressure between the heart and the eye, and pressure in the arteries entering the eye is 35–40 mm Hg lower than MAP as determined in the brachial arteries when we stand up. The pressure in the veins leaving the eye is almost the same as the IOP and for the eye the PP = (MAP − IOP). The relationship between blood flow (F), PP, and vascular resistance (R) is expressed as

$$F = (MAP - IOP)/R$$

Blood flow is reduced if MAP is reduced or IOP increased unless there is a concomitant change in R. In most tissues, such changes in perfusion pressure are compensated for by a change in R, and blood flow is kept at the same level despite moderate changes in PP. Regulation of the vascular resistance within the tissue is a local event and is called autoregulation. In the eye, blood flow through the retina is autoregulated (2,3), and one can estimate that in a healthy eye retinal blood flow is essentially unchanged up to an IOP of about 35 mm Hg. The same is true for blood flow through the optic nerve, both in monkey (4) and in human eyes (13). In addition, glucose consumption in the retina and the optic nerve is unaffected by moderate increments in IOP (14).

The situation is quite different for the choroid. In cats, monkeys, and dogs, increased IOP causes a concomitant reduction in choroidal blood flow (Fig. 1) (2,3,15). A reduction in PP by reducing MAP to about half by bleeding causes a similar reduction in choroidal blood flow in rabbits (16). The consequences for retinal metabolism are modest; at increased IOP the extraction rate of oxygen and glucose from choroidal blood is increased to compensate for the reduced blood flow (9), and the total amount extracted is on the same order as during normal IOP. The capacity of the retina for anaerobic glycolysis helps to protect the retina during moderate increments in IOP.

Autoregulation is the result of at least two mechanisms, one metabolic and one myogenic. The stimulus for the metabolic mechanism is the accumulation of vasodilatory metabolites. The high flow rate of the choroid prevents accumulation of vasodilatory metabolites, and the amount that diffuses from the retina is washed out by the choriocapillaris before it reaches the choroidal arteries. Therefore, one cannot expect a metabolic drive to be effective in the choroid. The results from the studies reported above indicate that the myogenic mechanism is also ineffective in the choroid under most circumstances, but a myogenic response has been elicited from the rabbit choroid during changes in arterial and venous pressures induced by hydraulic occluders placed on the thoracic descending aorta and inferior vena cava (17).

A reduction in MAP or an increase in venous pressure has the same effect on the PP, but the effect on local blood flow may vary. A marked reduction in blood pressure caused by, e.g., hemorrhage, will activate the sympathetic nerves. This is a protective mechanism aimed at distributing the remaining blood to tissues in which blood flow is most important for the function of the body, e.g., the brain. In other tissues, such as the gastrointestinal tract, sympathetic vasoconstriction will reduce blood flow beyond that caused by the reduction in the PP. No such mechanism appears to exist in the eye, and an acute hemorrhage does not activate the sympathetic nerves to the eye (16).

EFFECTS OF VASOACTIVE NERVES

Retinal blood flow is protected from systemic influences by a lack of vasoactive nerves. The same is true for the ONH, and stimulation of the cervical

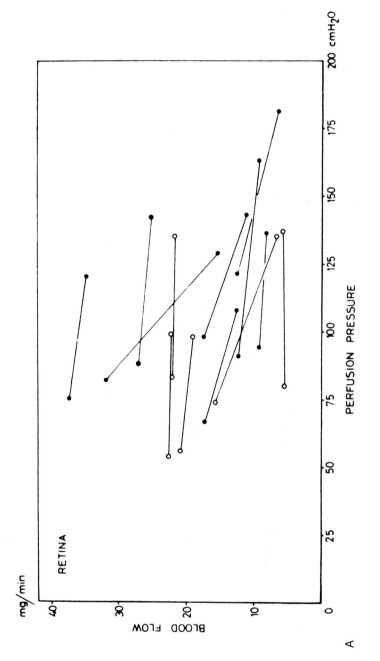

FIG. 1. Blood flow in the retina (**A**) and choroid (**B**) in cats at different perfusion pressures. One eye had its spontaneous intraocular pressure, the other eye had its pressure stabilized at a higher level. The rate of flow is plotted against the perfusion pressure, defined as the mean pressure in the femoral arteries minus the intraocular pressure and expressed in cm H_2O. Lines connect the points representing data for the two eyes of the same animal. From ref. 2.

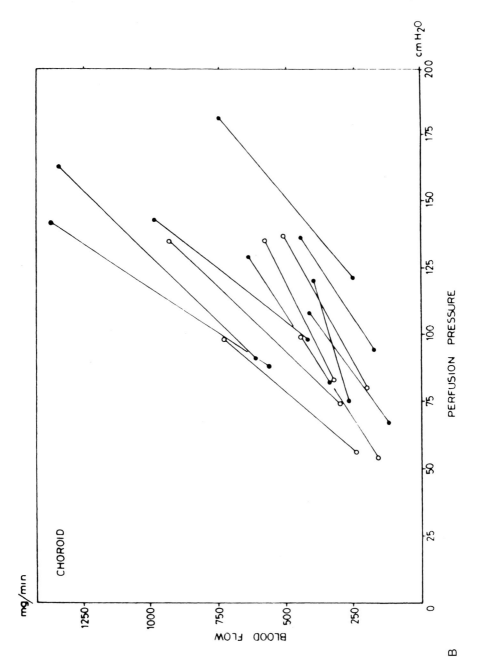

FIG. 1. *Continued.*

sympathetic chain in monkeys had no effect on blood flow through either retina or optic nerve head (18). The situation is quite different in the choroid, which is richly innervated by several vasoactive nerves. Therefore, stimulation of the sympathetic chain reduces choroidal blood flow in cats (19) and monkeys (18). Stimulation of the facial nerve also has an effect on choroidal blood flow, with marked vasodilatation in rabbits, cats, and monkeys (20). In rabbits this effect is mediated by NO at low frequencies (21), while vasoactive intestinal peptide (VIP) may be the transmitter released at high frequencies (22). It is possible that this neuronal pathway is involved in the reflective increase in choroidal blood flow induced by light (8). A ganglion cell plexus in the choroid of primates with a well-developed fovea has recently been described (23). These ganglion cells stain for NO synthase and for VIP. Their role in the regulation of choroidal blood flow is not known.

EFFECTS OF LIGHT

Light has some interesting effects on blood flow through the choroid, retina, and optic nerve. As pointed out above, light causes an initial increase of choroidal blood flow, possibly mediated by the facial nerve as a reflex intended to maintain a steady temperature at the photoreceptor level (8). Flickering light has an effect on the neuronal pathways, but there appear to be important species differences and differences among the various parts of the visual pathway. Flickering light increases blood flow markedly in the ONH of cats (24), whereas there is no or only a small effect in monkeys (25). In both species, flickering light induces a modest increase in retinal blood flow (25–27), whereas there is no effect on blood flow through the retrobulbar part of the optic nerve in cats (Table 3). Flickering light also increases the leukocyte velocity in the macular capillaries of the human retina (28). The increase in blood flow is caused by increased metabolic demands, and flickering light increases glucose consumption in the inner retina of monkeys (14).

TABLE 3. *Blood flow in $\mu l/min/mm^3$ tissue (mean $\pm$ SE, n = 7) through the retina, optic nerve head, and retrobulbar part of the optic nerve in dark-adapted eyes and eyes subjected to flickering light at 8 Hz; flow was determined in cats with no pretreatment and in cats pretreated with L-NAME (30–35 mg/kg bw)*

	No pretreatment		L-NAME	
	Dark-adapted	Flicker	Dark-adapted	Flicker
Retina	0.295 ± 0.026	0.417 ± 0.052*	0.339 ± 0.047	0.347 ± 0.038
Optic nerve head	0.040 ± 0.006	0.120 ± 0.019*	0.004 ± 0.003[†]	0.009 ± 0.004[†]
Optic nerve	0.041 ± 0.004	0.044 ± 0.004	0.035 ± 0.006	0.036 ± 0.005

From ref. 27.
* $p < 0.01$ compared to dark-adapted state.
[†] $p < 0.001$ compared to no pretreatment.

ENDOTHELIAL FACTORS

The vascular endothelium plays a key role in regulation of vascular tone. The effect of the vascular endothelium is twofold. In some tissues, such as the optic nerve, it is the barrier that prevents large substances and small water-soluble substances to reach the vascular smooth muscles. In this respect, the difference between the choroidal vessels and the vessels of the optic nerve is crucial. The permeable choriocapillaris will allow even large molecules to reach the extravascular space and the smooth muscles of the arterial walls, whereas only lipid-soluble blood-borne substances will reach the vascular smooth muscles of the central nervous system. In this respect, the lack of a blood–retinal barrier between the peripapillary choroid and the vessels of the ONH may be important. NO will pass through the barrier but ET cannot pass through the blood–retinal barrier and consequently cannot reach the vascular smooth muscles of the healthy retina or optic nerve. The possibility that the endothelium of a diseased vessel may constitute a less efficient barrier must be kept in mind.

The role of NO in regulation of blood flow is usually determined by studying the effect of a NO blocker, such as N^G-nitro-L-arginine methyl ester (L-NAME), on blood flow. Systemic administration of L-NAME has shown that NO is involved in maintaining a constant vasodilatory tone in the choroid in rabbits, dogs, and cats (29–33). In the rabbit choroid, NO is also released during low-frequency stimulation of the facial nerve (21), indicating a role in addition to maintainance of normal blood flow rates. The vasoconstrictive effect of L-NAME in the rabbit is partly dependent on intact sympathetic nerves (29). When NO is blocked by L-NAME, about half of the vasoconstrictive effect is lost if the eye is denervated, which indicates that L-NAME also activates the sympathetic vasoactive nerves or enhances the effect of the sympathetic tone on choroidal resistance vessels. This was seen only in the choroid and not in the retina as one might expect, because retinal blood flow is not influenced by sympathetic nerves.

In the retina, ONH, and optic nerve, the effect of NO is less straightforward. It is involved in regulation of normal flow rates but, once again, species differences and differences among various parts of the visual pathway exist. Therefore, administration of L-NAME reduces blood flow through the rabbit retina by 50% (29), whereas there is no clear effect on the dark-adapted retina of cats and monkeys (25,27). Normal blood flow through the ONH is markedly influenced by NO and is reduced by 50% in monkeys (25) and to about 10% of normal flow rates in cats, whereas flow through the retrobulbar part of the optic nerve in cats is not influenced by L-NAME (27). As pointed out above, flickering light increases blood flow through the retina in cats and monkeys. This effect is mediated by a release of NO in cats (27,34) but not in monkeys (25).

As expected, the effect of ET on retinal and ONH blood flow depends on whether it is applied inside or outside the blood–retinal barrier. When it is injected into the vitreous body, ET-1 causes vasoconstriction and blood flow reduction in the retina of cats (35,36) and in the ONH of rabbits (37). When given systemically, ET-1 caused a short-lasting increase in ONH blood flow of rabbits that was abolished by L-NAME, indicating that ET-1 releases NO from the vascular endothelium (36). The same is seen in the choroid. An intravenous injection of ET-1 has little effect on choroidal vascular resistance unless the cat is pretreated with L-NAME (35). After pretreatment with L-NAME there is marked vasoconstriction, indicating that a concomitant release of NO normally counteracts the vasoconstrictive effect of ET-1.

REFERENCES

1. Hayreh SS. The ophthalmic artery. III. Branches. *Br J Ophthalmol* 1962;46:212–47.
2. Alm A, Bill A. The oxygen supply to the retina. II. Effects of high intraocular pressure and of increased arterial carbon dioxide tension on uveal and retinal blood flow in cats: a study with labelled microspheres including flow determinations in brain and some other tissues. *Acta Physiol Scand* 1972;84:306–19.
3. Alm A, Bill A. Ocular and optic nerve blood flow at normal and increased intraocular pressures in monkeys (Macaca irus): a study with radioactively labelled microspheres including flow determination in brain and some other tissues. *Exp Eye Res* 1973;15:15–29.
4. Geijer C, Bill A. Effects of raised intraocular pressure on retinal, prelaminar, laminar, and retrolaminar optic nerve blood flow in monkeys. *Invest Ophthalmol Vis Sci* 1979;18:1030–42.
5. Auker CR, Parver LM, Doyle T, Carpenter DO. Choroidal blood flow. I. Ocular tissue temperature as a measure of flow. *Arch Ophthalmol* 1982;100:1323–6.
6. Parver LM, Auker C, Carpenter DO. Choroidal blood flow as a heat dissipating mechanism in the macula. *Am J Ophthalmol* 1980;89:641–6.
7. Parver LM, Auker CR, Carpenter DO, Doyle T. Choroidal blood flow. II. Reflexive control in the monkey. *Arch Ophthalmol* 1982;100:1327–30.
8. Parver LM, Auker CR, Carpenter DO. Choroidal blood flow. III. Reflexive control in human eyes. *Arch Ophthalmol* 1983;101:1604–6.
9. Törnquist P, Alm A. Retinal and choroidal contribution to retinal metabolism in vivo. A study in pigs. *Acta Physiol Scand* 1979;106:351–7.
10. Alder VA, Cringle SJ, Constable IJ. The retinal oxygen profile in cats. *Invest Ophthalmol Vis Sci* 1983;24:30–6.
11. Yancey CM, Linsenmeier RA. Oxygen distribution and consumption in the cat retina at increased intraocular pressure. *Invest Ophthalmol Vis Sci* 1989;30:600–11.
12. Wang L. In *Retinal glucose metabolism and blood flow. Effects of photic stimulation*. Acta Universitatis Upsaliensis (Thesis) 1997;674:1–31.
13. Riva CE, Grunwald JE, Sinclair SH. Laser Doppler measurement of relative blood velocity in human optic nerve head. *Invest Ophthalmol Vis Sci* 1982;22:241–8.
14. Bill A, Sperber G. Aspects of oxygen and glucose consumption in the retina: effects of high intraocular pressure and light. *Graefes Arch Clin Exp Ophthalmol* 1990;228:124–7.
15. Yu DY, Alder VA, Cringle SJ, Brown MJ. Choroidal blood flow measured in the dog eye in vivo and in vitro by local hydrogen clearance polarography: validation of a technique and response to raised intraocular pressure. *Exp Eye Res* 1988;46:289–303.
16. Bill A. Auswirkung einer akuten Blutung beim Kaninchen auf den Blutfuss im Auge und in einigen anderen Gewebe. Die Rolle der sympathischen Nerven. *Klin Mbl Augenheilk* 1984;184:305–7.
17. Kiel JW. Choroidal myogenic autoregulation and intraocular pressure. *Exp Eye Res* 1994;58:529–43.
18. Alm A. The effect of sympathetic stimulation on blood flow through the uvea, retina, and optic nerve in monkeys. *Exp Eye Res* 1977;25:19–24.
19. Alm A, Bill A. The effect of stimulation of the cervical sympathetic chain on retinal oxygen tension and on uveal, retinal, and cerebral blood flow in cats. *Acta Physiol Scand* 1973;88:84–94.

20. Nilsson SFE, Linder J, Bill A. Characteristics of uveal vasodilation produced by facial nerve stimulation in monkeys, cats, and rabbits. *Exp Eye Res* 1985;40:841–52.
21. Nilsson SFE. Nitric oxide as a mediator of parasympathetic vasodilation in ocular and extraocular tissues in the rabbit. *Invest Ophthalmol Vis Sci* 1996;37:2110–9.
22. Nilsson SFE, Bill A. Vasoactive intestinal peptide (VIP): effects on the eye and on regional blood flow. *Acta Physiol Scand* 1984;121:385–92.
23. Flügel-Koch C, Kaufman P, Lütjen-Drecoll E. Association of a choroidal ganglion cell plexus with the fovea centralis. *Invest Ophthalmol Vis Sci* 1994;35:4268–72.
24. Riva CE, Harino S, Shonat RD, Petrig BL. Flicker evoked increase in optic nerve head blood flow in anesthetized cats. *Neurosci Lett* 1991;128:291–6.
25. Kondo M, Wang L, Bill A. Vascular response in retina and optic nerve to L-NAME, a nitric oxide blocker, and flickering light in monkeys [Abstract]. *Invest Ophthalmol Vis Sci* 1995;36:S116.
26. Kiryu J, Asrani S, Shahidi M, Mori M, Zeimer R. Local response of the primate retinal microcirculation to increased metabolic demand induced by flicker. *Invest Ophthalmol Vis Sci* 1995;36:1240–6.
27. Kondo M, Wang L, Bill A. The role of nitric oxide in hyperaemic response to flicker in the retina and optic nerve in cats. *Acta Ophthalmol Scand* 1997;75:232–5.
28. Scheiner AJ, Riva CE, Kazahaya K, Petrig BL. Effect of flicker on macular blood flow assessed by the blue field simulation technique. *Invest Ophthalmol Vis Sci* 1994;35:3436–41.
29. Seligsohn E, Bill A. Effects of N^G-nitro-L-arginine methyl ester on the cardiovascular system of the anesthetized rabbit and on the cardiovascular response to thyrotropin-releasing hormone. *Br J Pharmacol* 1993;109:1219–25.
30. Mori Y. Effects of N(G)-monomethyl-L-arginine on choroidal circulation 1. General administration of N(G)-monomethyl-L-arginine. *Fol Ophthalmol Jpn* 194;45:1163–7.
31. Deussen A, Sonntag M, Vogel RL. Argentine-derived nitric oxide: a major determinant of uveal blood flow. *Exp Eye Res* 1993;57:129–34.
32. Vogel RM, Sonntag M, Deussen A. Effect of arginine-dependent nitric oxide synthesis on the regional perfusion of the eye in anesthetized dogs. *Ophthalmologe* 1994;91:763–7.
33. Mann RM, Riva CE, Stone RA, Barnes GE, Cranstoun SD. Nitric oxide and choroidal blood flow regulation. *Invest Ophthalmol Vis Sci* 1995;36:925–30.
34. Buerk DG, Riva CE, Cranstoun SD. Nitric oxide has a vasodilatory role in cat optic nerve head during flicker stimuli. *Microvasc Res* 1996;52:13–26.
35. Granstam E, Wang L, Bill A. Ocular effects of endothelin-1 in the cat. *Curr Eye Res* 1992;11:325–32.
36. Nishimura K, Riva CE, Harino S, Reinach P, Cranstoun SD, Mita S. Effects of endothelin-1 on optic nerve head blood flow in cats. *J Ocul Pharmacol Ther* 1996;12:75–83.
37. Maetani S, Sugiyama T, Oku H, Shimamura I, Shimizu K, Hamada J, Moriya S. Effect of systemic calcium antagonist on a model of ocular circulation disturbance induced by endothelin-1. *J Jpn Ophthalmol Soc* 1995;99:40–6.

Nitric Oxide and Endothelin in the Pathogenesis of
Glaucoma, edited by I. O. Haefliger and J. Flammer.
Lippincott–Raven Publishers, Philadelphia © 1998.

5

Nitric Oxide and Endothelin in Optic Nerve Head Blood Flow Regulation

Charles E. Riva

Institut de Recherche en Ophtalmologie, Sion, and University of Lausanne, Medical School, Lausanne, Switzerland

This article reports two investigations of optic nerve head (ONH) blood flow in cats: the role of nitric oxide (NO) in mediating the change in ONH blood flow (F_{onh}) during diffuse luminance flicker and the effect of endothelin-1 on F_{onh}. Large portions of text are directly borrowed from Buerk et al. (1) and from Nishimura et al. (2), with permission of the publishers.

NO AND F_{onh} DURING DIFFUSE LUMINANCE FLICKER

NO plays a key role in regulating vascular tone and blood flow in diverse organs (3,4). Coupling between neuronal activity and blood flow in the brain appears to be mediated by NO (5). NO plays a role in regulating basal blood flow to the eye in animals (6–10) and in increased retinal microcirculation of miniature pigs in response to flicker stimuli (11).

In vivo laser Doppler flowmetry (LDF) studies in the cat and human eye by Riva et al. (12–14) have shown that F_{onh} increases when the eye is stimulated by diffuse luminance flicker. These findings suggest that, like blood flow in the brain, F_{onh} and retinal blood flow are tightly coupled to neuronal activity. Further supporting this concept is the observation by Buerk et al. (15) that local K^+ ion concentration near the ONH, which reflects losses from neurons during propagation of action potentials, increases during flicker, and that both varied with the frequency and luminance of the stimulus.

To investigate whether NO mediates the increase in F_{onh} during increased neuronal activity induced by flickering light, Buerk et al. (1) determined NO concentration in the vitreous humor immediately in front of the ONH simultaneously with F_{onh}, at baseline and during flicker, both before and after systemic delivery of NOS inhibitors.

MATERIALS AND METHODS

Buerk et al. (1) used a pivoting microdrive (16) for positioning the NO micro-sensor in the eye and a microscope-mounted near-infrared LDF system (7,18) to obtain simultaneous F_{onh} and NO measurements. Experimental methods for F_{onh} measurements in the cat have been previously described (12–14). Protocols conformed to the ARVO Resolution on the Use of Animals in Research. For initial surgical procedures, cats (2–4 kg) were premedicated with atropine (0.04 mg/kg), then anesthetized with ketamine hydrochloride (HCl) (22 mg/kg) and acepromazine maleate (2 mg/kg). Catheters were placed in the femoral artery and vein and a tracheostomy was performed. Animals were then maintained on volatile anesthetics, mechanically ventilated with 21% O_2, 79% N_2, and 1.5–2.5% enflurane (Ethrane). End-tidal pCO_2, arterial blood pressure (BP), and heart rate (HR) were monitored throughout the experiment. Pancuronium bromide was delivered continuously (0.15 mg/kg/h) after an initial dose (0.2 mg/kg). A stain-less steel ring was sutured to the episcleral limbus to stabilize eye position. The pupil of the eye under study was dilated with 1% tropicamide and 10% phenylephrine, and a zero-diopter contact lens was placed on the cornea along with a drop of Healon. Nafion polymer (DuPont, Wilmington, DE)-coated re-cessed gold microsensors were fabricated from glass micropipettes with tip dimensions approximately 5 μm or less. Operational theory and construction details for recessed NO microsensors are described by Buerk et al. (1) and Buerk (19).

NO microsensors were positioned in the eye, avoiding visible blood vessels. Tips were placed very close to the surface of the ONH (<10 μm away, or in some cases actually touching the surface) within the spot where the laser beam was focused. Ambient light was reduced and the eyes were allowed to adapt to the dark for at least 30 min. The NO microsensor current (in picoamperes) was converted to concentration after calibration of each microsensor. Experimental F_{onh} and NO microsensor responses were measured during flicker at the maximal luminance from a photic stimulator (Model PS-22; Grass, Quincy, MA) delivered to the eye through the microscope by an optical fiber. The flash duration was 20 μs and the maximal luminance was approximately 8×10^{-5} μJ/cm^2/flash. The stimulus, usually 10 and sometimes 15 Hz, lasted for 1–2 min and elicited near-maximal F_{onh} responses. After control responses were obtained, NOS inhibitors were delivered intravenously ($n = 10$ cats). L-NNA was infused at 25 mg/min for 3–4 min for cumulative doses of 75–100 mg ($n = 5$ cats). N^G-nitro-L-arginine methyl ester (L-NAME) was delivered by sequential bolus injections (15–30 mg each). The cumulative dose of L-NAME was 60 mg ($n = 4$ cats), and one cat received a total of 90 mg. Measurements of flicker-induced F_{onh} responses were repeated after inhibiting NOS.

RESULTS

After dark adaptation, baseline NO concentrations near the ONH for normal conditions ($n = 6$ cats) ranged from 0.8 to 1.2 μM (0.3 and 0.5 Torr) (1).

Flickering light caused a small but significant increase in NO, ranging from 50 to 150 nM (0.02–0.06 Torr) above baseline. A representative example for the change in NO (top) and LDF (bottom) during flicker is shown in Fig. 1. With the onset of flicker at t = 0, there was a rapid rise in the NO current, with an average increase in NO concentration by 67 ± 1 nM during the final min of the flicker stimulus ($p<0.0001$). F_{onh} response also increased rapidly, particularly during the first 30 s. The average response was 32 ± 0.4% above baseline for the final minute of the flicker stimulus ($p<0.0001$). After stopping the flicker stimulus, both NO and F_{onh} returned to baseline levels.

Overall, NO increased during flicker by an average of 88 ± 23 nM (0.036 ± 0.009 Torr), significantly above baseline levels ($p<0.05$), and average F_{onh} increased by 44 ± 7.0% above baseline ($p<0.001$; n = 6 cats). Variable changes in baseline F_{onh} were observed after NOS inhibition. Individual changes are shown in Fig. 2A for the five L-NNA experiments. After beginning L-NNA infusion at t = 0 and delivering a cumulative dose of 75–100 mg, there was an overall decline in baseline F_{onh} with time. For four of the five cats, F_{onh} increased above baseline at some point. Similar variable changes in baseline F_{onh} were

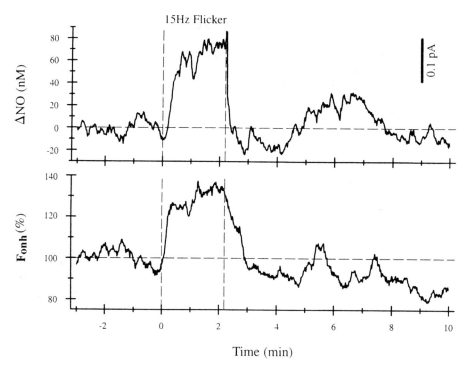

FIG. 1. Time course of changes in NO (*top*) and F_{onh} (*bottom*) under control conditions. At t = 0, the eye was stimulated with diffuse luminance flicker at 15 Hz for 2 min (stopping at second vertical dashed line). A scale for the NO microsensor current change in picoamperes is shown by the bar at upper right. From ref. 1.

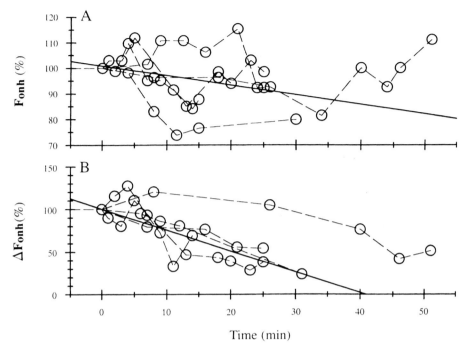

FIG. 2. Time course of F_{onh} changes after i.v. infusion (at t = 0) for cumulative dose of 75–100 mg of the NOS inhibitor L-NNA (n = 5). **A**: Changes in baseline F_{onh} (open circles) for individual cats (connected by dashed lines), with a small, overall decline (solid regression line, slope −0.37%/min, r = 0.35). The F_{onh}s were normalized with respect to the average F_{onh} baseline during control conditions. **B**: Changes in F_{onh} responses to flicker (10–15 Hz). The F_{onh} flicker responses were normalized with respect to the mean flicker responses during control conditions. For four cats, the response decreased by 50% within 21 min (solid regression line, slope −2.45%/min, r = 0.83), with a similar time trend after a 20–30-min delay in one cat. From ref. 1.

observed for the five cats in the L-NAME study. For some cats, there was a decrease in F_{onh} after the first dose (15 or 30 mg), followed by a modest increase of 2–5% in four cats after reaching a cumulative dose of 60 mg. Baseline F_{onh} was probably influenced by the increase in mean arterial pressure after NOS inhibition.

Changes in flicker responses after NOS inhibition were much more consistent, as shown in Fig. 2B for the five cats receiving L-NNA. F_{onh} responses became progressively smaller with time after infusion, except for one cat, in which there was a delay before declining. The time to fall to 50% of the control was less than 21 min. In all 10 experiments, there was an attenuation of the F_{onh} responses after i.v. administration of NOS inhibitors.

In Fig. 3, flicker-induced NO (top) and F_{onh} (bottom) responses are shown before and after L-NNA. Before L-NNA there was a rapid increase in NO by about 90 nM, with F_{onh} increasing by more than 50% above baseline after 1 min

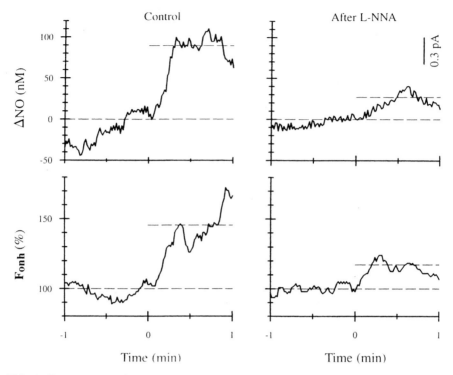

FIG. 3. F_{onh} responses (15 Hz, beginning at t = 0) for control conditions (*left*) and after i.v. infusion of L-NNA (*right*). Both NO and F_{onh} flicker responses are significantly higher than baseline levels ($p < 0.0001$). After L-NNA, both NO (*top right*) and F_{onh} (*bottom right*) responses to flicker were significantly attenuated. From ref. 1.

of flicker. Approximately 15 min after administration of the maximal dose of L-NNA, both NO and F_{onh} responses were significantly smaller than control responses ($p < 0.0001$). Similar results were obtained in the experiments before and after L-NAME (1). Approximately 30 min after the maximal cumulative dose of L-NAME (90 mg), there was a nonsignificant NO increase during flicker and the F_{onh} response was around 18%, significantly smaller ($p < 0.0001$) than the 50% increase before infusion of L-NAME.

Figure 4 shows all NOS inhibitor responses. Arterial blood pressure increased from 91.5 ± 3.7 to 118 ± 6 mm Hg ($p < 0.005$) after the maximal dose of NOS inhibitors. As shown in Fig. 4A, there was a decrease in the baseline NO concentration by 0.46 ± 0.04 μM ($p < 0.005$). NO levels after NOS inhibition were estimated to range between 0.3 and 0.7 μM. There was a nonsignificant 11.5% drop in F_{onh} from the control baseline.

Averaged control (open bars, $\pm$ SEM) and NOS inhibition results (shaded bars) for the F_{onh} and NO flicker responses are shown in Fig. 5B ($n = 6$ cats). The average increase in NO during flicker after NOS inhibition was 11 ± 3 nM,

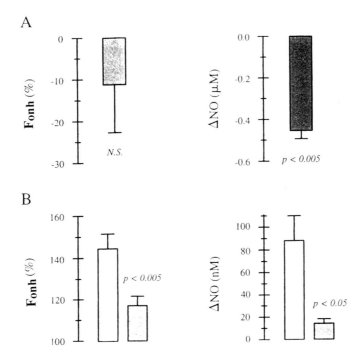

FIG. 4. Average results from NOS inhibition ($n = 6$). **A:** Although the mean decrease in baseline F_{onh} (*left*) was not significant, the baseline NO level (*right*) was significantly reduced ($p < 0.005$). **B:** Mean flicker responses showing increases in F_{onh} (*left*) and NO (*right*) for controls (open bars) and after inhibiting NOS (shaded bars). Both F_{onh} and NO flicker responses were significantly attenuated compared to control responses (p values from paired t tests are shown). From ref. 1.

significantly less than the control flicker response of 69 ± 16 nM ($p<0.05$). The mean NO response was 14 ± 4 nM, significantly below the average increase of 88 ± 23 nM for controls ($p<0.05$). Average F_{onh} during flicker for controls was $144 \pm 7\%$ of baseline and after NOS inhibition was significantly reduced to $117 \pm 5\%$ of baseline ($p<0.005$). The F_{onh} response to flicker was also significantly attenuated to 38% of the control response ($p<0.005$).

DISCUSSION

These results confirmed that both NOS inhibitors reduce the basal NO levels near the ONH and the amount of NO produced during flicker (1). These reductions paralleled the decrease of the F_{onh} responses after NOS inhibition and strongly implicate NO as a putative mediator of the coupling between blood flow and neuronal activity.

Recently, Donati et al. (11), who measured NO in the vitreous humor near the retinal surface of miniature pigs using a probe with tip diameter ≈ 100 μm, also found that NO increased during flicker. The changes were nearly 20-fold larger than those we found in the cat vitreous humor near the ONH. Intravenous infusion of L-NNA (20 mg/kg for 10 min) had no measurable effect on diameter (11), a result consistent with our measurements, in which NOS inhibition did not significantly reduce baseline F_{onh}. When 600 μM L-NNA was directly applied to arterioles by a puffer pipette, Donati et al. (11) observed a transient decrease in diameter (-45%) and concluded that basal NO production was important for controlling arteriolar tone in the retinal microcirculation. Most probably, basal NO has a similar role in the cat ONH.

The F_{onh} results of Buerk et al. (1) from the cat eye compare favorably with some aspects of the studies in primate optic nerve recently reported by Kondo et al. (7), who reported that flicker at 8 Hz increased optic nerve flow measured with microspheres by $\approx 13\%$ above baseline. These investigators also reported that cats had a threefold higher increase in flow with flicker and that L-NAME significantly reduced, by 52%, flow in the distal part of the ONH. After L-NAME, flicker caused a smaller increase in microsphere flow by $\approx 67\%$ of the normal response. In contrast to the primate, there was not a large decline in cat flow after NOS inhibition. The increase in mean arterial blood pressure may have been sufficient to offset vasoconstriction, or perhaps other autoregulatory mechanisms compensated for the effects of NOS inhibition in the cat ONH. Interestingly, microsphere ONH flow in primates still responded to flicker after NOS inhibition. The cat eye studies of Buerk et al. (1) also showed that neither F_{onh} nor the NO flicker responses were completely abolished for the cumulative doses used. In the cat, the reduction in average microsphere flow response to flicker after NOS inhibition was about 38% of the control flicker response. Differences in NO responses before and after inhibition were consistent with the cat F_{onh} changes.

The basal NO levels reported here for the vitreous humor near the ONH are similar to values reported for brain tissue but are lower than basal NO measured near arterioles in miniature pig retina (11), probably because in the former study (1) visible vessels were avoided. Donati et al. (11) found fairly steep NO gradients in the vitreous, with NO falling close to zero when the microprobe was withdrawn to ≈ 200 μm above the surface of the miniature pig retina. It is possible that measurements in the vitreous humor underestimate basal levels in ONH tissue.

Basal NO levels probably originate from two sources: vascular endothelium and NO-producing neurons. Buerk et al. (1) have hypothesized that neuronal sources of NO are responsible for the coupling of F_{onh} with increased neuronal activity. Donati et al. (11) present evidence that Müller cells in the retina may be another possible source of NO, because they have a significant rate of arginine biosynthesis. Therefore, the Müller cells around the periphery of the ONH might well be the sources of NO.

The study by Buerk et al. (1) is the first investigation that directly shows the coupling between F_{onh} and NO changes after NOS inhibition. Although these authors conclude that NO plays a key role in regulating F_{onh}, there are clearly other factors (e.g., pO_2, pH, pCO_2, K^+, circulating hormones) that can modify F_{onh} and vascular responses. K^+ has been shown to increase during flicker in the ONH (15). Further investigations are needed to elucidate the mechanism involved in this regulation.

EFFECT OF ENDOTHELIN-1 ON F_{onh}

Endothelin-1 is a potent vasoconstrictive peptide (20) that acts directly on vascular smooth-muscle cells. It produces a prolonged pressor response when injected i.v. and constricts the cerebral arteries when injected intracisternally (21). In addition to playing a role in blood pressure control, endothelin-1 induces cerebral vasospasm (22). In contrast, vasodilator responses to endothelin-1 have been also demonstrated in some blood vessels. These responses are believed to be due to the release of vasodilator substances, such as prostacyclin or endothelium-derived relaxing factor (EDRF:NO) (23) from endothelium (23–26).

In the eye, endothelin-1 injected intravitreally contracts retinal vessels in rabbits (27,28) and reduces retinal blood flow in cats (29). Therefore, this agent may play a role in the regulation of F_{onh}. To test this hypothesis, Nishimura et al. (2) have investigated the effects of i.v. and intravitreal injection of endothelin-1 on F_{onh} in anesthetized cats, using LDF.

MATERIALS AND METHODS

Twenty-five normal cats of either sex and weighing 2.5–4.0 kg were prepared as described above. Baseline F_{onh}, BP and HR were first recorded for at least 10 min. In the first type of experiment ($n = 12$ cats), endothelin-1 diluted in saline (50–2,500 pmol) was injected as a bolus of 50 μl through the pars plana into the vitreous close to the ONH with a 27-gauge needle. In the second type of experiment, endothelin-1 (0.004–0.4 nmol/kg) was injected i.v. ($n = 8$ cats). In another group of five cats, endothelin-1 was injected first, followed after 70–90 min by a bolus injection of 10 mg/kg of N^G-nitro-L-arginine methylester (L-NAME) or an infusion of 5 mg/kg/min L-NAME over 30 min. Endothelin-1 was injected again 15 min after starting the infusion of L-NAME or in combination with L-arginine HCl (50 mg/kg/min). The challenges of endothelin-1 were repeated at intervals of at least 2 h.

The preparation of endothelin-1 (10^{-4} M), L-arginine HCl, and N^G-nitro-L-arginine methyl ester (L-NAME) was described by Nishimura et al. (2). Bolus i.v. injections were given at a volume of 0.4 ml/kg, which were flushed in with 1 ml saline to wash out the dead spaces of the catheters. Infusions were given at a rate of 0.5 ml/min.

All data are expressed as mean $\pm$ SEM. Statistical significance was determined with Student's t test for either paired or unpaired variates or by Dunnett's multiple comparison test ($p<0.05$).

RESULTS

Effects of Intravitreal Injection of Endothelin-1

Figure 5a of Nishimura et al. (2) shows a typical recording of F_{onh} (Flow) after intravitreal injection of endothelin-1 (ET-1). Endothelin-1 (50–2,500 pmol)

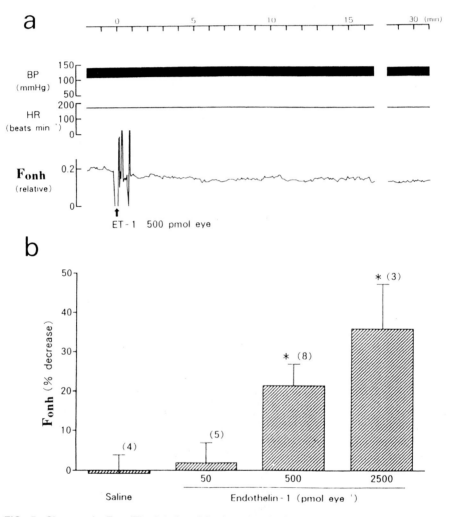

FIG. 5. Changes in F_{onh} (Flow) induced by intravitreal injection of endothelin-1 (ET-1) in anesthetized cats. **a**: A typical recording after the injection of ET-1 500 pmol per eye. **b**: The dose-related effects of ET-1 (50–2,500 pmol per eye) on F_{onh}. Data indicate the peak change from baseline. Figures in parentheses are the number of experiments. *$p < 0.05$ vs. baseline (Student's t test). From ref. 2.

produced a dose-related decrease in F_{onh} (Fig. 5b). The decreases in F_{onh} were significant at 500 pmol and 2,500 pmol ET-1 and were still present even after 30 min. BP and HR remained unaffected by these doses.

Effects of i.v. Injection of Endothelin-1

With i.v. bolus injections (Fig. 6), endothelin-1 (0.004–0.4 nmol/kg) produced a dose-related increase in F_{onh} (2). The increases were significant at 0.08 and 0.4 nmol/kg for F_{onh}. The increase in F_{onh} induced by endothelin-1 (0.4 nmol/kg) was short-lasting (Fig. 7a), and F_{onh} returned to its preinjection level 10 min after injection (2). Endothelin-1 produced a transient decrease in BP, followed by a more sustained increase. The transient decrease in BP was significant at 0.4 nmol/kg and the subsequent increase in BP was significant at 0.08 and 0.4 nmol/kg. Endothelin-1 produced no significant decrease in HR, except when injected at a dose of 0.4 nmol/kg.

Effects of i.v. Injection of Endothelin-1 in the Presence of L-NAME

At time $t = 0$, L-NAME was injected i.v. (5 mg/kg/min). Ten minutes later, BP was 143 ± 4 mm Hg ($n = 5$) compared with 89 ± 4 mm Hg at the start of the experiment. It was constant at 103 ± 4 mm Hg when endothelin-1 was injected. F_{onh} was not significantly affected by L-NAME (data not shown). The

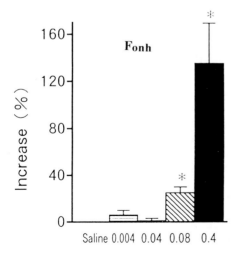

FIG. 6. Dose-related effects of i.v. injection of endothelin-1 on F_{onh}. The peak responses were obtained within 5 min after injection. Data indicate the peak change from baseline ($n = 8$). $p < 0.05$ vs. baseline (Student's t test). From ref. 2.

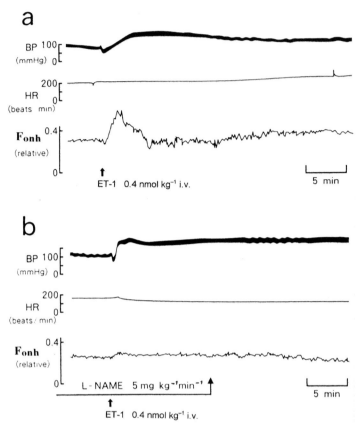

FIG. 7. Typical recordings of the effects of endothelin-1 (0.4 nmol kg^{-1}, i.v. in the absence
(**a**) or presence (**b**) of N^G-nitro-L-arginine methyl ester (L-NAME, 5 mg kg^{-1} min^{-1} i.v.) on blood
pressure (BP), heart rate (HR), and F$_{onh}$ (Flow). From ref. 2.

increase in F$_{onh}$ by endothelin-1 (Figs. 7 and 8) observed in the absence of L-
NAME was abolished in the presence of the inhibitor (2) and reversed in the
presence of L-NAME plus L-arginine. Pressor responses to endothelin-1 were
augmented in the presence of L-NAME, but the transient decrease in BP was
not affected (data not shown). The augmentation by L-NAME of the pressor
responses to endothelin-1 (Figs. 7 and 8) was abolished in combination with L-
arginine (2).

DISCUSSION

These results show that endothelin-1 has differential effects on F$_{onh}$. Injected into the vitreous body, it decreased F$_{onh}$, whereas it increased F$_{onh}$ when

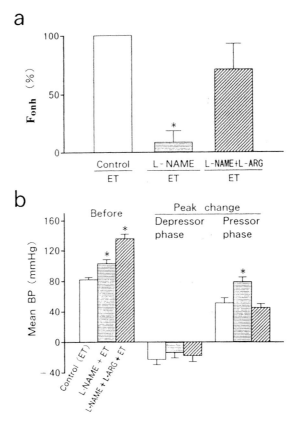

FIG. 8. Effects of L-NAME (5 mg/kg/min i.v.) and L-NAME plus L-arginine (L-ARG, 50 mg/kg/min i.v.) on the responses of F_{onh} (Flow) (**a**) and mean blood pressure (BP) (**b**) to endothelin-1 (ET, 0.4 nmol/kg i.v.) ($n = 5$). Endothelin-1 was injected three times at intervals of at least 2 h in each cat. (**a**) The peak increases in F_{onh}, which were obtained within 5 min, induced by the first endothelin-1 injection (control) were taken as 100%. Data are expressed as percent of the control response to endothelin-1. *$p < 0.05$ vs. control (Student's *t* test). (**b**) Depressor phase shows the initial peak decrease in mean BP, and pressor phase shows the subsequent peak increase in mean BP, which was obtained within 10 min after injection of endothelin-1. *$p < 0.05$ vs. control (Dunnett's test). From ref. 2.

injected i.v. These opposing effects could be due to the difference in the route of administration. It is possible that endothelin-1 acted first directly on the limiting membranes of the vascular smooth muscle surrounding the blood vessels when it was intravitreally injected. On the other hand, after i.v. injection it probably first interacted with the internal endothelial membranes facing the vascular lumen. However, systemic hemodynamic effects elicited by i.v. injection of endothelin-1 might also contribute to these responses.

Endothelin-1 is a potent vasoconstrictor peptide which acts directly on vascular smooth-muscle cells (20). Recent studies demonstrated that there are two distinct endothelin receptor subtypes in the vasculature, designated ET_A and ET_B (30,31). The ET_A subtype on the surrounding smooth-muscle cell membranes is responsible for contraction, whereas the ET_B subtype on endothelial cell membranes may be responsible for relaxation via the release of EDRF or prostacyclin (22,32). Our findings suggest that the reduction of F_{onh} induced by endothelin-1 is due to direct vasoconstriction, presumably by the ET_A subtype.

On the other hand, endothelin-1 can have a vasodilator action through stimulation of the ET_B subtype and the release of endogenous mediators, such as prostacyclin and/or NO, from endothelial cells. This notion is supported by our findings of an increase in F_{onh} induced by i.v. injection of endothelin-1, which could be completely inhibited in the presence of L-NAME. Therefore, it appears that endothelin-1 interacts with the ET_B subtype on endothelial cells to elicit vasodilatation through the release of NO when it is administered i.v.

It is generally accepted that the hypotensive response to endothelin-1 is induced by the release of a relaxing factor from the vascular endothelium. As others found in rats (24,26,33), we also observed that the initial hypotensive response to i.v. endothelin-1 was not affected by either L-NAME or indomethacin (data not shown), suggesting that the hypotensive response to endothelin-1 may be due to the release of some other vasodilator substances in addition to a cyclo-oxygenase product (prostacyclin) and NO.

We observed that the pressor response to i.v. endothelin-1 was increased in the presence of L-NAME. This augmentation indicates that endothelin-1 produced a direct vasoconstriction, which resulted in an elevation of total peripheral resistance as well as an opposing reduction in peripheral resistance caused by vasodilatation through L-NAME-sensitive NO release. Because L-NAME suppressed NO release, the net pressor response was enhanced. Our finding that an increase in F_{onh} induced by i.v. injection of endothelin-1 was absent in the presence of L-NAME, in spite of the L-NAME-induced increase in the pressor response, indicates that the increase in F_{onh} may not be caused by a hemodynamic effect. Furthermore, under this condition there was no decrease in F_{onh}. This result suggests that there is a blood–tissue barrier in the ONH blocking endothelin-1 access to the vascular smooth muscles or pericytes. If the blood–tissue barrier in the ONH is damaged, intravascular endothelin-1 could infiltrate the extravascular space of the ONH and thus gain access to vascular smooth muscles or pericytes, producing vasospasms or even vascular occlusions.

In conclusion, the results of Nishimura et al. (2) demonstrate that intravitreal injection of endothelin-1 decreases F_{onh} by its vasoconstrictive effect, probably through mediation of cell signaling pathways linked to stimulation of the ET_A subtype, whereas i.v. injection of endothelin-1 increases F_{onh} through NO release, presumably subsequent to stimulation of the ET_B subtype located on the endothelial cells.

ACKNOWLEDGMENTS

This research was supported by NIH grants EY-09269 and EY-08413 and by research grant #3200-043157.95 from Fonds National Suisse de la Recherche Scientifique, and by Loterie Suisse Romande.

REFERENCES

1. Buerk DG, Riva CE, Cranstoun SD. Nitric oxide has a vasodilatory role in cat optic nerve head during flickering stimuli. *Microvasc Res* 1996;52:13–26.
2. Nishimura K, Riva CE, Harino S, Reinach P, et al. Effects of endothelin-1 on optic nerve head blood flow in cats. *J Ocul Pharmacol* 1996;12:75–83.
3. Moncada S, Palmer RMJ, Higgs EA. The discovery of nitric oxide as the endogenous nitrovasodilator. *Hypertension* 1988;12:365–72.
4. Moncada S, Palmer RMJ, Higgs EA. Nitric oxide: physiology, pathophysiology, and pharmacology. *Pharmacol Rev* 1991;43:109–42.
5. Ladecola C, Pelligrino DA, Moskowitz MA, et al. Nitric oxide synthase inhibition and cerebrovascular regulation. *J Cereb Blood Flow Metab* 1994;14:175–92.
6. Deussen A, Sonntag M, Vogel R. L-Arginine-derived nitric oxide: a major determinant of uveal blood flow. *Exp Eye Res* 1993;57:129–34.
7. Kondo M, Wang L, Bill A. Vascular responses in retina and optic nerve to L-NAME, a nitric oxide blocker, and flickering light in monkeys [Abstract]. *Invest Ophthalmol Vis Sci* 1994;36:477.
8. Mann RM, Riva CE, Stone RA, et al. Nitric oxide and choroidal blood flow regulation. *Invest Ophthalmol Vis Sci* 1995;36:925–30.
9. Wang Y, Okamura T, Toda N. Mechanisms of acetylcholine-induced relaxation in dog external and internal ophthalmic arteries. *Exp Eye Res* 1993;57:275–82.
10. Yamamoto R, Bredt D, Snyder S, Stone R. The localization of nitric oxide synthase in the eye and related cranial ganglia. *Neuroscience* 1993;54:189–200.
11. Donati G, Pournaras CJ, Munoz J-L, et al. Nitric oxide controls arteriolar tone in the retina of the miniature pig. *Invest Ophthalmol Vis Sci* 1995;36:2228–37.
12. Riva CE, Harino S, Petrig BL, Shonat RD. Laser Doppler flowmetry in the optic nerve. *Exp Eye Res* 1992;55:499–506.
13. Riva CE, Harino S, Petrig BL, Shonat RD. Circulation of the optic nerve head: an investigation with laser Doppler flowmetry. In: Drance JM, van Buskirk EM, Neufeld AH, eds. *Pharmacology of glaucoma*. Baltimore: Williams & Wilkins, 1992:253–64.
14. Riva CE, Harino S, Shonat RD, Petrig BL. Flicker evoked increase in optic nerve head blood flow in anesthetized cats. *Neurosci Lett* 1991;128:291–6.
15. Buerk DG, Riva CE, Cranstoun SD. Frequency and luminance dependent blood flow and K^+ ion changes during flicker stimuli in cat optic nerve head. *Invest Ophthalmol Vis Sci* 1995;36:2216–27.
16. Poumaras CJ, Shonat RD, Munoz J-L, et al. New ocular micromanipulator for measurements of retinal and vitreous physiologic parameters in the mammalian eye. *Exp Eye Res* 1991;53:23–7.
17. Petrig BL, Riva CE. Near-IR retinal laser Doppler velocimetry and flowmetry: new delivery and detection techniques. *Appl Opt* 1991;30:2073–8.
18. Shonat RS, Riva CE, Petrig BL. New microscope based LDV camera. *Noninvas Assess Vis Syst* 1991;176–79.
19. Buerk DG. *Biosensors: theory and applications.* Lancaster, PA: Technomics, 1993.
20. Yanagisawa M, Kurihara H, Kimura S, et al. A novel potent vasoconstrictor peptide produced by vascular endothelial cells. *Nature* 1988;332:411–5.
21. Mima T, Yanagisawa M, Shigeno T, et al. Endothelin acts in feline and canine cerebral arteries from the adventitial side. *Stroke* 1989;20:1553–6.
22. Masaki T, Kimura S, Yanagisawa M, et al. Molecular and cellular mechanism of endothelin regulation. Implication for vascular function. *Circulation* 1991;84:1457–68.

23. Ignarro LJ, Buga GM, Wood KS, et al. Endothelium-derived relaxing factor produced and released from artery and vein is nitric oxide. *Proc Natl Acad Sci USA* 1987;84:9265–9.
24. De Nucci G, Thomas R, D'orleans-Juste P, et al. Pressor effects of circulating endothelin are limited by its removal in the pulmonary circulation and by the release of prostacyclin and endothelium-derived relaxing factor. *Proc Natl Acad Sci USA* 1988;85:9797–800.
25. Folta A, Joshua IG, Webb RC. Dilator actions of endothelin in coronary resistance vessels and the abdominal aorta of the guinea pig. *Life Sci* 1989;45:2627–35.
26. Fozard JR, Part ML. The role of nitric oxide in the regional vasodilator effects of endothelin-I in the rat. *Br J Pharmacol* 1992;105:744–50.
27. Sakaue H, Kiryu J, Takeuchi A, et al. Effects of endothelin on retinal blood vessels. *Acta Soc Ophthalmol Jpn* 1992;96:469–72.
28. Takei K, Sato T, Nonoyama T, et al. Analysis of vasoconstrictive responses to endothelin-I in the rabbit retinal vessels using an ET_A receptor antagonist and ET_B receptor agonist. *Life Sci* 1993;53:PL111–5.
29. Granstam E, Wang L, Bill A. Ocular effects of endothelin-I in the cat. *Curr Eye Res* 1992;11:325–32.
30. Arai H, Hori S, Aramori I, Ohkubo H, Nakanishi S. Cloning and expression of a CDNA encoding an endothelin receptor. *Nature* 1990;348:730–2.
31. Sakurai T, Yanagisawa M, Takuwa Y, et al. Cloning of a CDNA encoding a non-isopeptide-selective subtype of the endothelin receptor. *Nature* 1990;348:732–5.
32. Sakurai T, Yanagisawa M, Masaki T. Molecular characterization of endothelin receptors. *Trends Pharmacol Sci* 1992;13:103–8.
33. Gardiner SM, Compton AM, Kemp PA, et al. Regional and cardiac haemodynamic responses to glycerol trinitrate, acetylcholine, bradykinin and endothelin-I in conscious rats: effect of N^G-nitro-L-arginine methyl ester. *Br J Pharmacol* 1990;101:632–9.

Nitric Oxide and Endothelin in the Pathogenesis of Glaucoma, edited by I. O. Haefliger and J. Flammer. Lippincott–Raven Publishers, Philadelphia © 1998.

6

Modulation by Oxygen of Nitric Oxide–Induced Relaxation of Retinal Pericytes

Ivan O. Haefliger and *Douglas R. Anderson

*Laboratory of Ocular Pharmacology and Physiology, Department of Medicine, University of Basel, Basel, Switzerland; and *Department of Ophthalmology, Bascom Palmer Eye Institute, University of Miami School of Medicine, Miami, Florida*

In a vessel, blood flow is strongly modulated by changes in vascular diameter (1–3). Because of the relationship to the power four that exists between the vascular diameter and flow (Poiseuille's law), decreasing the diameter of a vessel by 50% will result in a drastic reduction of flow in this vessel by 94%. Conversely, increasing the diameter of this vessel by 50% will result in a huge increase of flow by more than 400%. These examples clearly illustrate the tremendous influence of a modification of the vascular diameter on local blood flow regulation.

Poiseuille's law is considered valid in the macrocirculation for vessels larger than 200 μm (whether it is an artery or a vein) and does not necessarily apply to the microcirculation because of the physical properties of blood in small vessels (e.g., viscosity, hematocrit, shear stress, large size of blood cellular elements compared to vessel diameter). Nevertheless, empirically when measurements were made in the microcirculation, a relationship close to the power four between the diameter and resistance, and therefore flow, could be observed in single unbranched vessels smaller than 60 μm (Fig. 1). (4). This remarkable observation implies that the size of the vascular diameter appears to have a similar influence on blood flow in both in the macro- and the microcirculation (5).

Although there is no doubt about the importance of precapillary resistance arteries in regulation of peripheral blood flow, this does not exclude the possibility that some modulation of blood flow can also take place in other vessels of the microcirculation, such as downstream in capillaries.

For ophthalmologists, and especially glaucomatologists, a possible modulation of flow within capillaries would certainly be an interesting concept, because the

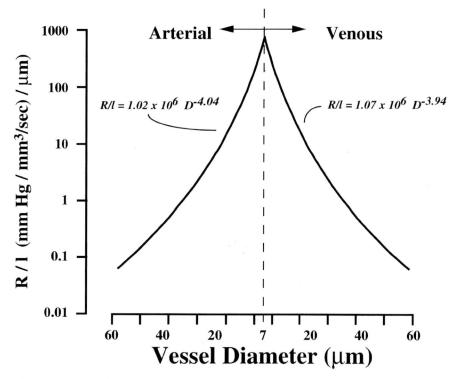

FIG. 1. Arteriovenous distribution of intravascular resistance per unit length measured in vivo in single unbranched vessels of the cat's mesenteric microcirculation. As blood traverses this network, as in larger vessels for the Poiseuille's law, it appears that the fourth power relationship of vessels' diameter the dominant factor in specifying intravascular resistance during normal flow. R/l, resistance (R) per unit length (l); D, vascular diameter. Modified from refs. 4 and 5.

vascular bed of the optic nerve head is essentially made of a dense capillary network, which is directly and continuously interconnected with the retinal capillary network (Fig. 2) (6).

To be plausible, this working hypothesis should at least imply that capillaries have the ability to modify their vascular diameter (7–9). Moreover, there is increasing evidence that, like larger vessels, capillaries also have vasoactive properties. Very schematically, capillaries are made of an internal lining of endothelial cells surrounded by a important layer of pericytes (Fig. 3). (10,11). Like the smooth-muscle cells of larger vessels, pericytes are contractile cells (12–28), which can be relaxed by nitric oxide (NO) (29). This chapter demonstrates that the relaxation induced by NO can be modulated by different concentrations of oxygen, not ignoring the important contribution of others but taking the opportunity to summarize some of the work we have done on NO effects in pericytes (30–32). The physiology of capillary blood flow regulation in the retina and optic nerve head may be relevant to glaucoma if one believes that a

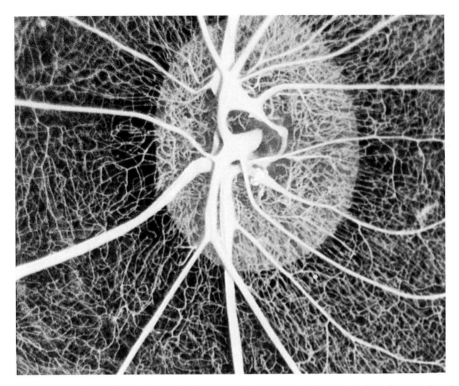

FIG. 2. Vascular casting showing the dense capillary network of a monkey's optic nerve head and its close interconnection with capillaries of the retinal circulation. From ref. 33.

Endothelial Cells

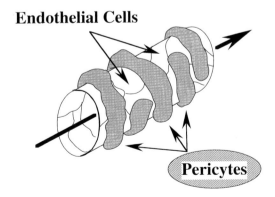

FIG. 3. Schematic and simplified drawing of a capillary illustrating the fact that this vessel is made of an internal lining of endothelium surrounded by a cover of contractile cells, the pericytes.

local dysregulation of blood flow is implicated in the pathogenesis of this disease (33).

To appreciate the potential importance of an interaction between NO and oxygen in the regulation of pericyte tone, two facts must be remembered concerning NO and oxygen in the eye. The first is the existence of a basal release of NO in the ophthalmic circulation, which maintains vessels in a constant state of mid-dilatation (34–37). The second is that the circulation of both the optic nerve head and the retina is regulated by oxygen (2,3,38). In hypoxia blood flow increases, whereas in hyperoxia blood flow decreases. Therefore, to determine if oxygen can modulate the NO-induced vasorelaxation of pericytes appears to be a logical and relevant question to address.

One convenient way to study pericytes is to culture them on a silicone membrane coating the bottom of a petri dish (30,39). By observing these cells with an inverted contrast microscope, it is possible to follow the contractile state of a single pericyte. By placing the petri dish in a closed chamber, it is possible by a suction–perfusion system to change the fluid above the cells and expose them to different drugs (29–32). With this experimental setup it is also possible

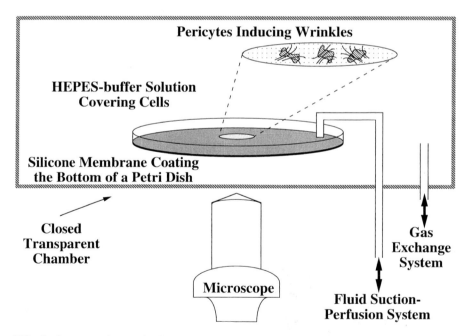

FIG. 4. Setup used to study changes in pericytes contractile tone. Pericytes were grown on a silicone membrane coating the bottom of a petri dish. Cells were observed by a phase-contrast inverted microscope. By a suction–perfusion system, the HEPES buffer solution covering the cells was exchanged and retinal pericytes exposed to different drugs. In addition, by a gas exchange system, the ambient air in the closed transparent chamber containing the petri dish could be saturated with 100% oxygen or 100% nitrogen (31,32).

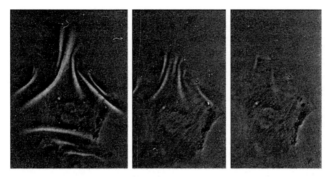

FIG. 5. Appearance of wrinkles induced by a single pericyte (×1,200) grown on a thin sheet of silicone and observed with a phase-contrast inverted microscope (*left*). After 10-min exposure to 3 and 100 μM of sodium nitroprusside, respectively, a marked loss of wrinkles could be observed (*middle* and *right*). From ref. 29.

to change the partial pressure of oxygen in the chamber and to study the effect of such changes on the tone of pericytes (Fig. 4) (31,32).

Figure 5 shows how, with this experimental setup, a pericyte appears before and after exposure to sodium nitroprusside (29). The relaxing effect of sodium nitroprusside is presented because sodium nitroprusside has the ability to release NO spontaneously. By increasing the concentration of sodium nitroprusside, it is possible to construct a dose–response curve (Fig. 6) (29). These two examples clearly demonstrate that pericytes are contractile cells and that they can be relaxed by a donor of NO, such as sodium nitroprusside.

To confirm that the relaxation caused by sodium nitroprusside was actually caused by the release of NO, the pericytes were relaxed with a single dose of sodium nitroprusside (3 μM) in the presence or absence of a scavenger of NO,

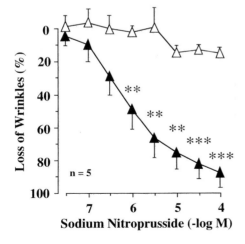

FIG. 6. Concentration–response curve of the relaxing effect of sodium nitroprusside (SNP) in comparison to time control experiments (open symbols). In a concentration-dependent manner, sodium nitroprusside evoked pericyte relaxation and thus a loss of wrinkles. $**p<0.01$; $***p<0.001$. From ref. 29.

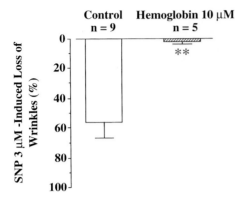

FIG. 7. Inhibitory effect of hemoglobin, a scavenger of nitric oxide, on the relaxation of retinal pericytes evoked by sodium nitroprusside. *$p<0.05$; **$p<0.01$. Modified from ref.30.

hemoglobin (10 μM). In the presence of hemoglobin, the relaxation to sodium nitroprusside was inhibited, demonstrating that the relaxation evoked by this drug is mediated by NO (Fig. 7) (30).

To further demonstrate that the relaxation evoked by the NO donor sodium nitroprusside involves the activation of a guanylate cyclase, the relaxation induced by SNP was inhibited by increasing concentrations of methylene blue, an inhibitor of guanylate cyclase (Fig. 8) (29). In other words, it appears that pericytes, which are the main contractile cells of capillaries, are relaxed by NO through activation of the guanylate cyclase pathway.

In the presence of different concentrations of oxygen, the relaxation evoked by the NO donor sodium nitroprusside (3 μM) was modulated (Fig. 9). In hyperoxia (100% oxygen), the relaxation induced by sodium nitroprusside was significantly more pronounced than in hypoxia (100% nitrogen) (32). In contrast to sodium nitroprusside, oxygen had no effect on the relaxation evoked by a drug such as forskolin (1 μM), which relaxes pericytes through activation of

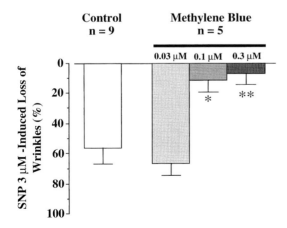

FIG. 8. Inhibitory effect of methylene blue, an inhibitor of guanylate cyclase, on the relaxation of retinal pericytes evoked by sodium nitroprusside. *$p<0.05$; **$p<0.01$. Modified from ref. 29.

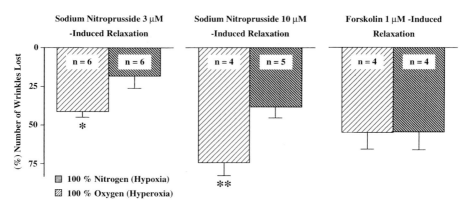

FIG. 9. Effect of 100% oxygen (hyperoxia) and 100% nitrogen (hypoxia) on the relaxation evoked by sodium nitroprusside, an NO donor that activates guanylate cyclase, or forskolin, an activator of adenylate cyclase. Relaxations evoked by sodium nitroprusside were more pronounced in hypoxia than in hyperoxia. Relaxations to forskolin were unaffected by hypoxia or hyperoxia. *$p<0.05$; **$p<0.01$. From ref. 32.

adenylate cyclase and an increase in cAMP (40). In addition, direct stimulation of membrane-bound guanylate cyclase by ANP, without NO or the intermediary, was unaffected by oxygen (32).

In conclusion it appears that, as in larger vessels, the diameter of vessels of the microcirculation (even of the size of capillaries) has a huge influence on the flow passing through these vessels (4,5). The capillaries of the retina, which form a continuous network with the capillaries of the optic nerve head (6), consist of a lining of endothelial cells surrounded by pericytes (10,11). These pericytes, which are contractile cells, can be relaxed by NO (29), and this relaxation is significantly more pronounced in hypoxia than in hyperoxia (31,32).

Because NO is present in the ophthalmic circulation (34–37) and because oxygen modulates the relaxation evoked by NO in the pericytes of capillaries (31,32), these results suggest that an interaction between oxygen and NO could participate in regulation of flow at the capillary level (33). It is the possible dysfunction of this regulation in glaucoma that we seek to understand better.

REFERENCES

1. Guyton AC. *Textbook of medical physiology.* 8th ed. Philadelphia: WB Sauders, 1991:150–7.
2. Alm A. Ocular circulation. In: Hart WM, ed. *Adlers's physiology of the eye.* 9th ed. St. Louis: Mosby–Year Book, 1992:198–227.
3. Haefliger IO, Anderson DR. Blood flow regulation in the optic nerve head. In: Ritch R, Shields MB, Krupin T, eds. *The glaucomas.* 2nd ed. St. Louis: Mosby–Year Book, 1996:189–97.
4. Lipowsky HH, Kolvalcheck S, Zweifach BW. The distribution of blood rheological parameters in the microvasculature of cat mesentery. *Circ Res* 1978;43:738–49.
5. Zweifach BW, Lipowsky HH. Pressure-flow relations in blood and lymph microcirculation. In:

American Physiological Society, ed. *Handbook of physiology. section 2. The cardiovascular system. Vol IV. Microcirculation.* Bethesda: American Physiological Society, 1984:251–307.

6. Anderson DR. Vascular supply to the optic nerve of primates. *Am J Ophthalmol* 1970;60:341–51.

7. Atkinson JLD, Anderson RE, Sundt TM. The effect of carbon dioxide on the diameter of brain capillaries. *Brain Res* 1990;517:333–40.

8. Buchanan RA, Wagner RC. Morphometric changes in pericytes—capillary endothelial cell associations correlated with vasoactive stimulus. *Microcirc Endothel Lymph* 1990;6:159–81.

9. Wallow IH, Bindley CD, Reboussin DM, Gange SJ, Fisher MR. Systemic hypertension produces pericyte changes in retinal capillaries. *Invest Ophthalmol Vis Sci* 1993;34:420–30.

10. Frank RN, Dutta S, Mancini MA. Pericyte coverage is greater in the retinal than in the cerebral capillaries of the rat. *Invest Ophthalmol Vis Sci* 1987;28:1086–91.

11. Frank RN, Turczyn TJ, Das A. Pericytes coverage of retinal and cerebral capillaries. *Invest Ophthalmol Vis Sci* 1990;31:999–1007.

12. Kelley C, D'Amore P, Hechtman HB, Shepro D. Vasoactive hormones and cAMP affect pericyte contraction and stress fibers in vitro. *J Musc Res Cell Motil* 1988;9:184–94.

13. Das A, Frank RN, Weber ML, Kennedy A, Reidy CA, Mancini MA. ATP causes retinal pericytes to contract in vitro. *Exp Eye Res* 1988;46:349–62.

14. Ramachandran E, Frank RN, Kennedy A. Effects of endothelin on cultured bovine retinal microvascular pericytes. *Invest Ophthalmol Vis Sci* 1993;34:586–95.

15. Dodge AB, Hechtman HB, Shepro D. Microvascular endothelial-derived autacoids regulate pericyte contractility. *Cell Motil Cytol* 1991;18:180–8.

16. Chakravarthy U, Gardiner TA, Anderson P, Archer DB, Trimble ER. The effect of endothelin-1 on the retinal microvascular pericyte. *Microvasc Res* 1992;43:241–54.

17. Joyce NC, DeCamilli P, Boyles J. Pericytes, like vascular smooth muscle cells, are immunocytochemically positive for cyclic GMP-dependent protein kinase. *Microvasc Res* 1984;28:206–19.

18. Joyce NC, Haire MF, Palade GE. Contractile proteins in pericytes. I. Immunoperoxidase localization of tropomyosin. *J Cell Biol* 1985;100:1379–86.

19. Joyce NC, Haire MF, Palade GE. Contractile proteins in pericytes. II. Immunocytochemical evidence for the presence of two isomyosins in graded concentrations. *J Cell Biol* 1985;100:1387–95.

20. Chan LS, Li W, Khatami M, Rockey JH. Actin in cultured bovine capillary pericytes: morphological and functional correlation. *Exp Eye Res* 1986;43:41–54.

21. DeNofrio D, Hoock TC, Herman IM. Functional sorting of actin isoforms in microvascular pericytes. *J Cell Biol* 1989;109:191–202.

22. Wallow IH, Burnside B. Actin filaments in retinal pericytes and endothelial cells. *Invest Ophthalmol Vis Sci* 1980;19:1433–41.

23. Herman IM, D'Amore PA. Microvascular pericytes contain muscle and nonmuscle actins. *J Cell Biol* 1985;101:43–52.

24. Nehls V, Drenckhahn D. Heterogeneity of microvascular pericytes for smooth muscle type alpha-actin. *J Cell Biol* 1991;113:147–54.

25. Davies P, Smith BT, Maddalo FB, et al. Characteristics of lung pericytes in culture including their growth inhibition by endothelial substrate. *Microvasc Res* 1987;33:300–14.

26. Helbig H, Kornacker S, Berweck S, Stahl F, Lepple-Wienhues A, Wiederholt M. Membrane potentials in retinal capillary pericytes: excitability and effect of vasoactive substances. *Invest Ophthalmol Vis Sci* 1992;33:2105–12.

27. Takahashi K, Brooks RA, Kanse SM, Ghatei MA, Kohner EM, Bloom SR. Production of endothelin-1 by cultured bovine retinal endothelial cells and presence of endothelin receptors on associated pericytes. *Diabetes* 1989;38:1200–2.

28. Berweck S, Thieme H, Lepple-Wienhues A, Helbig H, Wiederholt M. Insulin-induced hyperpolarization in retinal capillary pericytes. *Invest Ophthalmol Vis Sci* 1993;34:3402–7.

29. Haefliger IO, Zschauer A, Anderson DR. Relaxation of retinal pericytes contractile tone through the nitric oxide-cyclic GMP pathway. *Invest Ophthalmol Vis Sci* 1994;35:991–7.

30. Haefliger IO, Anderson DR. Pericytes and capillary blood flow modulation. In: Kaiser HJ, Flammer J, Hendrickson Ph, eds. *Ocular blood flow, new insights into the pathogenesis of ocular diseases.* Basel: Karger, 1996:74–8.

31. Haefliger IO, Anderson DR. Oxygen's effect on relaxation of retinal pericytes by sodium nitroprusside. *Graefes Arch Clin Exp Ophthalmol* 1997;235:388–92.

32. Haefliger IO, Anderson DR. Oxygen modulation of guanylate cyclase-mediated retinal pericyte relaxations to SIN-1 and ANP. *Invest Ophthalmol Vis Sci* 1997;38:1563–8.
33. Anderson DR. Glaucoma, capillaries and pericytes. 1. Blood flow regulation. *Ophthalmologica* 1996;210:257–62.
34. Haefliger IO, Flammer J, Lüscher TF. Heterogeneity of endothelium-dependent regulation in ophthalmic and ciliary arteries. *Invest Ophthalmol Vis Sci* 1993;34:1722–30.
35. Haefliger IO, Meyer P, Flammer J, Lüscher TF. The vascular endothelium as a regulator of the ocular circulation: a new concept in ophthalmology. *Surv Ophthalmol* 1994;39:123–32.
36. Meyer P, Flammer J, Lüscher TF. Endothelium-dependent regulation of the ophthalmic microcirculation in the perfused porcine eye: role of nitric oxide and endothelins. *Invest Ophthalmol Vis Sci* 1993;34:3614–21.
37. Donati G, Pournaras CJ, Munoz JL, Poitry S, Poitry-Yamate CL, Tsacopoulos M. Nitric oxide controls arteriolar tone in the retina of the miniature pig. *Invest Ophthalmol Vis Sci* 1995;36:2228–37.
38. Pournaras CJ. Autoregulation of ocular blood flow. In: Kaiser HJ, Flammer J, Hendrickson Ph, eds. *Ocular blood flow, new insights into the pathogenesis of ocular diseases.* Basel: Karger, 1996:40–50.
39. Harris AK, Wild P, Stopak D. Silicone rubber substrata: a new wrinkle in the study of cell locomotion. *Science* 1980;208:177–9.
40. Ferrari-Dileo G, Davis EB, Anderson DR. Effects of cholinergic and adrenergic agonists on adenylate cyclase activity of retinal microvascular pericytes in culture. *Invest Ophthalmol Vis Sci* 1992;33:42–7.

Nitric Oxide and Endothelin in the Pathogenesis of Glaucoma, edited by I. O. Haefliger and J. Flammer. Lippincott–Raven Publishers, Philadelphia © 1998.

7

Nitric Oxide–Synthesizing Cells in the Posterior Eye Segment

Ernst R. Tamm and *Elke Lütjen-Drecoll

*Laboratory of Molecular and Developmental Biology, National Eye Institute, National Institutes of Health, Bethesda, Maryland; and *Department of Anatomy, University of Erlangen–Nürnberg, Erlangen, Germany*

There is substantial evidence that nitric oxide (NO) plays an important role in various functional processes involving signal transduction in the posterior eye segment. As in other tissues (1), NO in the posterior eye is constitutively synthesized by two isoforms of nitric oxide synthase (NOS), neuronal NOS (NOS 1) and endothelial NOS (NOS 3). In addition, the other isoform, macrophage NOS (NOS 2), which is an inducible high-output enzyme that produces toxic amounts of NOS, may be involved under certain circumstances in pathologic processes of the posterior eye segment. Morphologic studies of the tissue-specific localization of the different isoforms of NOS have been made possible by the synthesis of specific antibodies. The neuronal isoform of NOS can also be identified using the NADPH-diaphorase (NADPH-d) reaction, an NADPH-dependent reduction of nitroblue tetrazolium to the dark-blue, water-insoluble dye nitroblue tetrazolium formazan (2). The NADPH-d reaction is also sensitive in detecting other isoforms of NOS. Its specificity, however, appears to be restricted to the neuronal isoform of NOS. In other cell types, other NADPH-dehydrogenating enzymes are present that can reduce nitroblue tetrazolium (2,3). The specificity of the NADPH-d reaction in identifying neuronal NOS can be increased by formaldehyde fixation, which inactivates some of the NADPH-d activity not related to NOS (2,4). Our knowledge about the localization and the origin of nitrergic nerves in the posterior segment of the human eye, which is the major subject of this review, has been obtained by a combination of NOS immunohistochemistry, NADPH-d histochemistry, and electron microscopy.

NO IN THE CHOROID

Choroidal arteries and arterioles that supply the avascular fovea and the outer parts of the retina, including the photoreceptors, are surrounded by a very dense perivascular neural network (Fig. 1). Some of the axons continue to the chorio-capillaries, where they appear to be in contact with pericytes. Recent studies have shown that a considerable number of the perivascular nerve fibers around choroidal vessels stain for NOS and NADPH-D and very probably use NO as neurotransmitter (Fig. 2a). In the human and Rhesus monkey eye, such choroidal nitrergic nerve fibers derive from a widespread plexus of similarly NOS- and NADPH-D–positive resident choroidal nerve cells (Figs. 1, 2b and c, and 3) (5,6). The cells appear either solitary or, more often, clustered in groups of 2 to 10 cells. In whole mounts of the human choroid, between 1,555 and 2,579 NOS/NADPH-D–positive ganglion cells were counted per eye (6). Choroidal ganglion cells are innervated because many varicose terminals are closely associ-ated with the perikarya of the cells (Fig. 2d). It is not clear whether these terminals derive only from the axons of other choroidal ganglion cells or from sources outside the eye. Such an extrinsic innervation might possibly come from one or more of the cranial autonomic ganglia that are known to project to the eye, i.e., the parasympathetic ciliary and pterygopalatine ganglia, the sympathetic superior cervical ganglion, and the sensory trigeminal ganglion. In this case, choroidal nerve cells would represent a third neuron in a rather complex nerve pathway. On the other hand, choroidal neurons might be postganglionic to neu-

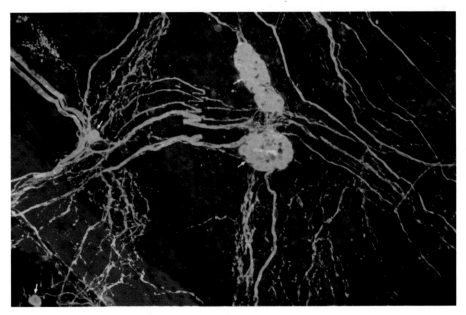

FIG. 1. Confocal microscopy of a whole mount from a Rhesus monkey choroid after staining of neural structures with the neuronal marker PGP 9.5. After immunostaining for PGP 9.5, choroidal axons and ganglion cells (*arrows*) express a green fluorescence. Groups of ganglion cells are connected by axon bundles. Choroidal arteries (*asterisk*) are densely surrounded by perivascular nerve fibers. × 200. From ref. 24.

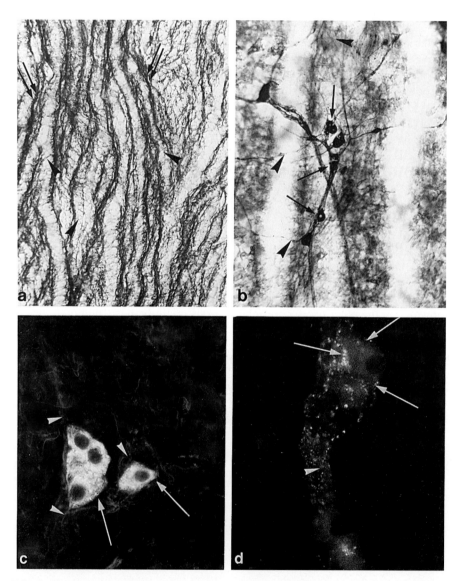

FIG. 2. Nitrergic innervation of the choroid. **a:** Whole mount of a rat choroid stained for NADPH-d. The temporal region in the vicinity of the optic nerve head is shown. Bundles of positively stained nerve fibers follow the course of the arterial vessels (*double arrows*). Small axons originate from these bundles, forming a delicate network around the vascular wall (*arrowhead*). × 80. **b:** Whole mount of a human choroid (temporal region) stained for NADPH-diaphorase. Positively stained ganglion cells are shown (*arrows*). These cells are connected with each other by stained axons (*asterisk*). Additional nerve fibers lead to the perivascular fiber network (arrowheads). × 51. **c:** Frozen tangential section of human choroid (temporal quadrant) stained immunocytochemically with antibodies against NOS. Strong positive labeling is seen in the cytoplasm of the ganglion cells (*arrows*). Very weak staining for NOS is also found for the axons of these nerve cells (*arrowheads*). × 220. **d:** Frozen tangential section through the temporal quadrant of a human choroid after incubation for anti-synaptophysin. Two ganglion cells are seen, which are surrounded by positively labeled varicosities (*arrows*). In addition, positive staining is also present in small vesicles lying in the cytoplasm of axons (*arrowhead*). × 270. From ref. 6.

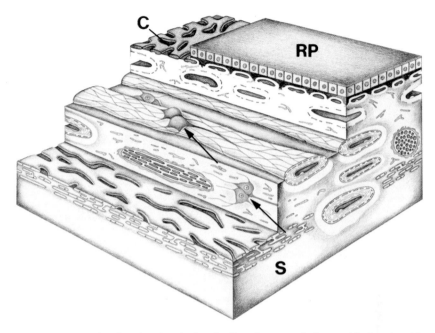

FIG. 3. Schematic drawing showing the localization of nerve cells (*arrows*) in the choroid and their association with choroidal arteries. C, choriocapillaries; RP, retinal pigment epithelium; S, sclera.

rons in the brainstem, e.g., in classical parasympathetic centers such as the nucleus of Edinger–Westphal or the superior salivatory nucleus.

Not all NOS-positive axons that innervate choroidal vessels in the human eye are derived from intrinsic choroidal ganglion cells. Because NOS-positive axons are already found in the wall of the short posterior ciliary arteries shortly after they penetrate through the sclera, a significant number of such axons appear to project to the human choroid from extraocular ganglion cells.

In addition to perivascular nerves and choroidal ganglion cells, NADPH-d activity is present in vascular endothelial cells of choroidal arteries and arterioles, albeit with considerably weaker intensity than in the choroidal perivascular nerves. No or only extremely weak NADPH-d activity is seen in the endothelial cells of the choriocapillaries. In addition, retinal vascular endothelial cells invariably show much stronger NADPH-d activity than choroidal vascular endothelial cells (Fig. 4). It appears reasonable to assume that the endothelial NADPH-d staining reflects the presence of the endothelial isoform of NOS and that this enzyme is more active in retinal than in choroidal vascular endothelial cells.

NO released by perivascular nerves relaxes vascular smooth muscle and has been shown to be responsible for nonadrenergic/noncholinergic (NANC) innervation in many parts of the circulation (7). Choroidal blood flow is also

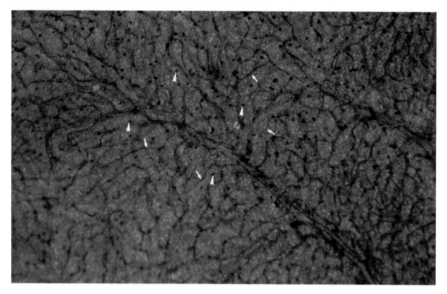

FIG. 4. NADPH-d–stained whole mount of the central retina from a normal rhesus monkey. In the foveal region, the capillaries are clearly stained (*arrows*). In addition, many amacrine cells (*arrowheads*) stain for NADPH-d. × 100.

modulated by such vasodilatory NANC nerves, which has been shown after intracranial stimulation of the facial nerve in rabbits, cats and monkeys (for review see ref. 8). Recent studies have provided evidence that choroidal nitrergic nerves are at least partly responsible for NANC vasodilatation. In pigs, electrical stimulation of the isolated long posterior ciliary artery that supplies the choroid, retina, and anterior uvea in this species caused a NANC vasodilatation that could be blocked with inhibitors of NOS (9). Similar results were reported for posterior ciliary arteries of humans (10). In rabbits, the increase in choroidal blood flow after stimulation of the facial nerve was shown to be reduced or abolished by NOS inhibition at low stimulation frequencies (11). In rabbits as in other species, including humans, the axons of the facial nerve synapse on nerve cells in the pterygopalatine ganglion that project with their axons to the eye (12,13). A very large number of pterygopalatine ganglion cells in rat, dog, pig, and monkey stain for NOS and/or NADPH-d (14–17). Pterygopalatine ganglionectomy in rats significantly reduces the number of peripheral NOS-IR nerve fibers in the eye (14). In humans, the pterygopalatine ganglion might also be the main source of those choroidal nitrergic axons that do not derive from the intrinsic choroidal ganglion cells but project from extraocular nerve cells to the choroid. We recently showed that approximately 70% of human pterygopalatine ganglion cells stain for NOS and NADPH-d, whereas in the human ciliary ganglion less than 1% of the neurons are NOS/NADPH-positive (18). In humans, another source for ocular nitrergic axons appears to be the trigeminal ganglion, because in the ophthalmic portion of this ganglion 17–19% of the ganglion cells are NOS- and NADPH-d–positive (18).

In summary, the human choroid appears to be under the influence of a basal release of NO, which maintains the vasodilatory tone of choroidal vessels, and it appears reasonable to assume that nitrergic choroidal nerve terminals contribute a substantial amount of it. The terminals derive from axons of intraocular intrinsic ganglion cells in the choroid and, in addition, most probably from extraocular ganglion cells in the pterygopalatine ganglion.

There is no doubt that the choroidal vasculature is of crucial importance for delivery of nutrients to the retina. Experiments in anesthetized cats and monkeys show that the amount of oxygen supplied by the choroid and consumed in the retina is about 80% and 65%, respectively (for review see ref. 8). In primates, the avascular fovea is totally dependent on supply from the choroid. Still, the physiologic role of the dense nitrergic vasodilatory innervation of choroidal vessels is less clear, because blood flow through the choroid is so extremely high that it exceeds the metabolic requirements. The oxygen extraction from choroidal vessels is low; the arteriovenous difference in oxygen concentration measures only 2 to 3% (8). Studies of the choroidal vasculature in cats and pigs indicate that the net extraction of oxygen and glucose is maintained at a normal level even after large alterations in choroidal blood flow (8). An intriguing possibility is that the physiologic role of the extremely high rate of choroidal blood flow is not so much the nutrition but more the prevention of a damaging increase in intraocular temperature (8,19). Such an increase might happen during observation of very bright objects emitting light with high intensity, especially in primates, in which the light is focused on the fovea. Under these conditions, the dense nitrergic vasodilative innervation might be important for a reflexive increase in choroidal blood flow (20).

In mammals, a dense network of choroidal ganglion cells is found only in humans and in higher monkeys, which have a fovea centralis comparable to that in humans (6). In contrast, other mammalian species without a fovea show dense nitrergic innervation of choroidal vessels but no or only very few choroidal ganglion cells (21). A possibility is that the presence of choroidal ganglion cells is related to the development of a centralized area of vision. Almost half of the ganglion cells in the human choroid are located in the central–temporal region of the choroid, adjacent to the fovea (6). The functional significance of an association between choroidal ganglion cells and fovea centralis remains to be established. The fovea centralis is supplied only by choroidal vessels, and the presence of a resident autonomous nerve cell plexus might be more advantageous in mediating vasodilatory reflexes when light is focused on the fovea. Another hypothesis is based on the fact that a fovea is only present in eyes of species with a well-developed accommodation system (21). In these eyes, a more sophisticated control of vasodilatory reflexes mediated by a choroidal ganglion cell plexus might be favorable, because changes in blood volume should change choroidal thickness, thereby influencing the position of the fovea centralis and, hence, visual acuity. In human eyes, the position of the fovea might also be modulated by a distinct network of choroidal nonvascular smooth muscle/ myofibroblast-like cells (22). These cells, which are most abundant in the choroid underneath the fovea, are in contact with autonomous nerve endings of yet unidentified nature.

Flügel et al. (6) reported that an age-related accumulation of lipofuscin granules in human choroidal ganglion cells is typically found in the central regions of the choroid, close to the fovea. This indicates that light intensity might be a factor that promotes aging in choroidal neurons. It would be interesting to know whether structural changes in choroidal ganglion cells are related not only to age but also to ocular diseases. A candidate might be diseases in which light exposure has been shown to be a contributing factor, such as age-related macular degeneration (23). In addition to age or light, other factors also might induce structural changes in choroidal ganglion cells. May et al. (24) recently demonstrated that in Rhesus monkeys with experimentally induced glaucoma [intraocular pressure (IOP) median 22–42 mm Hg], the number of choroidal ganglion cells was significantly reduced from the normal amount of approximately 600 in this species to 50–150 in glaucomatous eyes. The ganglion cell loss was associated with thinning of the choroid and structural changes in the choroidal vasculature. If high IOP also induces similar changes in human patients with glaucoma, the loss of choroidal ganglion cells might contribute to glaucoma-related changes in choroidal blood flow.

NO IN THE RETINA

In marked contrast to their abundance around choroidal vessels, autonomic perivascular NOS/NADPH-d–positive nerves are not present in the retina (14,24–26). The absence of NOS-positive autonomic nerves around vessels in the retina is not surprising, because in mammals (with the exception of the rabbit), retinal vessels beyond the surface of the optic disc are in general not supplied by any kind of autonomic vascular nerves (27,28). However, perivascular NADPH-d–positive nerve fibers have been demonstrated around the extraocular central retinal artery of dog, monkey, and human (29–31). In dogs, the source of these nerves appears to be the pterygopalatine ganglion (32). In vitro experiments have provided evidence that NO released from nitrergic nerves relaxes isolated strips of monkey and dog central retinal artery (29,30). In rabbits, stimulation of the facial nerve significantly increased retinal blood flow, an effect that could be abolished by NOS inhibition (11). In the dog, intra-arterial infusion of nicotine caused dilatation of arterioles in the fundus region, which could be abolished by hexamethonium and NOS inhibition, suggesting the involvement of nitrergic axons (29). Furthermore, nicotine does not dilate retinal arteries in dogs in which the pterygopalatine ganglion was damaged by ethanol injection, indicating that the pterygopalatine ganglion is the source of these axons (32). Taken together, these observations indicate that nitrergic nerves may influence retinal blood vessels by an effect on extraocular vessels.

In addition, NO might be released intraocularly in the retina from other sources than autonomic nerves. The endothelial cells of most of the retinal vessels in humans, rats, and rabbits stain for NOS and NADPH-d (Fig. 4) (14,24–26). RT-PCR experiments show the expression of mRNA for endothelial NOS in bovine retinal microvascular endothelial cells (25). In addition, some NOS-IR retinal nerve cells (mostly amacrine cells) in human and rat have been reported to associate closely with retinal capillaries (Fig. 4). Electron microscopy indicates that the processes of NOS-IR amacrine cells are in contact with the basal lamina that covers the endothelial cells and pericytes of retinal capillaries (33). If NO is synthesized in the perikarya of retinal nerve cells, it might easily diffuse to neighboring vascular cells. Therefore, a local mechanism coupled to intrinsic retinal activity would contribute to regulation of the retinal circulation. Such a functional coupling of amacrine-derived nerve processes and retinal vessels has already been suggested for the action of classical neurotransmitters and/or neuropeptides (28). Support for this hypothesis comes from comparison with the brain, in which neuronal processes associated with intraparenchymal capillaries are

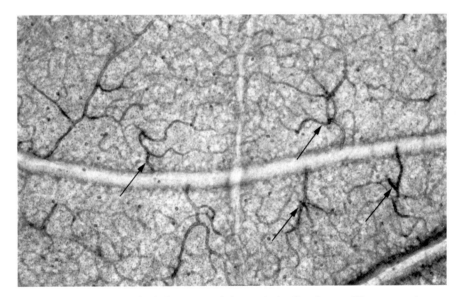

FIG. 5. NADPH-d–stained whole mount of the central retina from a Rhesus monkey eye suffering from experimentally induced glaucoma. In the glaucomatous eye, the retina shows intensely stained arterioles (*arrows*) and less intensely stained capillaries than the normal eye (Fig. 4). The number of NADPH-d–positive amacrine cells is reduced. Because the retina of the glaucomatous eye is considerably thinner than that of the normal eye, the bluish background stain of the NADPH-d reaction is less intense than in the whole mount of the normal retina (Fig. 4). × 100.

believed to regulate blood flow (34). Interestingly, flickering light increases blood flow in the cat and monkey retina and in the cat optic nerve head (ONH) (35,36) and formation of NO in the pig retina (37). NOS inhibition blocks the flicker-induced vasodilatation in the cat but not in the monkey (36).

Experimentally induced glaucoma in monkeys not only induced loss of NOS/NADPH-d−positive ganglion cells but also loss of NOS/NADPH-d−positive amacrine cells and structural changes in the retinal vasculature (24). The diameter of the retinal arterioles was reduced and the staining pattern of the vascular endothelial cells for NADPH-d was changed (Fig. 5). In the glaucomatous eye, arterioles stained more strongly than in controls, whereas the capillaries stained less intensely.

NO IN THE OPTIC NERVE HEAD

Similar to the short posterior ciliary arteries, the vessels that supply the ONH are surrounded by NOS and NADPH-d−positive perivascular nerve fibers. In addition, endothelial NOS (NOS 3) is present in vascular endothelia of vessels in the prelaminar region (37,38). This indicates that NO has also a vasodilatory function for blood flow in the ONH. Experiments in cat eyes support this hypothesis (35). In this species, ONH blood flow and NO levels in the vitreous humor in front of the ONH were increased after stimulation of neuronal activity with flickering light. In contrast, after NOS inhibition, blood flow and NO response to flicker were significantly attenuated. In the ONH of normal eyes, immunostaining for neuronal NOS (NOS 1) is also sparsely present in astrocytes (38). Neufeld and Hernandez (38) recently showed an increase in immunostaining of all three isoforms of NOS in the ONH of patients with primary open-angle glaucoma. In glaucomatous eyes, almost every astrocyte stained positively for neuronal NOS. This immunoreactivity was abundantly present throughout the prelaminar region and the lamina cribrosa and was localized inside the diminished nerve fiber bundles. In addition, macrophage NOS (NOS 2), which was not observed in normal ONH, was present in a few cells in the disorganized lamina cribrosa of the glaucomatous eyes. The authors suggest that this increase in immunostaining is due to increasing amounts of NOS. The increase in NOS might expose the ONH to excessive levels of NO which, in turn, could be neurodestructive to the axons of the retinal ganglion cells.

ACKNOWLEDGMENTS

Supported by grants from the Ria Freifrau von Fritsch-Stiftung of the University Erlangen-Nürnberg, Germany (ERT) and the Deutsche Forschungsgemeinschaft (ELD, Dr 124/6-3). ERT is the recipient of an Heisenberg-Award from the Deutsche Forschungsgemeinschaft (Ta 115/8-1).

REFERENCES

1. Förstermann U, Kleinert H. Nitric oxide synthase: expression and expressional control of the three isoforms. *Naunyn Schmiedebergs Arch Pharmacol* 1995;352:351–64.
2. Blottner D, Grozdanovic Z, Gossrau R. Histochemistry of nitric oxide synthase in the nervous system. *Histochem J* 1995;27:785–811.
3. Tracey WR, Nakane M, Pollock JS, Förstermann U. Nitric oxide synthases in neuronal cells, macrophages and endothelium are NADPH diaphorases, but represent only a fraction of total cellular NADPH diaphorase activity. *Biochem Biophys Res Commun* 1993;195:1035–40.
4. Matsumoto T, Nakane M, Pollock JS, Kuk JE, Förstermann U. A correlation between soluble brain nitric oxide synthase and NADPH-diaphorase activity is only seen after exposure of the tissue to fixative. *Neurosci Lett* 1993;155:61–4.
5. Bergua A, Jünnemann A, Naumann GOH. NADPH-D reactive choroidal ganglion cells in the human eye. *Klin Mbl Augenheilk* 1993;203:77–82.
6. Flügel C, Tamm ER, Mayer B, Lütjen-Drecoll E. Species differences in choroidal vasodilative innervation: evidence for specific intrinsic nitrergic and VIP-positive neurons in the human eye. *Invest Ophthalmol Vis Sci* 1994;35:592–9.
7. Sanders KM, Ward SM. Nitric oxide as a mediator of nonadrenergic noncholinergic neurotransmission. *Am J Physiol* 1992;262:G379–92.
8. Alm A. Ocular Circulation. In: Hart WMJ, ed. *Adler's physiology of the eye.* 9th ed. St. Louis: Mosby–Year Book, 1992:198–227.
9. Su E-N, Alder VA, Yu D-Y, Cringle SJ. Adrenergic and nitrergic neurotransmitters are released by the autonomic system of the pig long posterior ciliary artery. *Curr Eye Res* 1994;13:907–17.
10. Nyborg NCB, Nielsen PJ. Neurogenic nitric oxide accounts for the non-adrenergic noncholinergic vasodilation in human posterior ciliary arteries [Abstract]. *Invest Ophthalmol Vis Sci* 1994;34:1287.
11. Nilsson SFE. Nitric oxide as a mediator of parasympathetic vasodilation in ocular and extraocular tissues in the rabbit. *Invest Ophthalmol Vis Sci* 1996;37:2110–9.
12. Ruskell GL. The orbital distribution of the sphenopalatine ganglion in the rabbit. In: Rohen JW, ed. *The structure of the eye. II. Symposium.* Stuttgart: Schattauer-Verlag, 1965:355–68.
13. Ruskell GL. Facial parasympathetic innervation of the choroidal blood-vessels in monkeys. *Exp Eye Res* 1971;12:166–72.
14. Yamamoto R, Bredt DS, Snyder SH, Stone RA. The localization of nitric oxide synthase in the rat eye and related cranial ganglia. *Neuroscience* 1993;54:189–200.
15. Yoshida K, Okamura T, Kimura H, Bredt DS, Snyder SH, Toda N. Nitric oxide synthase-immunoreactive nerve fibers in dog cerebral and peripheral arteries. *Brain Res* 1993;629:67–72.
16. Sienkiewicz W, Kaleczyc J, Majewski M, Lakomy M. NADPH-diaphorase-containing cerebrovascular nerve fibres and their possible origin in the pig. *J Brain Res* 1995;36:353–63.
17. Yoshida K, Okamura T, Toda N. Histological and functional studies on the nitroxidergic nerve innervating monkey cerebral, mesenteric and temporal arteries. *Jpn J Pharmacol* 1994;65:351–9.
18. Tamm ER, Lütjen-Drecoll E. Functional morphology and origin of nitrergic nerves in the human eye [Abstract]. *Exp Eye Res* 1996;63(suppl):S.151.
19. Parver LM, Auker C, Carpenter DO. Choroidal blood flow as a heat dissipating mechanism in the macula. *Am J Ophthalmol* 1980;89:641–6.
20. Parver LM, Auker CR, Carpenter DO. Choroidal blood flow. III. Reflexive control in human eyes. *Arch Ophthalmol* 1983;101:1604–6.
21. Flügel-Koch C, Kaufman PL, Lütjen-Drecoll E. Association of choroidal ganglion cell plexus with the fovea centralis. *Invest Ophthalmol Vis Sci* 1994;35:4268–72.
22. Flügel-Koch C, May CA, Lütjen-Drecoll E. Presence of a contractile cell network in the human choroid. *Ophthalmologica* 1996;210:296–302.
23. Cruickshanks KJ, Klein R, Klein BE. Sunlight and age-related macula degeneration. *Arch Ophthalmol* 1993;111:514–8.
24. May CA, Hayreh SS, Ossoining K, Kaufman PL, Lütjen-Drecoll E. Choroidal ganglion cell plexus and retinal vasculature in laser-induced monkey glaucoma. *Ophthalmologica* 1997;211:161–71.

25. Chakravarthy U, Stitt AW, McNally J, Bailie JR, Hoey EM, Duprex P. Nitric oxide synthase activity and expression in retinal capillary endothelial cells and pericytes. *Curr Eye Res* 1994;14:285–94.
26. Perez MT, Larsson B, Alm P, Andersson KE, Ehinger B. Localisation of neuronal nitric oxide synthase-immunoreactivity in rat and rabbit retinas. *Exp Brain Res* 1995;104:207–17.
27. Laties AM. Central retinal artery innervation. Absence of adrenergic innervation to intraocular branches. *Arch Ophthalmol* 1967;77:405–9.
28. Ye X, Laties AM, Stone RA. Peptidergic innervation of the retinal vasculature and the optic nerve head. *Invest Ophthalmol Vis Sci* 1990;31:1731–7.
29. Toda N, Kitamura Y, Okamura T. Role of nitroxidergic nerve in dog retinal arterioles in vivo and arteries in vitro. *Am J Pathol* 1994;266:H1985–92.
30. Toda N, Toda M, Ayajiki K, Okamura T. Monkey central retinal artery is innervated by nitroxidergic vasodilator nerves. *Invest Ophthalmol Vis Sci* 1996;37:2177–84.
31. Bergua A. NADPH-diaphorase-positive innervation of the central retinal artery of the human optic nerve [Abstract]. *Exp Eye Res* 1996;63(suppl):S.142.
32. Toda N, Ayajiki K, Yoshida K, Kimura H, Okamura T. Impairment by damage of the pterygo-palatine ganglion of nitroxidergic vasodilator nerve function in canine cerebral and retinal arteries. *Circ Res* 1993;72:206–13.
33. Roufail E, Stringer M, Rees S. Nitric oxide synthase immunoreactivity and NADPH diaphorase staining are co-localised in neurons closely associated with the vasculature in rat and human retina. *Brain Res* 1995;684:36–46.
34. Lou HC, Edvinsson L, Mac Kenzie ET. The concept of coupling blood flow to brain function: revision required? *Ann Neurol* 1987;22:289–97.
35. Buerk DG, Riva CE, Cranstoun SD. Nitric oxide has a vasodilatory role in cat optic nerve head. *Microvasc Res* 1996;52:13–26.
36. Wang I, Kondo M, Bill A. Vascular responses to flickering light in the retina in cats and monkeys: effect of L-NAME [Abstract]. *Acta Physiol Scand* 1995;153:39A.
37. Donati G, Pournaras CJ, Munoz J-L, Poitry S, Poitry-Yamate CL, Tsacopoulos M. Nitric oxide controls arteriolar tone in the retina of the miniature pig. *Invest Ophthalmol Vis Sci* 1995;36:2228–37.
38. Neufeld AH, Hernandez MR. Nitric oxide synthase in the human glaucomatous optic nerve head [Abstract]. *Invest Ophthalmol Vis Sci* 1997;38:S161.

Nitric Oxide and Endothelin in the Pathogenesis of Glaucoma, edited by I. O. Haefliger and J. Flammer. Lippincott–Raven Publishers, Philadelphia © 1998.

8

Endothelin-1–Induced Optic Nerve Ischemia

Selim Orgül, *George A. Cioffi, *David R. Bacon, and *E. Michael Van Buskirk

*Department of Medicine, University of Basel, Basel, Switzerland; and *Ocular Microcirculation Unit, Devers Eye Institute and R.S. Dow Neurological Science Institute, Legacy Portland Hospitals, Portland, Oregon*

GLAUCOMATOUS OPTIC NEUROPATHY

Glaucoma has traditionally been defined as a disorder of increased intraocular pressure (IOP). Indeed, there is ample support for a pressure-induced optic neuropathy (3). However, a marked preponderance of an alteration of local and systemic physiologic parameters has been reported in glaucoma. Many of these parameters are related to vascular diseases (4). Moreover, about 20% of the glaucoma patients in the United States and Europe never have an IOP above the statistical norm, and almost 20% of the patients with glaucomatous optic neuropathy will still show a progression of the disease after the IOP has been lowered to within the statistical normal range. Because not all glaucoma patients suffer from increased IOP, the term ''low- or normal-tension glaucoma'' was introduced. Not to violate the pressure concept, an increased sensitivity to IOP was postulated in normal-tension glaucoma. However, current evidence suggests that there are no or only minor differences in optic nerve damage between patients with and those without elevated IOP. Furthermore, any separation according to a defined IOP level would be totally arbitrary. Therefore, it appears more reasonable to define glaucoma as a progressive degeneration of the optic nerve characterized by cupping and atrophy, i.e., glaucomatous optic neuropathy (16). This is basically a question of semantics. If glaucomatous damage is defined phenomenologically, summarizing all the diseases leading to progressive cupping of the optic nerve, the role of the clinician will be to inquire which risk factors can lead to such a clinical picture.

Laboratory data demonstrate that increased IOP impairs the axoplasmatic

79

flow and alters the composition of the extracellular matrix of the optic nerve. Furthermore, if IOP is increased in monkeys, the optic nerve develops an atrophy that mimics typical glaucomatous optic neuropathy in humans (14). Unfortunately, there are almost no laboratory non-pressure models for glaucomatous optic neuropathy. The purpose of the following studies was to attempt to develop an in vivo experimental model that would offer a titratable method to examine the effects of vascular insufficiency of the anterior optic nerve.

ENDOTHELIN

In the cardiovascular system, the endothelium lies in a strategic anatomic position between blood components and smooth-muscle cells and pericytes. The endothelial cells release vasoactive substances both spontaneously and after local stimulation. Such stimulation can be chemical, e.g., circulating hormones, or physical, e.g., shear stress or wall tension. The locally released mediators can be classified into vasodilators (endothelium-derived relaxing factors, EDRF) and vasoconstrictors (endothelium-derived constricting factors, EDCF). The most important constricting factor is endothelin-1 (ET-1).

ET-1 is a 21-residue peptide (6). ET-1 is among the most potent vasopressor substances yet discovered. In vivo, this peptide has been shown to produce localized vasoconstriction when injected directly into perivascular cerebral tissues, resulting in regional ischemic damage of the brain's neural tissues (15). It was hypothesized that an animal model of chronic optic nerve ischemia could be developed in a similar fashion, and that by chronically reducing the blood flow to the optic nerve the pathologic sequelae of ischemia could be examined.

Among the available vasoconstrictive compounds, ET-1 was used in the present experiments. It not only is the most potent vasoconstrictor known but also may play a role in some ischemic processes. In healthy young humans, the circulating levels of ET-1 are very low. In pathologic conditions, such as an ischemic cerebrovascular insult, the plasma level of ET-1 has been reported to be elevated (17). ET-1 is a strong vasoconstrictive agent of the ocular circulation as well, and the vasomodulating potency of endothelial mediators increases with decreasing diameters of the blood vessel (5). Moriya et al. (7) found a statistically significant increase in the levels of plasma ET-1 in patients with low-tension glaucoma compared to normal controls. These findings suggest that ET-1 might be involved in optic nerve pathology.

QUANTIFICATION OF VASOMOTOR EFFECTS IN VIVO

Measurements of optic nerve perfusion in laboratory animals are difficult because of the small volume of the tissue being studied and the fine caliber of the vessels. Vascular corrosion casting, by means of intra-arterial methylmethacrylate injection, allows formation of a three-dimensional replica of the ocular microvasculature. The castings of the ocular vasculature are obtained under controlled physiologic conditions. Batson's #17 methylmethacrylate injection medium, modified to reduce the viscosity to approximately 11 centipoise, is injected into the superior circulation through ascending branches of the aorta. After polymerization of the plastic, the eyes are corroded in 6 M potassium hydroxide to remove the tissue surrounding the vascular casts and are examined with a scanning electron microscope. This technique produces a precise replica of the microvasculature that appears to preserve the physiologic vascular tone at the moment of injection (2). Localized regions of arterial constrictions providing an anatomic basis for regional alterations in blood flow have been described (2). The arterial vessels display some degree of focal constriction compared to downstream vessel caliber at their branching points from the major feeding vessel in the ciliary body as well as in the optic nerve. The diameter at the constriction zone, seemingly a contractile cuff beyond the branching point of the vessel, can be compared to that of the same vessel about 50 μm downstream (Fig. 1). The difference between the diameters can be expressed as a percentage of the downstream vessel caliber. This approach provides a measure of focal vasoconstriction that is independent of the absolute vessel diameters. By averaging the focal vasoconstriction of many vessels, a measure of the local vasomotor effect is obtained.

To evaluate whether the corrosion-casting technique was robust enough to overcome potential methodologic artifacts to demonstrate a known physiologic effect, the effects of alterations of arterial blood gases on the arterial vessels supplying the optic nerve were examined. The blood gases were varied by manipulating the ventilation rate in albino rabbits before intraluminal injection of the casting medium. In these experiments, average relative arteriolar constriction values decreased with increasing pCO_2 (Fig. 2). In a regression analysis, a high correlation between pCO_2 and the average relative arteriolar constriction values has been demonstrated (9). This strong interrelationship between arterial pCO_2

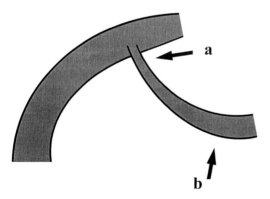

FIG. 1. Schematic representation of an arterial vessel that displays a focal zone of relative constriction near the branching point (*arrow a*), compared to downstream vessel caliber (*arrow b*).

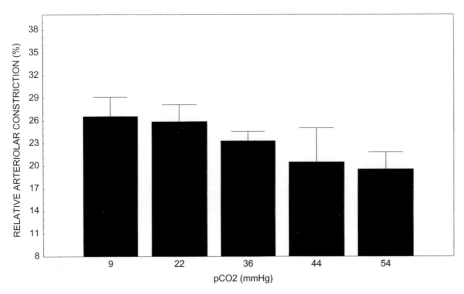

FIG. 2. Average (mean ± SEM) relative arteriolar constriction values measured by the corrosion-casting technique decreased with increasing pCO_2.

and anterior optic nerve arteriolar constriction confirms that the corrosion-casting technique is robust enough to overcome potential methodologic artifacts to demonstrate a known physiologic effect.

DOSE-DEPENDENT VASOCONSTRICTION OF THE OPTIC NERVE MICROVASCULATURE WITH ET-1

In an attempt to evaluate the effects induced by chronic microapplication of ET-1 on the anterior optic nerve microvasculature, variable dosages (range 4.69×10^{-4} to 9.0×10^{-1} μg/day) of ET-1 were delivered to the perineural region of the anterior optic nerve in albino rabbits via osmotically driven minipumps.

The minipump is a miniature osmotically driven pump (Alzet minipumps; Alza, CA) which continually delivers a test agent at a controlled flow rate. The pumps are oval capsules, approximately 2×0.4 cm, with a polyethylene delivery tube extending from one end. A predetermined dosage of any drug is delivered by varying the concentration of the drug within the minipump. A constant flow of 0.5 μl/h is delivered for the duration of the experiment. The capacity of the minipumps used in this experiment allowed a continuous delivery for up to 2 weeks. The minipumps were implanted in a subcutaneous space that was surgically created superior and nasal to the experimental eye. A polyethylene delivery tube was directed from the minipump through the upper eyelid into a surgically

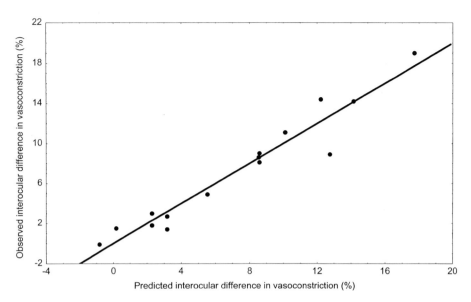

FIG. 3. Correlation between the effectively observed measurements and the predicted interocular difference in optic nerve vasoconstriction in a multiple regression analysis with the logarithm of the daily endothelin-1 dosage, the weight, and the sex of the rabbits (multiple $r^2 =$ 0.92; $p < 0.0001$).

created superiotemporal sub-Tenon's channel and was fixed in place using a scleral fixation suture adjacent to the optic nerve and its vascular supply.

The vasomotor effect was examined using the intraluminal microvascular corrosion-casting technique (see above). The average constriction was calculated for the endothelin-treated eyes and the untreated contralateral eyes. The interocular difference (between treated and untreated eyes) of the optic nerve vasoconstriction ranged from 0 to 19%. The interocular difference of the optic nerve vasoconstriction correlated highly with the logarithm of the daily ET-1 dosage, the weight, and the sex of the rabbits (Fig. 3), demonstrating a dose-dependent vasoconstriction with chronic local application of ET-1 in the vascular bed of the anterior optic nerve in albino rabbits (1). Consequently, this in vivo experimental model offers a titratable method with which the effects of chronic vasoconstriction and vascular insufficiency on the optic nerve can be examined.

QUANTIFICATION OF OPTIC NERVE BLOOD FLOW

Although a dose-dependent vasoconstriction with chronic local application of ET-1 in the vascular bed of the anterior optic nerve had been demonstrated, the amount of blood flow reduction with chronic local application of ET-1 still remained to be determined. In the animal model, many invasive techniques can be used to assess the blood flow and the microcirculation within the eye, including radioactively labeled microspheres, iodoantipyrine, hydrogen clearance, and laser Doppler velocity. These techniques have been employed for decades in various animal models and provide much of our baseline data by which newer, less invasive techniques are judged.

Since their introduction in blood flow research, intravascular radioactive microsphere injection techniques have been widely used as a measurement of ocular blood flow. Recently, a new method of microsphere blood flow assessment has been described in which nonradioactive colored microspheres (E-Z TRAC Ultraspheres; Interactive Medical Technologies, South Barrington, IL) are employed. These are injected in the same manner as radioactive microspheres. However, instead of analyzing tissue samples for radioactivity, the samples are digested and the number of actual microspheres contained within the tissue of interest are counted. This method obviates the expensive disposal of radioactive materials and the need for a multichannel gamma analyzer.

Application of the intravascular microsphere injection technique may not appear practical for studies on the eye. Because of the relatively small size of the optic nerve, one could expect that too few spheres would localize to the optic nerve vascular bed to permit flow determinations. To establish a reproducible technique to accurately assess blood flow in a small tissue such as the anterior optic nerve, the variability of the colored microsphere injection technique was evaluated. Colored microspheres 10.2 ± 0.23 μm in diameter were injected into the left atria of albino rabbits. The rabbits were divided into four groups, injected with 5, 10, 50, or 100 million microspheres, respectively. Microsphere quantification in the tissue was performed after postmortem dissection and alkaline corrosion of the anterior optic nerve. Analysis of the variability of the method was based on the assumption that the blood flow in the right and left anterior optic nerves should be fairly similar. The differences in the number of microspheres between the right and left optic nerves were analyzed with respect to the average number of microspheres recovered in both optic nerves. The rabbits injected with 100 million microspheres showed the highest average number of microspheres entrapped in the tissue (range 31.8–78.7 microspheres/mg optic nerve tissue). Furthermore, injection with 100 million microspheres yielded a significantly (Kruskal–Wallis test: $p = 0.0048$) lower relative interocular difference (range 2.3–12.8%) compared to the rabbits injected with 5, 10, or 50 million microspheres (range 15.3–162.8%). Consequently, the present experimental technique of optic nerve blood flow measurement is relatively inexpensive, highly reproducible, and obviates the need to dispose of radioactive materials (12).

OPTIC NERVE BLOOD FLOW REDUCTION AFTER LOCAL APPLICATION OF ET-1

To quantify the optic nerve ischemia induced by ET-1, blood flow was measured by the colored microsphere injection technique in rabbits and rhesus monkeys in which ET-1 was delivered to the perineural region of the anterior optic nerve.

ET-1 or balanced salt solution (BSS) was delivered to the perineural region of the anterior optic nerve via osmotically driven minipumps in five experimental and four control rabbits and in three experimental and three control rhesus monkeys (*Macaca mulatta*) (11, 13). After 14 days, ET-1 induced, independent of intraocular pressure, a statistically significant decrease in blood flow in the experimental eyes in both species. The average (mean ± SD) blood flow reduction in the experimental eyes was 37.8 ± 7.2% among the rabbits subjected to ET-1. Among the monkeys implanted with ET-1 minipumps, the average (mean ± SD) decrease in optic nerve blood flow in the experimental eye compared to the contralateral eye was 35.7 ± 9.1%. In both species, BSS did not influence blood flow.

IN VIVO QUANTIFICATION OF MORPHOLOGIC OPTIC NERVE CHANGES

According to the results reported above, ET-1 induces a dose-dependent arteriolar constriction in the vascular bed of the anterior optic nerve in rabbits and decreases anterior optic nerve blood flow in rabbits and monkeys. A further question that still needed to be addressed was whether optic nerve ischemia during an extended period of time would induce optic nerve atrophy. Previous studies with photographs or ophthalmoscopy have been unable to demonstrate convincingly morphologic optic nerve changes (preliminary experiments). Therefore a quantitative method to analyze the optic nerve topography was needed. The device chosen to quantify the morphology of the optic disc was the Heidelberg retina tomograph (HRT) (Heidelberg Engineering, Heidelberg, Germany). It appeared reasonable to use this method because previous experi-

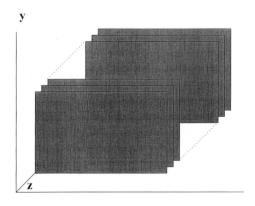

FIG. 4. Principle of confocal imaging. Thirty-two successive images are obtained from different focal planes. Confocal optics guarantee that no light from outside the imaged focal plane will reach the objective. The height for each imaged point is set at the level of the focal plane with the highest measured intensity of the reflected light. These measurements allow a determination of the topography of the structure of interest, i.e., the optic disc.

ments have shown a comparable reproducibility of the topometric data obtained in rabbits with the HRT, compared to humans (10).

The HRT is a laser-scanning ophthalmoscope that utilizes confocal optics, designed for three-dimensional measurements of the retinal surface topography (Fig. 4). It produces three-dimensional topographic images and calculates topometric variables of the optic nerve and peripapillary region. Sequential topographic images can be analyzed with respect to the same region of interest, and changes in the topography can be quantified.

MORPHOLOGIC CHANGES AFTER 2 MONTHS OF OPTIC NERVE ISCHEMIA

The morphologic changes after optic nerve ischemia were evaluated in albino rabbits that were implanted with osmotic minipumps filled with ET-1 (flow rate 0.1 μg/day). These rabbits were observed for 8 weeks. Because the capacity of the minipumps used in this study allowed delivery for only 2 weeks, a new minipump was implanted every 2 weeks. Only the reservoir was replaced, whereas the delivery tube was left undisturbed.

Topographic images were obtained before minipump implantation, after 4 weeks of local ET-1 administration, and at the end of the 8-week observation period. The topometric data obtained indicated an increase in optic nerve cupping in the experimental eyes after 8 weeks of local administration of ET-1 compared to that of the control eyes (Fig. 5). This effect could not be explained by

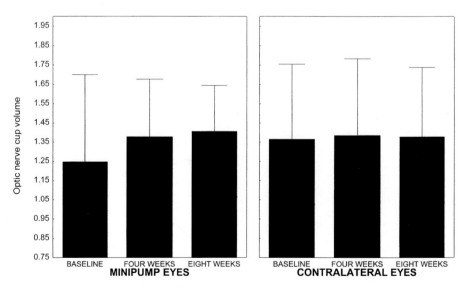

FIG. 5. The experimental eyes showed a progressive increase in optic nerve cup volume (ANOVA $p=0.0078$).

differences in IOP. Furthermore, definite histopathologic changes were observed in a masked evaluation of the experimental optic nerves. These abnormalities included loss of myelin and gliosis of the prelaminar portion of the optic nerve (13). The observed demyelination is in agreement with results obtained in peripheral nerves (8).

CONCLUSION

The potential role of vascular insufficiency in glaucoma has been debated for over a century and remains controversial. It has been difficult to settle these controversies with current experimental techniques. Indeed, there has not been any previous experimental model that could be used to examine the effects of vascular insufficiency on the optic nerve. Experimental optic nerve atrophy similar to that seen in glaucoma patients can be induced by increased IOP (14). However, increased IOP cannot account for the changes observed in the current study. Because these experiments were performed in rabbits, their significance for human optic neuropathies must be considered cautiously, and the present model of optic nerve ischemia needs to be tried in a primate model to allow more reliable comparisons with conditions observed in the human eye.

REFERENCES

1. Cioffi GA, Orgül S, Onda E, Bacon DR, Van Buskirk EM. An in vivo model of chronic optic nerve ischemia: the dose-dependent effects of endothelin-1 on the optic nerve microvasculature. *Curr Eye Res* 1995;14:1147–53.
2. Fahrenbach WH, Bacon DR, Morrison JC, Van Buskirk EM. Controlled vascular corrosion casting of the rabbit eye. *J Electron Microsc Tech* 1988;10:15–26.
3. Fechtner R, Weinreb RN. Mechanisms of optic nerve damage in primary open-angle glaucoma. *Surv Ophthalmol* 1994;39:23–42.
4. Flammer J. To what extent are vascular factors involved in the pathogenesis of glaucoma? In: Kaiser HJ, Flammer J, Hendrickson P, eds. *Ocular blood flow. New insights into the pathogenesis of ocular diseases*. Basel: Karger; 1996:12–39.
5. Haefliger IO, Flammer J, Lüscher TF. Heterogeneity of endothelium-dependent regulation in ophthalmic and ciliary arteries. *Invest Ophthalmol Vis Sci* 1993;34:1722–30.
6. Lüscher TF, Boulanger CM, Dohi Y, Yang ZH. Endothelium-derived contracting factors. *Hypertension* 1992;19:117–30.
7. Moriya S, Sugiyama T, Shimizu K, Hamada J, Tokuoka S, Azuma I. Low-tension glaucoma and endothelin (ET-1). *Folia Ophthalmol Jpn* 1992;43:554–9.
8. Myers RR, Heckman HM, Galbraith JA, Powell HC. Subperineurial demyelination associated with reduced nerve blood flow and oxygen tension after epineural vascular stripping. *Lab Invest* 1991;65:41–50.
9. Orgül S, Cioffi GA, Bacon DR, Onda E, Van Buskirk EM. Optic nerve vasomotor effects of arterial blood gases. *J Glaucoma* 1995;4:322–6.
10. Orgül S, Cioffi GA, Bacon DR, Van Buskirk EM. Reproducibility of topometric data with a scanning laser ophthalmoscope in rabbits. *Jpn J Ophthalmol* 1995;39:438–42.
11. Orgül S, Cioffi GA, Bacon DR, Van Buskirk EM. An endothelin-1 induced model of chronic optic nerve ischemia in rhesus monkeys. *J Glaucoma* 1996;5:135–8.

12. Orgül S, Cioffi GA, Bacon DR, Van Buskirk EM. Measurement of optic nerve blood flow with nonradioactive colored microspheres in rabbits. *Microvasc Res* 1996;51:175–86.
13. Orgül S, Cioffi GA, Wilson DJ, Bacon DR, Van Buskirk EM. An endothelin-1 induced model of optic nerve ischemia in the rabbit. *Invest Ophthalmol Vis Sci* 1996;37:1860–9.
14. Quigley HA, Hohman RM, Addicks EM. Chronic experimental glaucoma in primates. II. Effect of extended intraocular pressure elevation on optic nerve head and axonal transport. *Invest Ophthalmol Vis Sci* 1980;19:137–52.
15. Sharkey J, Ritchie IM, Kelly PAT. Perivascular microapplication of endothelin-1: a new model of focal cerebral ischemia in the rat. *J Cardiovasc Pharmacol* 1993;13:865–71.
16. Van Buskirk EM, Cioffi GA. Glaucomatous optic neuropathy. *Am J Ophthalmol* 1992;113:447–52.
17. Ziv I, Fleminger G, Djaldetti R, Achiron A, Meland E, Sokolovsky M. Increased plasma endothelin-1 in acute ischemic stroke. *Stroke* 1992;23:1014–6.

Nitric Oxide and Endothelin in the Pathogenesis of Glaucoma, edited by I. O. Haefliger and J. Flammer. Lippincott–Raven Publishers, Philadelphia © 1998.

9

Vasoactive Stimuli and Visual Field Modulations

Lutz E. Pillunat

Universitäts Augenklinik und Poliklinik, Hamburg, Germany

The amount of glaucomatous optic nerve damage that is caused by a given level of intraocular pressure (IOP) is highly variable from one individual to another (1,2). Therefore, an increased IOP cannot be regarded as the only risk factor for glaucoma damage.

Besides additional risk factors such as age or diabetes, an impaired blood supply to the optic nerve may be of pathogenic importance. This vascular theory was first proposed by von Graefe (17) and Magitot (28). There is now substantial evidence that hemodynamic factors are of pathogenic importance (27), especially in normal-pressure glaucoma (7, 34). An association of normal-pressure glaucoma has been found with migraine (31), excessive thermal vasoreactivity of the digits (8), decreased blood pressure (22), increased prevalence of myocardial ischemia (23), reduced ciliary perfusion pressures (35), and low basal flow velocities in the ophthalmic artery (39). In addition to hemodynamic parameters, however, progression of visual field loss must be regarded as the most important issue in glaucoma follow-up. Therefore, vasoactive stimuli that can modulate visual function might be of therapeutic relevance, especially in normal-pressure glaucoma.

CARBON DIOXIDE

In neurology, cerebral vasospastic disorders are diagnosed and cerebral reserve capacity in arteriosclerotic diseases is measured by a carbon dioxide test (4,5). Vasodilatation is induced by breathing increased carbon dioxide concentrations and cerebral blood flow is measured by transcranial ultrasound. Because optic nerve vessels are comparable to central nervous system vessels, the carbon dioxide test was applied in this study to patients suffering from normal-pressure glaucoma.

Previous studies showed that an increased inspiratory carbon dioxide concentration increases ocular pulse volumes and improves the central visual field in some patients suffering from normal-pressure glaucoma (33,37). In other normal-pressure glaucoma patients, however, no improvement occurred with increased inspiratory carbon dioxide concentrations. These results suggest that in some patients a preexisting ocular vasospasm might be relaxed by applying carbon dioxide as a potent cerebral vasodilator.

This observation was confirmed by measuring retrobulbar hemodynamics using color Doppler imaging (21). In 10 normal-pressure glaucoma patients the end-diastolic velocities were significantly lower and the resistance index was significantly higher compared to age-matched controls. When PCO_2 was increased, control subjects remained unchanged. However, it increased end-diastolic velocities in normal-pressure glaucoma patients and abolished the difference in resistance index between the two groups. It appears to be important, however, to determine whether medical therapy might prolong these acute carbon dioxide effects. Therefore, drugs that relax preconstricted ocular vessels, as in ocular vasospasm are of potential interest.

ACETAZOLAMIDE

Flammer et al. (9,10), as early as 1983, demonstrated an improvement of the visual field in glaucoma patients after administration of acetazolamide. The differential threshold of the visual field improved significantly in nine glaucoma patients by 14%. It is well known that acetazolamide causes acidosis, which leads to an increase in blood flow in the brain and in the choroid due to vasodilatation. In monkeys, choroidal blood flow increases by 75% after acetazolamide administration. It therefore appears possible that the improvement in visual function is due to improved blood flow to the optic nerve, which might be the result of decreased vascular resistance, very similiar to the action of carbon dioxide.

CALCIUM-CHANNEL BLOCKERS

It is widely accepted that calcium-channel blockers are appropriate therapy for vasospasm. In a retrospective review of normal-pressure glaucoma patients treated with nifedipine, less visual field decay occured than in a matched control group (29). Furthermore, Kitazawa et al. (26) showed that after an oral application of nifedipine the visual field defect (mean deviation) decreased by 22% in 12 eyes suffering from normal-pressure glaucoma (26). Because nifedipine lowers systemic blood pressure and the pathogenic importance of low blood pressure is a controversial issue (22), a centrally acting calcium-channel blocker (nimodipine) that has no known systemic side effects may have theoretically advantages.

Bose et al. (4) showed that contrast sensitivity improved acutely in normal-pressure glaucoma patients and in healthy volunteers after a single administration of nimodipine. The authors assume that this effect might be due to an increased blood supply to the optic nerve head (ONH), because Riva et al. (38) found increased optic nerve blood flow in cats after i.v. administration of nicardipine.

Experimental studies showed that nimodipine crosses the blood–brain barrier easily and in considerable amounts (24). The local flow of cerebral blood, which is profoundly reduced after middle cerebral artery occlusion, was increased in animals treated with nimodipine (16,48). On isolated preconstricted ciliary arteries, nimodipine showed a significantly stronger vasodilating effect than nifedipine (30).

MATERIALS AND METHODS

Patients

A total of 33 patients with normal-pressure glaucoma were included in the study. All patients underwent a complete neurologic examination, including physical examination, EEG, carotid artery Doppler, and CT of the skull to exclude a neurologic origin of the visual field defects. Bilateral normal-pressure glaucoma was present in all patients, and one eye of each subject was randomly selected. Glaucomatous optic nerve cupping corresponding to the visual field defect was present in all patients. Visual field defects were defined as at least six adjacent test points in the Humphrey 30-2 visual field that showed more than -6 dB depth. In no patient did IOP exceed 21 mm Hg. IOP measurements were performed at least at three visits, and included one measurement during the night and one in a supine position. None of the patients included in the study was receiving systemic β-blockers, calcium-channel blockers, or antihypertensive therapy. All topical drugs were withdrawn 8 weeks before the start of the study. Except for mild cataracts, all patients showed no evidence of ophthalmologic diseases except normal-pressure glaucoma. Five patients included in the study suffered from age-related diabetes mellitus type II without any ocular manifestations. There were 20 women and 13 men in the study. The mean age was 61.9 years.

In keeping with the tenets of the Declaration of Helsinki, informed consent was obtained and documented in writing after the nature of the study was explained to the subjects.

Ocular Pulse Amplitudes and Ocular Pulse Volumes

To measure ocular pulse amplitudes (OPA), oculo–oscillo-dynamography (OODG) was used. OODG (42,44,45) represents a similiar but more sensitive method than oculo–pneumoplethysmography (OPG) described by Gee (14). To measure OPA, two calibrated suction cups were applied at the temporal side of the sclera on both eyes. The exterior rim was located 0.5–1 mm from the limbus. By applying a suction of 30 mm Hg, the IOP was raised by approximately 6

mm Hg. The OODG was switched to the constant mode to register pulse amplitudes of a comparable height. The suction cups were connected to a highly
sensitive capacitive electrostatic transducer. The pulse-dependent oscillations of
each eye were amplified and finally plotted on a strip chart recorder.

To calculate ocular pulse volumes from the measured pulse amplitudes, an
external calibration signal representing 1 μl is given on every original registra-
tion. By measuring the height of 15 recorded pulse amplitudes and by comparing
their average height to the given magnitude of the external calibration signal,
the individual ocular pulse volume is derived.

Carbon Dioxide

Through a partially closed mask system, carbogen gas (95% oxygen and 5%
carbon dioxide) was administered. Because of the partially closed system, the
patient had to rebreathe a portion of expired air. Therefore, the end-tidal carbon
dioxide concentration was approximately 0.5% higher compared to breathing
pure carbogen. The mask system was connected to a carbon dioxide monitor
(Datex Normocap Oxy) and end-tidal carbon dioxide concentrations were measured continuously.

Visual Fields

All patients were experienced in performing automated visual fields. In all
patients and in all parts of the study, Humphrey 30-2 central visual fields were
used. As a stable baseline field, at least two stable visual fields, i.e., ± 1 dB
mean deviation, were regarded as a prerequisite to enter the study. After obtaining
a valid baseline field, a central visual field was performed while the patient
breathed ambient air or increased carbon dioxide concentrations. The order was
selected at random and the patient was masked with regard to the actual condition. The visual fields were analyzed with the Humphrey Statpac program.

In addition, IOP, systemic blood pressure, and heart rate were measured while
patients were breathing room air and during carbon dioxide exposure. Mean
blood pressure (BP) was calculated according to Wezler and Böger s formula
(47): $BP_{mean} = BP_{diast.} + 0.42 (BP_{syst.} - BP_{diast.})$.

According to results in healthy volunteers, patients were divided into carbon
dioxide responder and non-carbon dioxide responder subgroups. Previous studies
(36,37) showed that healthy subjects demonstrate a mean increase in ocular
pulse volumes of 0.14 ± 0.03 μl during breathing carbogen compared to breathing ambient air. Eyes of normal-pressure glaucoma patients, that showed a higher
increase of OPV during carbon dioxide exposure than the mean increase (plus
twice the SD) in healthy subjects (>0.2 μl) were defined as carbon dioxide
responders. All patients received 30 mg nimodipine twice daily. Mean follow-
up was 18 months.

The OODG recordings and the visual fields were analyzed without knowledge concerning the actual experimental condition, i.e., breathing ambient air, rebreathing carbogen, or nimodipine treatment.

RESULTS

The results of 31 patients were evaluated. One patient was excluded from the study because a change in systemic medication was necessary. Another patient did not show up after 3 months of therapy and was therefore excluded.

Mean brachial arterial pressure dropped slightly, but not significantly, during nimodipine treatment. There was no change in heart rate during the entire treatment period. IOP dropped during application of increased carbon dioxide concentrations, but these changes proved not to be statistically significant. During nimodipine treatment the IOP did not change compared to baseline.

Mean ocular pulse amplitudes and ocular pulse volumes changed statistically significantly from 4.92 mm (0.29 μl) to 8.57 mm (0.52 μl) during exposure to increased carbon dioxide concentration. When these changes were analyzed individually, it was obvious that the group of normal-pressure glaucoma patients could be subdivided into two subgroups. In a previous study (36), 30 healthy subjects showed a mean OPV increase of 0.14 $\pm$ 0.3 μl during carbon dioxide exposure. According to these results, 13 patients (13 eyes) showed a remarkably higher increase in ocular pulse amplitudes and ocular pulse volumes than the remaining 18 eyes. Thirteen eyes showed an increase in OPV that was significantly higher than the mean increase in healthy subjects, including twice the SD. By comparing the changes in both subgroups, the differences proved to be statistically significant ($p = 0.0012$). Other than age differences, there were no systemic or ophthalmologic factors, such as systemic diseases, a difference in the amount of visual field defect, or differences in mean IOP, that could be correlated with the higher increase of OPV during carbon dioxide exposure (Table 1). The carbon dioxide responders appeared to be younger and exhibited

TABLE 1. *Demographic data of the carbon dioxide responder subgroup compared to the non-carbon dioxide responder subgroup*

	CO$_2$ responder	Nonresponder
n	13	18
Age	58.5 years	63.6 years
Male	5	7
Female	8	11
Visual field defect	−9.4 dB	−8.88 dB
c/d ratio	0.61	0.73
Mean blood pressure	105.3 mm Hg	106.4 mm Hg
Heart rate	79.8/min	79.1/min
Intraocular pressure	15.5 mm Hg	14.9 mm Hg
History of vasospasm (migraine, cold hands, cold feet)	8	9

less optic nerve damage. However, these changes were not significantly different between the two subgroups examined.

After 3 months of nimodipine therapy, the ocular pulse volumes decreased by approximately 7%, and MD, PSD, and CPSD decreased by approximately 10% in subgroup I compared to the carbon dioxide condition. This decrease was not statistically significant. Comparing the results after 3 months of treatment to baseline, however, shows significant ($p < 0.05$) improvements (Fig. 1). In

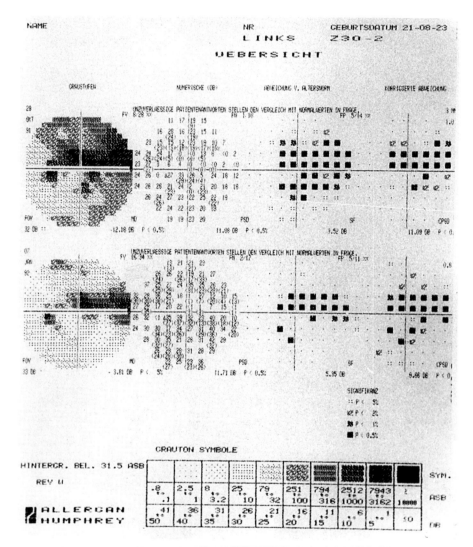

FIG. 1. Comparison of the visual field of a 69-year-old woman with NPG (CO_2 responder) during breathing ambient air (*upper field* −12.18 dB) and after 3 months of nimodipine therapy (*lower field* −3.81 dB).

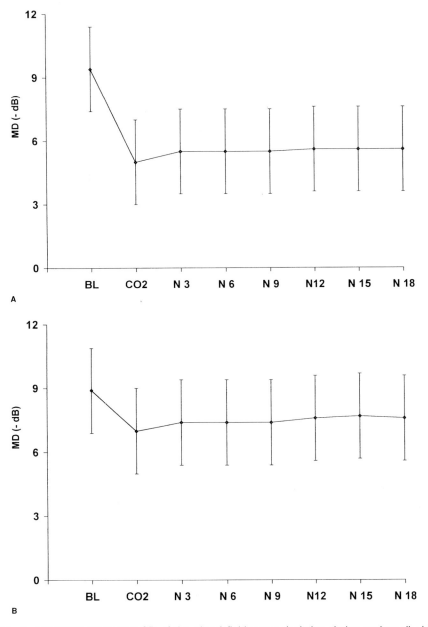

FIG. 2. Arithmetic mean and SD of the visual field mean deviation during carbon dioxide exposure (CO_2) and nimodipine treatment. **A**: Carbon dioxide responder subgroup (I). **B**: Non-carbon dioxide responder subgroup (II). N3–N18, month 3–month 18; BL, baseline; dB, decibels; MD, mean deviation.

subgroup II, ocular pulse volumes, MD, PSD, and CPSD also showed a slight decrease after 3 months of therapy that was not significant compared to the carbon dioxide condition. The visual field indices in subgroup II improved during therapy by approximately 15% compared to baseline. In contrast to subgroup I, however, these changes were not statistically significantly different ($p = 0.085$).

During the entire treatment period of 18 months, the visual field indices (Fig. 2A,B) and ocular pulse volumes remained stable. In subgroup I (carbon dioxide responders), the mean improvement of the mean deviation, PSD, and CPSD indices after 18 months of therapy were still significantly different from baseline. In subgroup II (nonresponders), the mean visual field indices were not significantly different from baseline.

The results in subgroup I, however, were slightly correlated ($r = 0.56$) when the increase of OPV and the decrease in the mean deviation of the visual fields were compared. Under nimodipine treatment, the correlation became even stronger in subgroup 1 ($r = 0.69$ after 6 months of nimodipine therapy) whereas no change was observed in subgroup II.

DISCUSSION

As various experimental and clinical studies have shown (11,32,36,37,41), total ocular blood flow increases during exposure to increased carbon dioxide concentrations. By recording ocular pulse amplitudes it was shown that in healthy subjects a statistically significant increase of 39% was found during rebreathing carbogen (36). Compared to these results, the overall effect on ocular pulse volumes in patients suffering from normal-pressure glaucoma was found to be stronger. The results of this and previous studies (37) show that not all patients suffering from normal-pressure glaucoma present the same ocular carbon dioxide reactivity. These findings suggest that some patients are more susceptible to induced vasodilatation as provoked by exposure to carbon dioxide breathing. Furthermore, these changes are correlated with an improvement in visual function. Therefore, the results suggest that some patients with normal-pressure glaucoma suffer from a hemodynamic disorder that can be relieved by induced ocular vasodilatation with carbon dioxide. These observations are supported by color Doppler imaging studies (21) that lead to similar conclusions.

Regulation of the constrictive tone in small vessels is controlled, in addition to other factors, by the calcium content of smooth-muscle cells in the vessel wall. Therefore, some authors are treating ocular vasospasm, i.e., a disorder of ocular hemodynamics, in the same way as peripheral vasospasm in Raynaud's phenomenon, with calcium-channel blockers (12,13). Kitazawa et al. (26) showed statistically significant improvements in the visual field in normal-pressure glaucoma patients after administration of nifedipine. In 12 patients, the mean deviation improved by 22% during treatment. By comparing this observation to the results presented in this study, the overall effect appears to be similar.

Taking the mean deviation of all visual fields in all patients examined ($n = 31$), the visual field improved by 25%. By separating the patients according to the carbon dioxide test, the results are different.

The visual field (MD) in normal-pressure glaucoma patients who showed a high susceptibility to carbon dioxide (subgroup I) improved significantly more (41%) compared to the nonresponders (subgroup II) (14%) after 18 months of nimodipine treatment. Therefore, the carbon dioxide test appears to help identify patients with normal-pressure glaucoma who suffer from ocular vasospasm and who may benefit from administration of a centrally acting calcium-channel blocker.

The experimental design of the carbon dioxide test was derived from the setup that is used routinely in neurology to diagnose cerebral hemodynamic disorders (5). Because high oxygen concentrations, as used in the present study, may partially counteract the effect of carbon dioxide on ocular vessels (11,18,20,41), further studies are needed to show whether the results presented might be improved and/or reproduced by the administration of similiar carbon dioxide concentrations mixed with lower oxygen concentrations, i.e., room air (32). Nevertheless, the current experimental design seems to be sensitive enough to identify patients who benefit from the administration of a centrally acting calcium-channel blocker.

Breathing different gas mixtures affects the circulation in different parts of the entire body as well as the ocular circulation. The improvement of the visual fields in patients suffering from normal-pressure glaucoma during exposure to carbon dioxide, however, does not appear to be a systemic effect, because heart rate and blood pressure remained constant. Administration of a centrally acting calcium-channel blocker and exposure to carbon dioxide affect the cerebral circulation. However, it seems unlikely that the observed improvement of visual fields in some normal-pressure glaucoma patients is due to changes in cerebral circulation. The visual fields correspond to the glaucomatous appearance of the optic disc, i.e., the field defects were not due to cerebral disorders. Furthermore, there was a significant correlation with an increase in ocular pulse volumes, indicating that visual field improvement might be due to changes in ocular hemodynamics.

Ocular pulse amplitudes and ocular pulse volumes are hemodynamic parameters that reflect the circulation of the entire eye and are therefore mainly due to choroidal pulsations (14,44). Because retinal and optic nerve blood flow are only a small part of the entire ocular circulation, the observed changes in OPA and OPV do not necessarily reflect changes in retinal or optic nerve hemodynamics. However, the results suggest that some patients with normal-pressure glaucoma may suffer from a hemodynamic disorder such as ocular vasospasm, which can be released by provoked vasodilatation due to breathing CO_2 or by the administration of nimodipine. From the results of this and previous studies, it does not appear possible to determine where this hemodynamic disorder may be located—whether it is an extraocular vasospasm of the ophthalmic artery or an intraocular hemodynamic disorder of retinal, choroidal, or optic nerve circulation. Therefore, studies are needed in which optic nerve blood flow (38) and retinal blood flow (19,43) are investigated.

Previous results using color Doppler imaging during carbon dioxide exposure suggest that extraocular blood flow, i.e., flow velocity of the ophthalmic artery, is improved in normal-pressure glaucoma patients (21). In this previously published study by Harris and co-workers (21), however, the flow velocity in the ophthalmic artery was lower and the resistance index higher in normal-pressure glaucoma patients compared to healthy controls. In the study presented here and in previous other studies, the baseline OPVs were comparable between healthy subjects and normal-pressure glaucoma patients as well as between the carbon dioxide responder subgroup and the nonresponder group. These results may be due to a higher sensitivity of CDI measurements compared to ocular pulse amplitude measurements. Because the CDI results were significantly different only in the ophthalmic artery and not in the ciliary or retinal arteries, it is also possible that measuring ocular pulse amplitudes reflects intraocular hemodynamics to a higher degree.

Testing of visual fields and judging changes always carries the risk of evaluating artifacts, such as practice effects, and short-term and long-term fluctuations. Obviously, it is not possible to rule out these effects completely. However, for inclusion in the study the patients had to be experienced with visual field testing. Furthermore, two comparable visual fields were a requirement before entering the study. The performance during visual field testing was comparable between both subgroups. The mean deviation as well as the pattern SD and the corrected pattern SD improved in the carbon dioxide responder subgroup. During the first part of the study, the patients were masked to the actual gas condition. Breathing higher carbon dioxide concentrations might be unpleasant, and therefore the masking of the patient to the actual condition could not be guaranteed. However, no patient complained or stopped the examination. Therefore, it appears unlikely that the observed significant improvements of the central visual field in subgroup I during carbon dioxide exposure or nimodipine treatment are due to learning effects or to any other uncontrolled circumstances. According to the literature available, there are no reports in which the influence of increased carbon dioxide concentrations on visual field defects has been investigated. Kitazawa et al. (26), however, showed that after oral administration of nifedipine the mean visual field defect decreased by 22% in 12 eyes suffering from normal-pressure glaucoma. Netland and co-workers (29) showed that long-term treatment with nifedipine might be beneficial in normal-pressure glaucoma but not in high-pressure glaucoma. In this retrospective study, less visual field deterioration occurred in normal-pressure glaucoma patients who were receiving nifedipine treatment. In addition, Flammer and co-workers (9,10) demonstrated a threshold improvement of 14% in nine glaucomatous eyes after oral administration of acetazolamide. The different amount of visual field improvement (41% in this study in subgroup

I) may be due to the patients selected or to the different pharmacologic actions of nifedipine/acetazolamide and carbon dioxide/nimodipine.

Increased carbon dioxide is clearly the most potent vasodilator of cerebral circulation (3,25,40). It is an established standard by which vasodilator reactivity is calibrated in physiology and neurology (6). Carbon dioxide apparently exerts its actions on both cerebral arterioles and small arteries apparently by releasing NO from the vascular endothelium in a manner similiar to either perivascular or intracellular pH changes (46). These pH changes may also lead to additional vasodilatation beyond that of nimodipine. Carbon dioxide leads to a 10% higher increase of OPV and improvement of the visual fields compared to nimodipine. Experimental studies demonstrated that nimodipine relaxes preconstricted isolated ciliary arteries better than nifedipine (30). Bose et al. (4) showed that contrast sensitivity improved acutely in normal-pressure glaucoma patients after a single administration of nimodipine. Furthermore, nimodipine proved to be beneficial after cerebral ischemia. Patients with stroke showed more functional improvements after nimodipine treatment compared to placebo (15). The results of the present study indicate that therapy with oral nimodipine maintains the acute carbon dioxide effect for at least 18 months without lowering blood pressure or changing IOP. Even the non-carbon dioxide responders whose visual fields did not improve during nimodipine therapy remained stable during the treatment period. To confirm the results described in this study, multicenter studies are needed.

REFERENCES

1. Anderson DR. The posterior segment of glaucomatous eyes. In: Luetjen-Drecoll, ed. *Basic aspects of glaucoma research.* Stuttgart: Schattauer, 1982:167–90.
2. Anderson DR. The mechanisms of damage of the optic nerve. In: Krieglstein GK, Leydhecker W, eds. *Glaucoma update II.* Heidelberg: Springer-Verlag, 1983:89–93.
3. Archer LNJ, Evands DH, Patton JH, Levene MI. Controlled hypercapnia and neonatal cerebral artery Doppler ultrasound waveforms. *Pediatr Res* 1986;20:218–22.
4. Bose S, Piltz JR, Breton ME. Effect of nimodipine, a centrally active calcium channel blocker, on spatial contrast sensitivity in normal tension glaucoma. *Ophthalmology* 1992;99:132.
5. Widder B. Der CO_2-Test zur Erkennung haemodynamisch kritischer Carotisstenosen mit der transkraniellen Dopplersonographie. *Dtsch Med Wschr* 1985;110:1553–61.
6. Widder B, Paulat K, Hackspacher J, Mayr E. Transcranial doppler CO_2 test for the detection of hemodynamically relevant carotid artery stenosis and occlusion. *Eur Arch Psychiatr Neurol Sci* 1986;236:162–8.
7. Drance SM. Some factors in the production of low tension glaucoma. *Br J Ophthalmol* 1972;56:229–42.
8. Drance SM, Douglas GR, Wijsman K, Schulzer M, Britton RJ. Response of blood flow to warm and cold in normal and low-tension glaucoma patients. *Am J Ophthalmol* 1988;105:35–9.
9. Flammer J, Drance SM. Reversibility of glaucomatous visual field defects after acetacolamide. *Can J Ophthalmol* 1983;18:139–41.
10. Flammer J, Drance SM. Effect of acetacolamide on the differential threshold. *Arch Ophthalmol* 1983;101:1378–80.
11. Frayser R, Hickham JB. Retinal vascular response to breathing increased carbon dioxide and oxygen concentrations. *Invest Ophthalmol Vis Sci* 1964;3:427–31.

12. Gasser P, Flammer J. Influence of vasospasm on visual function. *Doc Ophthalmol* 1984;66: 3–18.
13. Gasser P, Flammer J. Blood-cell velocity in the nailfold capillaries of patients with normal-tension and high-tension glaucoma. *Am J Ophthalmol* 1991;111:585–8.
14. Gee W, Oller DW, Homer LD, Bailey CR. Simultaneous bilateral determination of the systolic artery pressure of the ophthalmic artery by ocular pneumoplethysmography. *Invest Ophthalmol Vis Sci* 1977;16:86–92.
15. Gelmers HJ, Gorters K, de Weerdt CJ, Wiezer HJA. A controlled trial of nimodipine in acute ischemic stroke. *N Engl J Med* 1988;318:203–7.
16. Gotoh O, Mohammed AA, McCulloch J, Graham DI, Harper AM. Nimodipine and the hemodynamic and histopathological consequences of middle cerebral artery occlusion. *J Cereb Blood Flow Metab* 1986;6:321–31.
17. Graefe A, von. Ueber die glaucomatoese Natur der Amaurose mit Sehnervenexkavation und ueber die Classifikation der Glaukome. *Graefes Arch Clin Exp Ophthalmol* 1862;8:271–97.
18. Grunwald JE, Riva CE, Brucker AJ, Sinclair SH, Petrig BL. Altered retinal vascular response to 100% oxygen breathing in diabetes mellitus. *Ophthalmology* 1984;91:1447–52.
19. Grunwald JE, Riva CE, Stone RA, Keates EU, Petrig BL. Retinal autoregulation in open-angle glaucoma. *Ophthalmology* 1984;91:1690–4.
20. Harris A, Malinovsky VE, Cantor LB. Isocapnia blocks exercise induced reductions in ocular tensions. *Invest Ophthalmol Vis Sci* 1992;33:2229–32.
21. Harris A, Sergott RC, Spaeth GL, Katz JL, Shoemaker JA, Martin BJ. Color doppler analysis of ocular vessel blood velocity in normal tension glaucoma. *Am J Ophthalmol* 1994;118: 642–9.
22. Hayreh SS, Zimmerman MB, Podhajski P, Alward WLM. Nocturnal arterial hypotension and its role in optic nerve head and ocular ischemic disorders. *Am J Ophthalmol* 1994;117:603–24.
23. Kaiser HJ, Flammer J. Silent myocardial ischemia in glaucoma patients. *Ophthalmologica* 1993;207:6–8.
24. Kerkhoff W van den, Drewes LR. Transfer of the calcium antagonists nifedipine and nimodipine across the blood brain barrier and their regional distribution in vivo. *J Cereb Blood Flow Metab* 1995;5:459–60.
25. Kety SS, Schmidt CF. The effect of altered tensions of carbon dioxide and oxygen and cerebral blood flow and cerebral oxygen consumption in young men. *J Clin Invest* 1948;27:484–512.
26. Kitazawa Y, Shirai H, Go FJ. The effect of Ca-antagonists on the visual field in low tension glaucoma. *Graefes Arch Clin Exp Ophthalmol* 1989;227:408–12.
27. Lee SS, Schwartz B. Role of the temporal cilioretinal artery in retaining central visual field in open angle glaucoma. *Ophthalmology* 1992;99:696–9.
28. Magitot A. *Contribute a l'étude de la circulation arterielle et lymphatique du nerf optique et du chiasme.* Thesis. Paris, 1908.
29. Netland PA, Chaturvedi N, Dreyer EB. Calcium channel blockers in the management of low-tension and open-angle glaucoma. *Am J Ophthalmol* 1993;115:608–13.
30. Nyborg NCB, Nielsen PJ. Comparison of the vasodilator effect of nifedipine and nimodipine in bovine isolated ocular arteries [Abstract]. *Proc Eur Glaucoma Soc* 1992;186.
31. Phelps CD, Corbett JJ. Migraine and low-tension glaucoma. A case-control study. *Invest Ophthalmol Vis Sci* 1985;26/8:1105–8.
32. Pillunat LE, Harris A, Anderson DR, Knighton RW, Joos KM. Effect of varying inspired oxygen and carbon dioxide on optic nerve blood flow in humans by laser doppler flowmetry. *Invest Ophthalmol Vis Sci* 1994;35:1255.
33. Pillunat LE, Lang GK. Ocular carbon dioxide reactivity in normal pressure glaucoma. *Invest Ophthalmol Vis Sci* 1992;33:1279.
34. Pillunat LE, Stodtmeister R, Wilmanns I. Pressure compliance of the optic nerve head in low tension glaucoma. *Br J Ophthalmol* 1987;71:181–7.
35. Pillunat LE, Stodtmeister R, Marquardt R, Mattern A. Ocular perfusion pressures in different types of glaucoma. *Int Ophthalmol* 1989;13:37–42.
36. Pillunat LE, Lang GK. Ocular carbon dioxide reactivity in healthy volunteers: effect of age and CO_2 concentration applied. *Germ J Ophthalmol* 1992;1:254.
37. Pillunat LE, Lang GK, Harris A. The visual response to increased ocular blood flow in normal pressure glaucoma. *Surv Ophthalmol* 1994;38:139–49.

38. Riva CE, Harino S, Petrig BL, Shonat RD. Laser Doppler flowmetry in the optic nerve. *Exp Eye Res* 1992;55:499–506.
39. Rojanapongpun R, Drance SM, Morrison BJ. Ophthalmic artery flow velocity in glaucomatous and normal subjects. *Br J Ophthalmol* 1993;77:25–30.
40. Severinghaus JW, Lassen N. Step hypocapnia to seperate arterial from tissue PCO_2 in the regulation of cerebral blood flow. *Circ Res* 1967;20:272–91.
41. Sponsel WE, DePaul K, Zetlan SR. Retinal hemodynamic effects of carbon dioxide, hyperoxia, and mild hypoxia. *Invest Ophthalmol Vis Sci* 1992;33:1864–9.
42. Stodtmeister R, Hornberger M, Hoefer M, Pillunat LE, Gaus W. Okulo-oszillo-dynamographie nach Ulrich: Ergebnisse bei Augengesunden. *Klin Monatsbl Augenheilk* 1988;192:219–33.
43. Tanaka T, Riva C. Blood velocity measurements in human retinal vessels, *Science* 1974;186:830–1.
44. Ulrich WD, Ulrich C. Oculo-oscillo-dynamography: a diagnostic procedure for recording ocular pulses and measuring retinal and ciliary arterial blood pressures. *Ophthal Res* 1985;17:308–17.
45. Ulrich WD, Ulrich C. Okulooszillodynamographie, ein neues Verfahren zur Bestimmung des Ophthalmikablutdruckes und zur okulaeren Pulskurvenanalyse. *Klin Mbl Augenheilk* 1985; 186:385–8.
46. Wang Q, Paulson OB, Lassen NA. Effect of nitric oxide blockade by NG-nitro-L-arginine on cerebral blood flow response to changes in carbon dioxide tensions. *J Cereb Blood Flow Metab* 1992;12:947–63.
47. Wezler K, Böger A. Die Dynamik des arteriellen Systems. *Erg Physiol* 1939;41:292–314.
48. White RP, Cunningham, MP, Robertson JT. Effect of the calcium antagonist nimodipine on contractile responses of isolated canine basilar arteries induced by serotonin, prostaglandin F2a, thrombin and whole blood. *Neurosurgery* 1982;10:344–8.

Nitric Oxide and Endothelin in the Pathogenesis of
Glaucoma, edited by I. O. Haefliger and J. Flammer.
Lippincott–Raven Publishers, Philadelphia © 1998.

10

Peripheral Microcirculatory Responses to Vasoconstrictors in Glaucoma Patients

*†Walter E. Haefeli, *Lilly Linder, ‡Andreas Gass,
*‡Silvana C. Romerio, ‡Paul Gasser, and ‡Josef Flammer

*Division of Clinical Pharmacology, Department of Internal Medicine, University
Hospital, Basel; †Department of Pharmacy, University of Basel, Basel; and
‡Department of Ophthalmology, University of Basel, Basel, Switzerland

More than a single pathogenic factor appears to cause nerve fiber loss and excavation of the optic nerve head (ONH) with corresponding visual field defects in patients with open-angle glaucoma. In addition to the elevation of intraocular pressure (IOP) that is an established risk factor for visual field defects, increasing evidence suggests that further factors determine onset, severity, course, and outcome of the disease. In particular, the finding that glaucomatous lesions may also occur in patients with IOP values that are consistently in the normal range (normal-tension glaucoma) points to other mechanisms potentially contributing to the occurrence of visual field defects. It therefore appears likely that local perfusion rather than IOP alone determines the severity of the disease. In theory, any anatomic or functional factor that reduces blood supply below a critical minimum may ultimately cause local ischemia of the ONH and promote glaucomatous damage (Fig. 1). Therefore, factors that reduce local perfusion pressure [e.g., arterial hypotension, elevated IOP (5)] are potential risk factors for glaucomatous damage that should be identified and corrected. One major cause of reduction in blood flow is transient vasospasms of vessels supplying a vascular bed. These spasms may occur in different arterial beds and may therefore result in different symptoms, depending on the anatomic area involved. For example, Raynaud's phenomenon and vasospastic angina are believed to be caused by a predisposition of the vasculature to vasospasms (38), and in migraine patients vasospasms or vascular dysregulation may play a certain role (13,43), although it is currently believed that migraine attacks are not a primary vascular phenomenon (34,42). Interestingly, in patients with vasospasms in one vascular bed similar events often occur in other areas of the circulation (vasospastic syndrome)

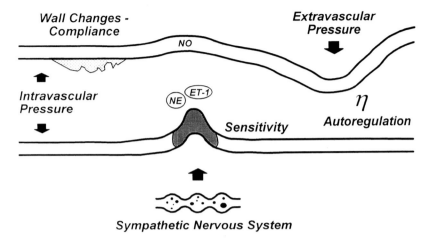

FIG. 1. Factors that modify perfusion of the optic nerve head. In addition to intraocular pressure, blood viscosity, and systemic arterial pressure, autoregulatory mechanisms, including the amount of circulating and locally released vasoactive compounds (e.g., ET-1, endothelin-1; NE, norepinephrine) and the spontaneous release of vasodilators (e.g., NO, nitric oxide) could modulate local flow in the optic nerve head.

(38,39,53), and in patients with vasospastic manifestations in two circulatory beds, spasms are more likely to occur in additional vascular areas (39).

In the past, a number of studies in patients with normal-tension glaucoma revealed indirect evidence for the involvement of the vasculature in the disease. A high prevalence of migraine (40), silent myocardial ischemia (30), digital spasms after exposure to cold water (13,18,20), and immunologic diseases (7) have been reported in patients with normal-tension glaucoma, suggesting that these patients may suffer from a more generalized multifocal disease also affecting the ocular circulation. Moreover, lower arterial blood pressure values (14,31), particularly at night with nocturnal episodes of hypotension (29), have been found, and orthostatic blood pressure dysregulation is more prevalent than in patients with primary open-angle glaucoma (12). Both the fact that visual field defects increase after spasmogenic stimuli, such as immersion of one hand in cold water (22), and the fact that drugs that improve the perfusion characteristics in the peripheral circulation also improve visual function further argue for a pathophysiologic link between certain forms of glaucoma and vasospasms (19).

The reason for the vascular propensity for vasospasms remains to be elucidated. As illustrated in Fig. 1, the causes for the reduction in ocular perfusion pressure are multifaceted. They include elevations in IOP, decreases in blood pressure, changes in rheologic characteristics of the blood, and structural alterations in the vascular wall. Moreover, functional changes with decreases in basal or stimulated endothelium-dependent vasodilatation or increases in the vascular sensitivity to locally released or circulating vasoconstrictors might also change the perfusion of the ONH. Depending on the vasculature studied and the nature of the underlying disease, multiple changes in local vascular responsiveness have been reported, but thus far no unifying concept of vascular disturbances in patients with vasospastic syndromes has been presented. Patients with vaso- spasms differ from control subjects in several important aspects concerning the sensitivity of the vasculature to vasoactive compounds and the regulation of vascular tone. The response of the endothelium-dependent vasodilator bradykinin was markedly reduced in superficial hand veins of patients with Raynaud's disease (3), whereas the effect of the endothelium-independent nitric oxide (NO) donor sodium nitroprusside was similar to controls, as was the venoconstrictor effect of norepinephrine. Moreover, in patients with vasospastic angina attacks (syndrome X) endothelium-dependent vasodilatation was only one-third of con- trol values, and the response to the endothelium-independent vasodilator papav- erine was also markedly reduced (8), suggesting that the functional changes extend beyond the endothelial layer. In contrast to those findings in human capacitance vessels and in the coronary microcirculation, large intracranial arter- ies were supersensitive to endothelium-independent relaxation with nitroglycerin in patients with migraine (47). Because inhibition of NO formation results in a supersensitivity of the vasculature to nitroglycerin, the findings of Thomsen and co-workers (47) may provide indirect evidence for disturbed release of NO in migraine patients. Moreover, patients with Raynaud's phenomenon (54), normal- tension glaucoma (46), acute migraine attacks (16), and variant angina (48) all have been reported to have elevated circulating endothelin-1 (ET-1) concentra- tions. In addition, the release of ET-1 after stimuli such as cold pressor testing was markedly increased in the venous outflow of the cold-challenged limb (54), and postural increases in ET-1 concentrations appeared blunted in patients with normal-tension glaucoma compared to patients with open-angle glaucoma or controls (32). Many in vitro and in vivo studies have clearly shown that ET-1 also has profound vasoconstrictor effects in the ocular circulation (24,25,37), including the optic nerve, where it may provoke ischemia (9).

Vascular tone may therefore be modulated by changes in circulating vasocon- strictors and vasodilators, by changes in locally released vasoactive compounds, and by alterations of the sensitivity of the vascular wall to respond to these agonists. In addition to endothelium-derived vasodilators, vasoconstrictor agents may critically modulate vascular tone and are involved in the maintenance of resting vascular tone. In the human forearm catecholamines, ET-1 (36) and its precursor peptide "big" ET-1 (28), and NO (49) contribute to the maintenance of vascular tone, as shown in several studies using specific receptor antagonists and enzyme inhibitors. In contrast, prostacyclin does not appear to control base- line tone (33,50).

Substantial evidence suggests that in some patients with vasospasms the vascu- lar bed of the human forearm is also involved (13,18). It therefore appears necessary to study vascular responses in this vasculature. Because of the hetero- geneity of responses in different vascular beds in patients with different diseases, the methods should be suitable to quantify agonist-induced changes in the arterial, microvascular, and venous forearm circulation.

Responsiveness to locally administered agonists has been extensively studied in resistance arteries (4,21) and hand veins of the human forearm circulation (1,2). This vascular bed rarely develops severe atherosclerosis, but the extent of structural changes in the brachial artery correlates with the degree of atherosclerotic lesions in critical vascular beds in humans, such as carotid and coronary arteries (44). Moreover, in comparative studies in human hand veins and in the systemic circulation, vasoconstrictor responses were linearly correlated, indicating that the sensitivity determined in hand veins reflects the response observed after systemic administration (51). Hence, both the arterial and the venous circulation of the human forearm may serve as surrogates for vascular responses in other circulatory beds that are not readily accessible in pharmacologic studies. Finally, using laser Doppler flowmetry it is also possible to assess vascular responsiveness in the microcirculation of the human forearm (6) after intra-arterial administration of small amounts of vasoactive compounds (17).

RESULTS

To assess the sensitivity of the peripheral microcirculation to vasoconstrictors, we have recently studied microvascular responsiveness of cutaneous blood vessels of the human forearm circulation to ET-1 (0.005–25 ng/min/100 ml tissue; Clinalfa, Läufelfingen, Switzerland) and to the selective full α_1-agonist phenylephrine (0.3–10 μg/min/100 ml tissue; Neo-Synephrine, Sanofi-Winthrop, Münchenstein, Switzerland) in 16 glaucoma patients (nine patients with primary open-angle glaucoma, seven with normal-tension glaucoma) and 16 age- and sex-matched controls (17). In these studies, vasoconstrictor dose–response curves were constructed using laser Doppler flowmetry during agonist administration into the human brachial artery. The technical details have previously been described (17,23). Group comparisons were done with the Mann–Whitney U test, dose–response curves of the two groups were compared with ANOVA for repeated measurements, and the vasoconstrictor effects were related to resting intra-arterial blood pressure with linear regression analysis.

As expected for an effect mediated through an endothelial vasodilator receptor (ET_B) and receptors on vascular smooth-muscle cells mediating constriction (mainly through ET_A receptors), ET-1 dose–response curves were biphasic in all but one patient. At lower dose rates, ET-1 induced vasodilatation; at higher dose rates vasoconstriction prevailed (Fig. 2). These curves were not significantly different among patients with normal-tension glaucoma, open-angle glaucoma, and controls. Similarly, there were no differences in the responses to phenylephrine (Fig. 3). Analysis of the relationship of the constrictor responses to blood pressure revealed significant correlations with ET-1–induced effects, whereas there was no correlation with phenylephrine-induced vasoconstriction in any of

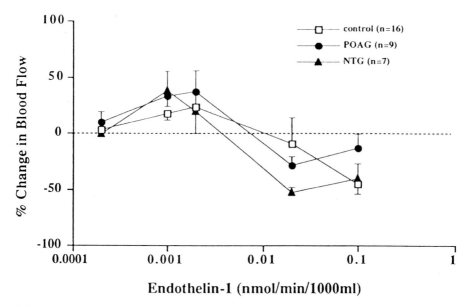

FIG. 2. Dose–response curves in the cutaneous microcirculation to intra-arterially administered endothelin-1 in 16 patients with glaucoma and 16 healthy age- and sex-matched controls. At lower dose rates, endothelin-1 induced vasodilatation, and at higher dose rates vasoconstriction.

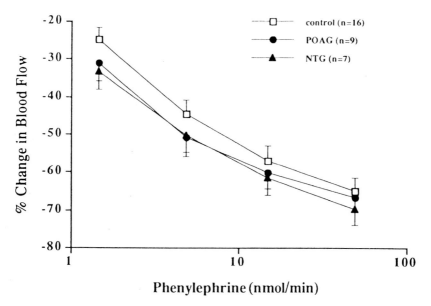

FIG. 3. Dose–response curves in the cutaneous microcirculation to intra-arterially administered phenylephrine in 16 patients with glaucoma and 16 healthy age- and sex-matched controls.

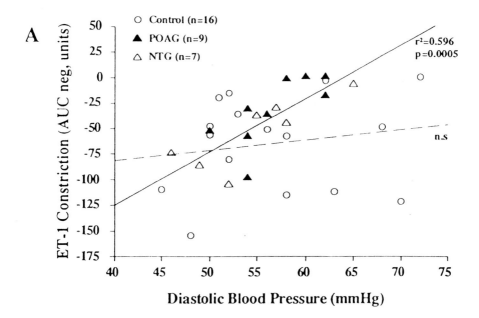

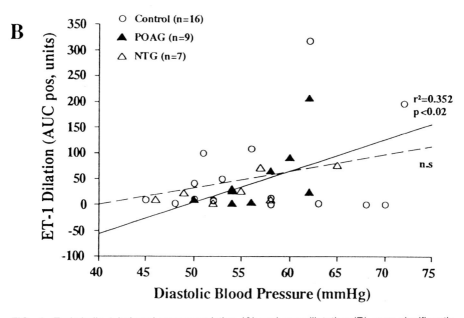

FIG. 4. Endothelin-1 induced vasoconstriction (**A**) and vasodilatation (**B**) were significantly correlated with resting blood pressure values in patients with glaucoma, whereas there was no correlation in the 16 healthy age- and sex-matched controls (○).

the groups. To account for the biphasic shape of the curve, ET-1 effects were expressed as absolute effect values or in area under the curve (AUC) values. In glaucoma patients, all these responses were correlated with diastolic and systolic blood pressure values that were measured intra-arterially, immediately before administration of vasoconstrictors (Fig. 4). Moreover, when individual AUCs were divided into a positive area (representing vasodilatation) and a negative area (vasoconstriction), the correlation was still present (Fig. 4). In contrast, there was no correlation between ET-1 responses and blood pressure in the control group (Fig. 4).

DISCUSSION

The results of this study are remarkable with respect to the relationship between intra-arterial blood pressure and ET-1 responses in the cutaneous microcirculation of the human forearm in glaucoma patients, which was not found in controls. A relationship between venous ET-1 responses and blood pressure has previously been described in patients with arterial hypertension and in controls (26). Interestingly, in this previous study in which the constrictor effects of ET-1 were measured in superficial hand veins, the slopes of the regression curves were opposite in patients and controls. With increasing mean arterial pressure values the constrictor effect of ET-1 increased, whereas in healthy controls the opposite was the case, and in the subjects with the lowest blood pressure values ET-1 was more efficacious. In our study evaluating ET-1 effects in the microcirculation no such correlation was found in healthy controls, although they had mean blood pressure values similar to those of glaucoma patients. In contrast, the correlation found in glaucoma patients was comparable to the relationship observed in healthy controls in the study by Haynes and co-workers (28). Several mechanisms can potentially modulate the vasoconstrictor responses of ET-1.

First, increases in local ET-1 release may reduce endothelin binding sites and/or downregulate ET-1 receptors (10), which may ultimately result in reduced responses to ET-1. To date there is no published evidence that changes in blood pressure may modulate local ET formation. In contrast, in several studies in patients with vasospastic syndromes, elevated plasma ET concentrations at rest (16,46,48,54) and after stimulation (54) have been found, suggesting that ET is somewhat enhanced, particularly in patients with lower blood pressure values (i.e., normal-tension glaucoma patients).

Second, chronic changes in NO production have been shown to modulate the expression and sensitivity of ET receptors to the agonist (41). Stimulation of NO and cGMP formation by various agonists resulted in a stimulation of the expression of ET_A receptors in vascular smooth-muscle cells and in increased vasoconstrictor responses to ET-1 in rat mesenteric arteries. Thus far there is no published evidence for increased production of NO in glaucoma patients, and other patients with peripheral vasospasm (Raynaud) have been shown to have a blunted response to bradykinin-induced venodilatation (3), which is mediated to a significant extent via NO (45).

Third, reduced production of endothelium-derived vasodilators (e.g., NO, prostacyclin) could also enhance the vasoconstrictor effects of ET-1. Although some authors found blunted NO effects (after stimulation with acetylcholine) with increasing blood pressure (35), such a relationship has been questioned by others (11). The effect of blood pressure on *baseline* NO production is still not entirely clear. On the other hand, indirect evidence suggests that, at least in superficial veins, prostacyclin potently modulates ET-1-induced constriction and that blockade of prostacyclin production with acetylsalicylic acid potentiates ET-induced venoconstriction (27).

Fourth, ET-1 may modulate the effect of α-adrenoceptor agonists (52), and ET responses are modulated by the sympathetic nervous system (26). The latter could be the cause for the inverse relationship between ET-1 venoconstriction and arterial blood pressure in hypertensive patients. The pattern observed in glaucoma patients more closely resembled the relationship observed in healthy controls (26), in whom those with the lowest blood pressure values had the profoundest venoconstriction. It can therefore be speculated that, in patients with glaucoma, lower blood pressure values result in higher activity of the sympathetic nervous system, which has not been evaluated thus far. However, microneurographic studies in patients with Raynaud's phenomenon revealed no evidence for increased sympathetic outflow (15).

In summary, ET-1-mediated microcirculatory effects in the human forearm of glaucoma patients are related to intra-arterial blood pressure values, whereas no correlation was found in a carefully matched control group of healthy subjects. The reason for these differences in ET-1 responses could reflect differences in ET receptor expression or sensitivity, differences in the release of counteracting vasodilators (e.g., prostacyclin), or differences in the activity of the sympathetic nervous system.

REFERENCES

1. Aellig W. Clinical pharmacology, physiology and pathophysiology of superficial veins-1. *Br J Clin Pharmacol* 1994;38:181-96.
2. Aellig W. Clinical pharmacology, physiology and pathophysiology of superficial veins-2. *Br J Clin Pharmacol* 1994;38:289-305.
3. Bedarida GV, Kim D, Blaschke TF, Hoffman BB. Venodilation in Raynaud's disease. *Lancet* 1993;342:1451-4.
4. Benjamin N, Calver A, Collier J, Robinson B, Vallance P, Webb D. Measuring forearm blood flow and interpreting the responses to drugs and mediators. *Hypertension* 1995;25:918-23.
5. Bill A. Some aspects of the ocular circulation. *Invest Ophthalmol Vis Sci* 1985;26:410-24.
6. Bircher A, de Boer EM, Agner T, Wahlberg JE, Serup J. Guidelines for measurement of cutaneous blood flow by laser Doppler flowmetry. A report from the Standardization Group of the European Society of Contact Dermatitis. *Contact Dermatitis* 1994;30:65-72.
7. Cartwright MJ, Grajewski AL, Friedberg ML, Anderson DR, Richards DW. Immune-related disease and normal-tension glaucoma. *Arch Ophthalmol* 1992;110:500-2.
8. Chauhan A, Mullins PA, Taylor G, Petch MC, Schofield PM. Both endothelium-dependent and

endothelium-independent function is impaired in patients with angina pectoris and normal coronary angiograms. *Eur Heart J* 1997;18:60–8.

 9. Cioffi GA, Orgül S, Onda E, Bacon DR, Van Buskirk EM. An in vivo model of chronic optic nerve ischemia: the dose-dependent effects of endothelin-1 on the optic nerve microvasculature. *Curr Eye Res* 1995;14:1147–53.

10. Clozel M, Löffler B-M, Breu V, Hilfiger L, Maire J-P, Butscha B. Downregulation of endothelin receptors by autocrine production of endothelin-1. *Am J Physiol* 1993;265:C188–92.

11. Cockcroft JR, Chowiencyk PJ, Benjamin N, Ritter JM. Preserved endothelium-dependent vasodilation in patients with essential hypertension. *N Engl J Med* 1994;330:1036–40.

12. Demailly P, Cambien F, Plouin PF, Baron P, Chevallier B. Do patients with low tension glaucoma have particular cardiovascular characteristics? *Ophthalmologica* 1984;188:65–75.

13. Drance SM, Douglas GR, Wijsman K, Schulzer M, Britton RJ. Response of blood flow to warm and cold in normal and low-tension glaucoma patients. *Am J Ophthalmol* 1988;105:35–9.

14. Drance SM, Sweeney VP, Morgan RW, Feldman F. Studies of factors involved in the production of low tension glaucoma. *Arch Ophthalmol* 1973;89:457–65.

15. Fagius J, Blumberg H. Sympathetic outflow to the hand in patients with Raynaud's phenomenon. *Cardiovasc Res* 1985;19:249–53.

16. Färkkilä M, Palo J, Saijonmaa O, Fyhrquist F. Raised plasma endothelin during acute migraine attack. *Cephalalgia* 1992;12:383–4.

17. Gass A, Flammer J, Linder L, Romerio SC, Gasser P, Haefeli WE. Inverse correlation between endothelin-1-induced vasoconstriction and blood pressure in glaucoma patients. *Graefes Arch Clin Exp Ophthalmol* 1997;235 (in press).

18. Gasser P, Flammer J. Influence of vasospasm on visual function. *Doc Ophthalmol* 1987;66:3–18.

19. Gasser P, Flammer J. Short- and long-term effect of nifedipine on the visual field in patients with presumed vasospasm. *J Int Med Res* 1990;18:334–9.

20. Gasser P, Flammer J. Blood-cell velocity in the nailfold capillaries of patients with normal-tension and high-tension glaucoma. *Am J Ophthalmol* 1991;111:585–8.

21. Greenfield ADM, Whitney RJ, Mowbray JF. Methods for the investigation of peripheral blood flow. *Br Med Bull* 1964;19:101–9.

22. Guthauser U, Flammer J, Mahler F. The relationship between digital and ocular vasospasm. *Graefes Arch Clin Exp Ophthalmol* 1988;226:224–6.

23. Haefeli WE. Assessment of peripheral vascular responsiveness in patients with glaucoma. In: Drance SM, ed. *Vascular risk factors and neuroprotection in glaucoma—update.* Amsterdam: Kugler Publications, 1996.

24. Haefliger IO, Flammer J, Lüscher TF. Nitric oxide and endothelin-1 are important regulators of human ophthalmic artery. *Invest Ophthalmol Vis Sci* 1992;33:2340–3.

25. Haefliger IO, Flammer J, Lüscher TF. Heterogeneity of endothelium-dependent regulation in ophthalmic and ciliary arteries. *Invest Ophthalmol Vis Sci* 1993;34:1722–30.

26. Haynes WG, Hand MF, Johnstone HA, Padfield PL, Webb DJ. Direct and sympathetically mediated venoconstriction in essential hypertension. *J Clin Invest* 1994;94:1359–64.

27. Haynes WG, Webb DJ. Endothelium-dependent modulation of responses to endothelin-1 in human veins. *Clin Sci* 1993;84:427–33.

28. Haynes WG, Webb DJ. Contribution of endogenous generation of endothelin-1 to basal vascular tone. *Lancet* 1994;344:852–4.

29. Hayreh SS, Zimmerman B, Podhajsky P, Alward WLM. Nocturnal arterial hypotension and its role in optic nerve head and ocular ischemic disorders. *Am J Ophthalmol* 1994;117:603–24.

30. Kaiser HJ, Flammer J, Burckhardt D. Silent myocardial ischemia in glaucoma patients. *Ophthalmologica* 1993;207:6–8.

31. Kaiser HJ, Flammer J, Graf T, Stümpfig D. Systemic blood pressure in glaucoma patients. *Graefes Arch Clin Exp Ophthalmol* 1993;231:677–80.

32. Kaiser HJ, Flammer J, Wenk M, Lüscher T. Endothelin-1 plasma levels in normal-tension glaucoma: abnormal response to postural changes. *Graefes Arch Clin Exp Ophthalmol* 1995;233:484–8.

33. Kilboom Å, Wennmalm Å. Endogenous prostaglandins as local regulators of blood flow in man: effect of indomethacin on reactive and functional hyperaemia. *J Physiol* (Lond) 1976;257:109–21.

34. Lance JW. Current concepts of migraine pathogenesis. *Neurology* 1993;43(suppl 3):S11–5.

35. Linder L, Kiowski W, Bühler FR, Lüscher TF. Indirect evidence for release of endothelium-derived relaxing factor in human forearm circulation in vivo. Blunted response in essential hypertension. *Circulation* 1990;81:1762–7.
36. Love MP, Haynes WG, Gray GA, Webb DJ, McMurray JJV. Vasodilator effects of endothelin-converting enzyme inhibition and endothelin ET_A receptor blockade in chronic heart failure patients treated with ACE inhibitors. *Circulation* 1996;94:2131–7.
37. Meyer P, Flammer J, Lüscher TF. Endothelium-dependent regulation of the ophthalmic microcirculation in the perfused porcine eye: role of nitric oxide and endothelins. *Invest Ophthalmol Vis Sci* 1993;34:3614–21.
38. Miller D, Waters DD, Warnica W, Szlachcic J, Kreeft J, Théroux P. Is variant angina the coronary manifestation of a generalized vasospastic disorder? *N Engl J Med* 1981;304:763–6.
39. O'Keeffe ST, Tsapatsaris NP, Beetham WP. Increased prevalence of migraine and chest pain in patients with primary Raynaud disease. *Ann Intern Med* 1992;116:985–9.
40. Phelbs CD, Corbett JJ. Migraine and low-tension glaucoma. A case control study. *Invest Ophthalmol Vis Sci* 1985;26:1105–8.
41. Redmond EM, Cahill PA, Hodges R, Zhang S, Sitzmann JV. Regulation of endothelin receptors by nitric oxide in cultured rat vascular smooth muscle cells. *J Cell Physiol* 1995;166:469–79.
42. Silberstein SD. Advances in understanding the pathophysiology of headache. *Neurology* 1992;42(Suppl 2):6–10.
43. Skyhoj-Olsen T, Friberg L, Lassen NA. Ischemia may be the primary cause of the neurologic deficits in classic migraine. *Arch Neurol* 1987;44:156–61.
44. Sorensen KE, Kristensen IB, Celermajer DS. Atherosclerosis in the human brachial artery. *J Am Coll Cardiol* 1997;29:318–22.
45. Strobel WM, Lüscher TF, Simper D, Linder L, Haefeli WE. Substance P in human hand veins in vivo: tolerance, efficacy, potency, and mechanism of venodilator action. *Clin Pharmacol Ther* 1996;60:435–43.
46. Sugiyama T, Moriya S, Oku H, Azuma I. Association of endothelin-1 with normal tension glaucoma: clinical and fundamental studies. *Surv Ophthalmol* 1995;39(Suppl 1):S49–56.
47. Thomsen LL, Iversen HK, Brinck TA, Olesen J. Arterial supersensitivity to nitric oxide (nitroglycerin) in migraine sufferers. *Cephalalgia* 1993;13:395–9.
48. Toyo-oka T, Aizawa T, Suzuki N, et al. Increased plasma level of endothelin-1 and coronary spasm induction in patients with vasospastic angina pectoris. *Circulation* 1991;83:476–83.
49. Vallance P, Collier J, Moncada S. Effects of endothelium-derived nitric oxide on peripheral arteriolar tone in man. *Lancet* 1989;2:997–1000.
50. Van der Ouderaa FJ, Buytenhek M, Nugteren DH, Van Dorp DA. Acetylation of prostaglandin endoperoxide synthetase with acetylsalicylic acid. *Eur J Biochem* 1980;109:1–8.
51. Vincent J, Blaschke TF, Hoffman BB. Vascular reactivity to phenylephrine and angiotensin II: comparison of direct venous and systemic vascular responses. *Clin Pharmacol Ther* 1992;51:68–75.
52. Yang Z, Richard V, von Segesser L, et al. Threshold concentrations of endothelin-1 potentiate contractions to norepinephrine and serotonin in human arteries. A new mechanism of vasospasm? *Circulation* 1990;82:188–95.
53. Zahavi I, Chagnac A, Hering R, Davidovich S, Kuritzky A. Prevalence of Raynaud's phenomenon in patients with migraine. *Arch Intern Med* 1984;144:742–4.
54. Zamora MR, O'Brien RF, Rutherford RB, Weil JV. Serum endothelin-1 concentrations and cold provocation in primary Raynaud's phenomenon. *Lancet* 1990;336:1144–7.

Nitric Oxide and Endothelin in the Pathogenesis of Glaucoma, edited by I. O. Haefliger and J. Flammer. Lippincott–Raven Publishers, Philadelphia © 1998.

11

Free Radicals in the Pathogenesis of Ocular Diseases

Harald Schempp and Erich F. Elstner

Lehrstuhl für Phytopathologie, Technische Universität München, Weihenstephan, Germany

All organelles in aerobic cells are exposed to activated oxygen species and thus to oxygen stress. A well-balanced antioxidative strategy has been elaborated over billions of years in both plants and animals. This review discusses the basic reactions that are operant during oxidative stress situations in which certain pro-oxidative situations and antioxidative processes in ocular compartments occur.

For and understanding of the role of oxygen in certain ocular diseases, general mechanisms and rules of oxygen activation are first discussed.

OXYGEN ACTIVATION

Aerobic life started some 3.5 billion years ago. The precursors of our cyano-bacteria developed photosynthetic oxygen evolution at the expense of water by photosystem II, slowly rendering the atmosphere aerobic and thus making possible respiratory processes and the development of heterotrophic organisms.

Molecular oxygen is an unreactive molecule in the triplet ground state ($^3O_2$). It must be activated to react with atoms or molecules in the (''normal'') singlet ground state, thus circumventing spin-forbidden reactions. The most important reactions concerning this subject are briefly adressed below.

Homolytic and Heterolytic Reactions: How Are Free Radicals Created?

During heterolytic reactions (a), electron pairs are transferred, either utilizing or creating ions:

$$A - B \leftrightarrow A^+ + B^- \tag{a}$$

Homolytic reactions (b) extinguish or create radicals through the transfer of single electrons, represented as a dot:

$$A - B \leftrightarrow A^{\bullet} + B^{\bullet} \tag{b}$$

A radical is a compound containing an unpaired electron. There are stable and unstable radicals. Most free radicals are highly reactive and create new radicals, thus initiating chain reactions. This is especially true for lipids (unsaturated fatty acids) in membranes.

Mechanisms of Oxygen Activation

Light Reactions and Their Consequences: The Formation of Secondary Oxygen Radicals

Oxygen activation can be achieved by photodynamic reactions through pigments via activated states, where P represents a pigment (mostly aromatic or heterocyclic compounds) in its ground state and P* is its light-activated form:

$$P + light \rightarrow P^* \text{ (excitet pigment)}$$
$$P^* + O_2 \rightarrow {}^1O_2 + P \text{ (exciton transfer forming singlet oxygen)} \tag{I}$$

Reaction I represents a photodynamic reaction classified as Photodynamic Reaction Type II.

Singlet oxygen, in contrast to atmospheric oxygen, is not subject to the spin rule and reacts rapidly with most organic molecules (RH), especially at double bonds of unsaturated fatty acids, producing hydroperoxides:

$$RH + {}^1O_2 \rightarrow ROOH \tag{II}$$

Reaction II can also be catalyzed by lipoxygenases utilizing triplet ground state oxygen and peroxidizing unsaturated fatty acids, yielding conjugated diene hydroperoxides:

$$R-CH=CH-CH_2-CH=CH-R + {}^3O_2$$
$$\rightarrow R-CH_2(-OOH)-CH=CH-CH=CH-R \tag{IIa}$$

ROOH, in turn, can be reduced by single-electron donors (E^-) such as reduced transition metal ions (Fe^{2+} or Cu^+), semiquinones, heme- and nonheme proteins, isoalloxazines, or pteridines yielding alkoxyl ($RO^{\bullet}$) − radicals:

$$E^- + ROOH \rightarrow E^{\bullet} + RO^{\bullet} + OH^- \tag{III}$$

$$Fe^{2+} + ROOH \rightarrow Fe^{3+} + RO^{\bullet} + OH^- \text{ (Fenton reaction)} \tag{IIIa}$$

These $RO^{\bullet}$ radicals may react further, co-oxidizing other molecules (co-oxidative bleaching of carotenoids) or initiating chain reactions:

$$RO^{\bullet} + RH \rightarrow R^{\bullet} + ROH \tag{IV}$$

$$OH^{\bullet} + RH \rightarrow R^{\bullet} + H_2O \tag{IVa}$$

In analogy, the organic radical $R^{\bullet}$ can also be produced from unsaturated fatty acids by OH radicals or Fenton-type oxidants, thus starting the chain reaction of lipid peroxidation.

The organic radical $R^{\bullet}$ is able to add atmospheric oxygen ($^3O_2$ is a biradical), yielding peroxyl radicals, $ROO^{\bullet}$:

$$R^{\bullet} + O_2 \rightarrow ROO^{\bullet} \qquad\qquad (V)$$

$ROO^{\bullet}$, in turn, can initiate chain reactions analogous to alkoxyl radicals (reaction IV):

$$ROO^{\bullet} + RH \rightarrow ROOH + R^{\bullet} \qquad\qquad (VI)$$

Photodynamic reactions not involving physical transfer of excitation energy via $P*$ and $^1O_2$ but undergoing charge separation within the excitet pigment are called Photodynamic Reactions Type I:

$$P + light \rightarrow P*$$

$$P* \rightarrow {}_+P^- \text{ (charge separation)} \qquad\qquad (VII)$$

$${}_+P^- + O_2 \rightarrow {}_+P + O_2^{\bullet-} \text{ (superoxide formation)}$$

$_+P$ may represent the photo-oxidized (bleached) pigment, or an oxidant initiating co-oxidations which, in the presence of an appropriate electron donor, can be restored for the next cycle.

Photodynamic reactions type II can be converted into type I in the presence of an appropriate electron donor for the photoactivated pigment. Therefore, we must envisage mixed-type mechanisms, because a vast number of cellular components are assumed to act as potential electron donors. This has been shown for the artificial dye rose bengal, the complex quinoid compounds hypericin (an ingredient of the herb *Hypericum perforatum*), and the fungal toxin cercosporin. In ocular problems, riboflavin, heme derivatives, or tryptophan or its oxidation product, *N*-formyl kynurenin, and a vast number of drugs (69) may be of current interest as initiators of photodynamically induced or enhanced problems (cataract) (see below and refs. 25 and 26).

Reductive Oxygen Activation: The Formation of Primary Oxygen Radicals

In the presence of reductants (E_1) with sufficient affinity for oxygen and an appropriately negative redox potential (E_0' of the redox pair $O_2/O_2^{\bullet-} = -330$ mV), superoxide may be formed from atmospheric oxygen:

$$E_1^- + O_2 \rightarrow E_1^{\bullet} + O_2^{\bullet-} \text{ (superoxide formation)} \qquad\qquad (VIII)$$

Superoxide dismutates at neutral pH in aqueous media with a rate constant $k = 2 \times 10^5$ ($L \cdot mol^{-1} s^{-1}$), yielding hydrogen peroxide:

$$O_2^{\cdot -} + O_2^{\cdot -} + 2\ H^+ \rightarrow H_2O_2 + O_2 \text{ (dismutation)} \qquad \text{(IX)}$$

$$O_2^{\cdot -} + Fe^{3+} \rightarrow O_2 + Fe^{2+} \qquad \text{(IXa)}$$

Superoxide may reduce Fe^{3+}, yielding Fe^{2+} (IXa).

In analogy to reaction III, hydrogen peroxide can be monovalently reduced by the already mentioned electron donors (E^-), yielding the extremely reactive hydroxyl radical $OH^{\cdot}$:

$$H_2O_2 + E^- \rightarrow E^{\cdot} + OH^- + OH^{\cdot} \qquad \text{(X)}$$

$$H_2O_2 + Fe^{2+} \rightarrow Fe^{3+} + OH^- + OH^{\cdot} \text{ (Fenton reaction; see IIIa)} \qquad \text{(Xa)}$$

The combination of reaction IXa and Xa is called the Haber–Weiss reaction. $OH^{\cdot}$ has a very positive redox potential (close to $+2$ V) and a lifetime of approximately 1 μs, thus reacting close to the site of its generation and producing site-specific oxidative damage. The oxygen species $OH^{\cdot}$ is the major target of the antioxidative power of phenolics because, owing to its kinetic properties (see above), it is a reactive oxygen species and is not under the control of specific enzymes and/or detoxification chains (see below).

OXYGEN ACTIVATION IN DIFFERENT COMPARTMENTS OF CELLS

All compartments of cells possess enzymic and nonenzymic tools for oxygen activation, some only after exogenous initiation such as injury, infection, UV radiation, cold or heat treatment, or toxicity. Mechanisms of oxygen activation in different compartments of cells have recently been reviewed (25,28).

Mitochondria

Mitochondria represent an important site of oxygen activation, forming superoxide and its successors. Under stress conditions (intensive strain, such as active sports participation) or aging, an alternative pathway that does not include the cyanide-sensitive cytochrome c/a pathway may be induced.

Superoxide and peroxide are formed close to reaction complexes I and II, i.e., in the proximity of the ubiquinol–flavoprotein–nonheme–iron complex oxidizing NADH and/or in the neighborhood of cytochrome b. Cytochrome c peroxidase and Mn-SOD cooperatively appear to detoxify reactive oxygen species. Superoxide production may amount up to 2–5% of overall electron flow.

Microsomes

Microsomes are derived from the endoplasmic reticulum and represent an electron transport system that reductively activates the heme iron protein P_{450} at the expense of NAD(P)H via flavin-dependent reductases, nonheme iron ''redox-ins,'' and/or a b-type cytochrome. After induction by several intrinsic or xenobi-otic metabolites, this electron transport system may cause peroxidation by the overshoot phenomenon, damaging its own membrane lipids after cessation of its hydroxylating task. Several anticancer drugs (e.g., daunorubicin, adriamycin) and redox toxins have been shown to couple at these reductases, initiating redox cycling and thus production of reactive oxygen species (ROS).

Peroxisomes

Peroxisomes, unlike mitochondria, are compartments with a single unit mem-brane, containing xanthine oxidase as an $O_2^{\cdot-}$ and H_2O_2-producing enzyme in addition to glycolate oxidase and fatty acid β-oxidases as H_2O_2-producing en-zymes. High concentrations of catalase and peroxidase in addition to SOD are involved in detoxification of ROS. Inhibition of xanthine oxidase by agents such as allopurinol, or by certain flavonoids such as quercitin (25), may play a regula-tory role in this context.

Plasma Membranes

Plasma membranes contain NAD(P)H oxidases that are more or less specific for their electron acceptors, acting similar to diaphorases. Under certain circum-stances, these flavoproteins may be rendered auto-oxidizable, coupling to co-factors such as quiniones or cytochrome b, as shown for leukocyte activation and after hypersensitive responses in infected plants. Especially in the presence of auto-oxidizable acceptors such as certain quinones, superoxide and its deriva-tives are produced which may function as cellular messengers.

OXIDATIVE VASCULAR DAMAGE

Diseases of the vascular system and damage to organs by ROS, manifested as failure of function, have recently been excessively dealt with (60,73). In this context, the activity of leukocytes and therefore of nonspecific immunity are also associated with ROS production. Both negative and positive effects of ROS are associated with each other in the sense that, on the one hand, they can act as second messenger molecules but, on the other hand, can cause damage to the heart, kidneys, liver, pancreas, brain, eyes, and nervous system.

Today it appears beyond doubt that regulatory functions of ROS and the damage caused by ROS are closely associated and can only be differentiated or influenced by very carefully selected and specific manipulations. It is therefore not surprising that many workers regard this field as a ''cross-talk'' of oxidants and antioxidants, minutely regulated by a wealth of enzymes, hormones, cytokines, and small regulatory or antioxidative molecules (33). Some new perspectives have been added by the finding (2) that hypertonus is influenced by oxidative processes (stress) via the regulation of certain transcriptional factors such as vascular cell adhesion molecule-1 (VCAM-1), which regulates the recruitment of monocytes and thus (indirectly?) the growth of smooth-muscle cells in the blood vessels, which in turn is coupled to changes in vessel properties and arterial inflammatory processes.

REACTIVE OXYGEN SPECIES

Which Is the Finally Damaging Species, and Where?

Oxygen activation is biologically necessary (25,35). Of great importance, however, are the cellular compartment in which it occurs and the extent of activation.

In biochemical experiments, evaluation of an oxidative event or situation is always dependent on the model used and on the currently accepted theory. This is the basis of biochemistry and physiologic chemistry and also of classical academic medicine.

Local and/or organ-specific ischemia or hypoyxia followed by reperfusion constitutes a model for study of the generation of ROS and the damage caused by them. For example, focal cerebral ischemia in brain tissue leads to demonstrable formation of OH$^\bullet$ in the striatum of rats and appears to be responsible for the sensitivity of this brain region to hypoxia (46). Because of their relatively high reproducibility and their medical importance, these ischemia–reperfusion models have been intensively studied. Two extremely important points should be kept in mind, however. First, there are forms of ROS that are concerned with the regulation of intermediary metabolism and also with induction of immune responses. These processes are under metabolic control. Symptoms such as change in color, edema, or pain may be considered as warnings of potential loss of metabolic control and therefore of the need for medical intervention. Swelling of a tissue with visible rubor is also an antioxidative mechanism, because extravasation of blood plasma introduces albumin, an excellent antioxidant, into this region. Second, there are also ROS that escape metabolic control by intrinsic scavenger systems, and therefore inevitably cause tissue destruction (see below).

The first category comprises superoxide, hydrogen peroxide, organic peroxides (leukotreine and prostaglandin precursors) and also nitric oxide (NO; formerly called endothelium-derived relaxation factor, EDRF). The second category comprises diffusion-controlled reactions based on the extremely site-specific escape of strong oxidants of the OH$^{\bullet-}$ type from "solvent cages" (12,27,66,89).

The subcellular areas concern only a few nanometers because both site-specific production and destruction of neighboring molecules occur at an identical location. For at least three reasons these reactions are no longer under the control of the otherwise responsible regulators and antioxidative defense chains. First, these species react extremely rapidly with most biomolecules. Second, their localization is extremely limited because they can diffuse only very small distances. Finally, the most important scavenger enzymes, such as superoxide dismutases (SOD), catalase (CAT), and glutathione peroxidase(s) (GSH-POD) are ineffective because they are too slow. In the case of the hormone relaxin, for example, Li et al. (48) showed that in a strongly localized reaction, i.e., in the intimate neighborhood of an activating metal center, oxidation may occur that is no longer accessible to endogenous protective enzymes. Such oxidation may cause primary molecular damage, mostly to proteins or membrane lipids, which can be repaired by cooperatively working enzymic processes. These processes include proteases and lipases, which excise damaged amino or fatty acids, and reinstallation of de novo–synthesized molecules.

Aerobic cells cannot establish mechanisms for avoiding or eliminating such oxidative damage, for simple chemical reason. If molecules or atoms react with other molecules or atoms in a diffusion-controlled manner, i.e., with reaction constants faster than $k = 10^8$ L/mol/s (and this is true of OH radical-type oxidants), enzyme catalysis is not efficient because free diffusion of the reaction products, rather than thermodynamic or kinetic parameters, is rate-limited at the active sites. To control these reactions, only small Kamikaze-type molecules have a chance to interact with the final oxidant directly at the point of its formation, i.e., the "solvent cage." During this process, these small molecules act as single-electron donors. This reaction is followed either by destruction of the donor molecule or by its repair via secondary donors. Primary donors are mostly phenols such as tocopherol, ubiquinol, probucol, butylated derivatives of hydroxytoluene (BHT) or hydroxianisole (BHA), flavonoids, cumarins, purins, or tryptophane, to mention just a few. These primary donors are converted into more or less stable oxygen- or nitrogen-centered radicals in which phenoxyl radicals play an outstanding role. As secondary donors that "repair" the single-electron deficiency, ascorbic acid or glutathione may predominately operate. These, in turn, are repaired, at the expense of NAD(P)H, by their corresponding reductases. Repair is not always efficient. Therefore, most of these compounds must be continuously supplied with the food (vitamins).

This antioxidative system follows a certain "pecking order." By repairing the primary damage, it thus helps to avoid visible or measurable secondary damage that takes the form of disease symptoms (11,20).

Natural antioxidants, such as those mentioned above, usually operate cumulatively and interdependently (32), but they can be individually characterized during their actions. We know today that only strongly electropositive solvent cages (see below), with their functional crypto OH· (and at acidic pH under 4.8 also the perhydroxyl radical $HO_2^·$ ($O_2^{·-} + H^+ \leftrightarrow HO_2^·$; pKs = 4.8), can initiate lipid peroxidation (c.f. reactions IV–VI), and therefore membrane damage, when functional loss of compartmentalization occurs.

The following section summarizes the currently most widely accepted biochemical hypotheses concerning the primary oxidant in cell, organ, or blood vessel damage.

The beginning of the oxidative cascade (finally ending in loss of function and/ or tissue necrosis) is characterized by hypoxia (ischemia), extreme metabolic stress, extreme or chronic nutritional deficiency, loss of regulatory functions, or by injury or toxicity. These primary events cause enzyme induction (xanthine oxidase, NAD(P)H oxidases, NO synthase) that lead to formation of the abovementioned strong oxidants (51). In subsequent reactions, activation of leukocytes enhances this process via several pathways, including cytokines and calcium translocations into the cellular plasma compartment and thus via induction of other complex processes, such as the arachidonic acid cascade.

The balance between effective cellular extent of regulation and the velocity of the damage-evoking reaction cascade is finally determined by whether repair mechanisms govern the scenario or a progress of perturbation takes over (scheme 1).

Scheme 1: Repair or Progress of Damage?

Hypoxia or other effectors → oxygen activation → repair mechanisms (desirable) such as toxins or injury (infections) → oxygen activation → subsequent reactions under (OH˙) formation (not desirable)

It would therefore not be desirable to block the induction of necessary repair pathways by nonspecific scavengers. Similarly, administration of high doses of ascorbic acid after traumatic processes may enhance rather than reduce deleterious reaction sequences, thus supporting rather than delaying tissue necrotization. This is because of ascorbic acid's capacity to reduce Fe^{III+} or Cu^{2+}, forming the toxic Fe^{II+} or Cu^+. Likewise, enhanced iron administration may overwhelm the control of iron homeostasis, yielding an iron "overload," as is known from genetic diseases such as thalassemia or sideroblastic anemia (and others; see also below). This also holds true for alcohol- or diet-dependent secondary hemochromatoses, in which the formation of OH˙ radicals has been shown (40).

Which reactions have to be envisaged as main producers of strongly electropositive reacting substances as the OH˙-radical? The most important ones are summarized in Table 1.

TABLE 1. *Potential sources of OH radicals*

Reaction, source	Reference
Xanthine oxidase, Fenton-type oxidants	26
Activated leukocytes	26
NAD(P)H oxidases	61
Decay of peroxynitrite	66
Reaction of hypochlorite with superoxide	17, 18

For the first two reactions or sources, transition metal catalysis is required, but for the other three this is apparently not necessary. This observation has tremendous consequences for the evaluation and estimation of potential locations of OH˙ formation.

The Xanthine Oxidase System

Xanthine oxidase (XO, E.C.1.2.3.1.) is found in several cell types, such as endothelial cells, and is mostly present as xanthine dehydrogenase (XDH, "D-enzyme" oxidizing hypoxanthine, xanthine, or certain aldehydes via NAD reduction) (25). During certain stress reactions, however this D-enzyme is converted (e.g., protease-catalyzed; c.f. ref. 37) into xanthine oxidase ("O-enzyme") which reacts with the same electron donors but reduces oxygen instead of NAD^+, thus producing superoxide and hydrogen peroxide.

Impurities of or deliberately added iron ions create strong oxidants, which can be identified very sensitively via several appropriate methods (25). After reperfusion of hypoxic liver, XO penetrates the blood stream and finally reaches the alveolar capillary membranes, changing their tonus or inducing extravasation of plasma components (25,82).

The activity of XO (and also that of the closely related if not identical enzyme aldehyde oxidase, E.C.1.2.3.2.) (25) can be strongly up- or downregulated by other molecules, yielding extremely complicated and confusing situations. In the presence of the iron transport molecule ferritin and of catecholamines, the formation of OH˙ is strongly stimulated (3). Nitrogen monoxide (NO), which can be formed in all types of leukocytes and in endothelial cells from L-arginine catalyzed by the enzyme NO synthase (NOS; see below), presumably by binding to sulfhydryl centers, is able to inhibit XOD (37) but may also react extremely rapidly with superoxide formed by XO, thus forming the strongly oxidizing solvent cage {HO-NOO} (see below). There are indications that the interactions of XO and NOS may create a "common enemy" in toxicity induced by viral infections and efficiently treated with a combination of XO and NOS inhibitors and with antioxidants such as omega-3 fatty acids, vitamin E, nicotinamide, β-carotene and ascorbic acid, here acting as the reducing stabilizer for vitamin E.

The case becomes even more complicated with the knowledge that aldehyde oxidase (AO), in the presence of both iron ions and the ubiquitous adenosine diphosphate (ADP), generates oxidants of the OH˙ radical type, initiating lipid peroxidation and thus setting the scene for cellular necrosis (54). Through the oxidation of ethanol by alcohol dehydrogenase, which yields the substrate for AO (acetaldehyde), this process is inevitably connected with alcoholism.

This example clearly shows that coupling of more than one different processes is essential for necrosis and blood vessel damage, i.e., a primary initiator, such as ethanol (3), and the reductive liberation of iron from its transport molecules. This process also can be initiated by infections via bacterial proteases, which cause the liberation of iron from transferrin. This appears to dominate endothelial damage after infection with *Pseudomonas aeruginosa* (53). Experimentally, vascular endothelial cells can be damaged by infusion with modified hemoglobin molecules and subsequent activation of the cellular enzyme hemoxigenase, also via iron liberation (57). Another such process is the formation of a strong oxidant that is reactive enough to initiate lipid peroxidation. Finally, as a result of the latter step, the attack of biomolecules (sugars, unsaturated fatty acids, amino acids) by OH• radicals forms new radicals, thus initiating chain reactions that finally destroy tissues by necrotization.

Many natural antioxidants, such as certain flavonoids and cumarins and other phenolic compounds, interact only or exclusively at the final step, thus ameliorating the situation at the right place and at the right time and avoiding perturbation of biologic equilibrium.

Leukocytes

The last four mechanisms listed in Table 1 correspond to possibilities expressed in the plasma space as well as in the membranes of activated leukocytes (25,26).

For catalysis of the formation of OH• radicals, again both primary and secondary enzyme catalyses are necessary, in which both NAD(P)H oxidase complexes and peroxidases are responsible for the production of precursors of OH• formation. The NAD(P)H-oxidases primarily produce superoxide and hydrogen peroxide. The formation of OH• is a secondary effect dependent on the catalysis mainly of iron (Haber–Weiss, Fenton reaction; see reaction Xa), where the metal ion is essentially derived from storage or transport proteins or from hemoglobin (see above). Another principle of the production of strong oxidants is the oxidation of halides (X^-) with hydrogen peroxide by myeloperoxidase (MPO), producing hypohalides (OX^-; c.f. ref. 30). These, in turn, may be converted into OH• in the presence of superoxide or Fe^{II+}. MPO of neutrophils catalyzes the formation of hypochloric acid at the expense of hydrogen peroxide and chloride ion, while the eosinophile peroxidase (EPO; c.f. ref. 52) catalyzes an analogous reaction much more rapidly with bromide. Both types can utilize the pseudohalide rhodanide (SCN^-) as a substrate.

The sum of the above mentioned reactions can be stated as follows, where X^- stands for the halide (17,18):

$$H_2O_2 + X^- \rightarrow \text{MPO or EPO} \rightarrow HOX + OH^- \qquad (XI)$$

$$HOX + O_2^- \rightarrow OH^• + O_2 + X^- \qquad (XII)$$

$$HOX + Fe^{II+} \rightarrow OH^• + X^- + Fe^{III+} \qquad (XIII)$$

Reactions XII and XIII represent new reaction mechanisms unknown until very recently.

Interaction of NO and Superoxide: the Production of Peroxynitrite

Another principle for the generation of OH· is the decay of peroxynitrite, formed from NO (c.f. ref. 43) and superoxide according to the reaction:

$$NO + O_2^{\cdot -} \rightarrow ONOO^- \qquad (XIV)$$

Activated leukocytes (e.g., by lipoxin A_4, LXA_4) produce NO (which should actually be written NO· because it is a free radical, just like nitrogen dioxide, $NO_2^{\cdot}$) from the amino acid arginine catalyzed by the enzyme NO synthase (NOS; E.C.1.14.13.39) according to the generalized formula:

$$R(NH_2)C{=}NH + 1.5\ (NADPH + H^+) + 2\ O_2 \rightarrow$$
$$RC{=}O + NO^{\cdot} + 1.5\ NADP^+ + 2\ H_2O \qquad (XV)$$

It has been suggested that the first product of reaction XV might not be NO· but NO^-, which is subsequently converted to NO· by SOD (70). According to another very recent report, NOS not only produces NO but at low arginine concentrations also superoxide, possibly explaining why under certain conditions NO synthesis causes cellular damage and under other conditions does not (9,87).

Mechanisms of Damage by Peroxynitrite

Experiments with model reactions and inhibitors (13) demonstrated that only in the presence of both radicals, NO· and $O_2^{\cdot -}$ and through their interaction could damage of endothelial cells occur. Very similar results were obtained by Lamarque and Whittle (45), who showed that in the simultaneous presence of both NO donors, such as sodium nitroprusside, and superoxide generators, such as XO, gastric mucosal cells become damaged. Volk et al. (81) concluded that the strong inhibition of a model reaction by catalase indicates an interaction between NO and H_2O_2, which results in damage to liver endothelial cells.

A controversial but in some details similar observation was made by Mohsen et al. (55), who observed damage to cardiomyocytes by H_2O_2, which was prevented, however, in the presence of NO or catalase. Other authors (81) used several NO generators such as S-nitroso-N-acetyl-DL-penicillamin (SNAP), sodium nitroprusside, or 3-morpholinosydnonimine-N-ethylcarbamide (SIN-1), where SIN-1 produces simultaneously both NO and $O_2^{\cdot -}$. SIN-1 was also used by Inoue and Kawanishi (39). These authors concluded that the damage to calf thymus DNA, measured as the formation 8-hydroxy-deoxyguanosine (8-OHdG) by SIN-1, was due to the formation of an OH·-like oxidant. This strong oxidant, which is produced in a slightly acidic mileau ($\sim pK_a$ for ONOOH = 6.8), corresponds to the "free" OH· radical (66) formed according to:

$$ONOOH \rightarrow \{ONO^{\cdot}\ {}^{\cdot}OH\} \rightarrow NO_2^{\cdot} + OH^{\cdot} \qquad (XVI)$$

Even if the percentage of free OH˙ (relative to other generated radicals, as calculated by electron paramagnetic resonance, EPR) appears to be as little as 1–4% of total ONOOH (65), the effect may be again due to the site-specificity of the "cage" {ONO˙ ˙OH} and especially to the escaping OH˙ in immediate proximity to the locus of its formation.

Depending on the locus and chemical environment in direct proximity to the cage, this species can apparently act more or less as a toxin. This may explain why in certain models in which ROS are formed (activated leukocytes; xanthine oxidase and others), NO, which is present in arterial walls in a concentration of 100–400 nmol/L (56) increases toxicity, whereas in other models it acts similar to an antioxidant or protectant.

If Haber–Weiss (or Fenton-type) reactions are predominating, NO might act as an antioxidant by binding O_2^- and thus avoiding both the formation of hydrogen peroxide via dismutation and reduction of Fe^{III+} (see reaction IXa).

There are still other mechanisms that independently of OH˙, lead to an increase in vascular or neurologic pathogenesis. The first of these is the nonenzyme-catalyzed formation of vasoconstrictory F_2 isoprostanes from arachidonic acid (AA; ca. 10% of all unsaturated fatty acids in LDL are AA), via oxidation by ONOOH (formed from SIN-1) (56). This process might simultaneously lead to oxidative modification of LDL and thus induce atherogenic processes. The second is the SOD-catalyzed formation of the highly reactive nitronium ion ($O{=}N^+{=}O$) from peroxynitrite according to:

$$ONOO^- \cdots SOD{-}Cu^{2+} \rightarrow SOD{-}Cu^{1+}O^- \cdot \cdot O{=}N^+{=}O˙ \quad (XVII)$$

which is able to nitrify, e.g., tyrosine (Tyr) residues in proteins (5) and thus to compete with signal chains in which tyrosine phosphorylations have central regulatory functions (protein kinases):

$$SOD{-}Cu^{1+} \cdot \cdot O^- \cdot \cdot O{=}N^+{=}O + Tyr \rightarrow$$
$$SOD{-}Cu^{2+} + OH^- + NO_2{-}Tyr \quad (XVIII)$$

An excellent review of these extremely complex interactions between NO and ROS and their effects on vascular endothelia, especially with regard to regulatory processes, has been given by Marin and Rodriguez-Martinez (50).

GENERAL MECHANISMS OF OXYGEN DETOXIFICATION

Because activated oxygen is toxic, it must be continuously under strict control by integral detoxification processes, detoxificating enzymes, and organic antioxidants. One principal way to deal with oxygen toxicity is "avoidance," i.e., circumventing one- or two-electron–donating processes toward oxygen. This can be achieved by strong coupling of electron transport chains operating at the electronegative region of oxygen activation or by stoichiometric coupling of oxygen-activating processes with utilization of activated oxygen. Another possibility is the inhibition or inactivation of oxygen-activating processes or enzymes. This has been shown for XO, lipoxygenases, prostaglandin cyclase, NAD(P)H oxidases, and other enzymes by a wealth of compounds used in medicine. The so-called nonsteroidal anti-inflammatory drugs (NSAIDs) and several flavonoids are good examples of this principle.

Integral Detoxification Processes

Integral detoxification processes connect elementary reactions of intermediary metabolism with detoxification of ROS or their derivatives. This can be achieved by activation of enzymes or induction of isoenzymes, such as peroxidases, DT-diaphorase, or members of the P_{450}-group, by coupling of peroxide utilization with NADPH oxidation via ascorbate or glutathione peroxidases, or by the "peroxidized-membrane repair team," including phosoplipase(s) and glutathione peroxidases, thus in concert opening membrane positions of peroxidized fatty acids to renewal activity. Phenolic compounds play an important role in this context, acting as antioxidants, inducers of enzymes, and co-factors for regulation of enzymic activities.

Detoxification therefore, in a wider sense, also concerns the replacement of damaged molecules such as DNA, proteins, and membrane lipids by a complex "crew" of integrated repair enzymes and replacement processes. A continuous involvement of these repair processes, however, would render them inactive, because they also continuously function as targets for these reactive oxidants. Therefore, another batch of first-aid molecules, such as phenolics, is biologically more than logical. The only "help" for the final repair teams are small molecules with "Kamikaze-type" virtues, representing antioxidants with or without a chance to be metabolically "repaired" themselves. A review on screening for such compounds for pharmacologic purposes has recently appeared (11).

Detoxifying Enzymes

As already mentioned, detoxification by enzymic processes is only possible if the reaction constant of the oxygen species under question is reasonably low under physiologic conditions so that the enzymic reaction allows at least one k-order of magnitude between the reaction under enzyme catalysis and the noncatalyzed spontaneous reaction between the oxygen species and any reaction partner in its "molecular" neighborhood. Therefore, the reactions of OH˙, $^1O_2$, RO˙, ROO˙, and HOO˙ are not under enzymic control. Their reaction constants with potential reaction partners in their typical "environments" are too rapid (generally $k \geqslant 10^8$) for enzyme catalysis. Therefore, the reactions of biomolecules with these oxygen species have to be "mended" after their reaction, i.e., damage.

In order not to "flood" these repair processes, the above-mentioned antioxidative molecules serve as scavengers and quenchers of activated states.

Enzyme-catalyzed detoxification mainly concerns superoxide, peroxides and epoxides (produced by P_{450} activity) as more or less "stable" reduced oxygen species. In most aerobic cells, catalase (CAT), SODs, ascorbate peroxidase, mono- or dehydro-ascorbate reductases, glutathione peroxidase(s) (GSH-POD), glutathione reductase, and different peroxidases (PODs) either individually or cooperatively remove stable reactive oxygen species. Different individual physiologic parameters or "stresses" may induce different enzymes.

Superoxide dismutases (SODs), containing copper–zinc, manganese, or iron in their active centers, catalyze reaction XIX and, under physiologic conditions, accelerate the spontaneous reaction by a factor of 10^4, thus removing superoxide from corresponding equilibria;

$$O_2^{\cdot-} + O_2^{\cdot-} + 2 H^+ \rightarrow H_2O_2 + O_2 \text{ (see reaction IX)} \qquad \text{(XIX)}$$

Catalases are heme–iron proteins and disproportionate hydrogen peroxide–forming oxygen and water.

$$2 H_2O_2 \rightarrow 2 H_2O + O_2 \qquad \text{(XX)}$$

Peroxidases are also heme–iron proteins, catalyzing H_2O_2-dependent oxidation of a wide spectrum of substrates (SH_2), such as phenolics (guaiacol), according to:

$$SH_2 + H_2O_2 \rightarrow S + 2 H_2O \qquad \text{(XXI)}$$

Glutathione peroxidases (GSH-POD) are mainly selenoenzymes (GSH-POD I) and utilize both organic (GSH-POD II; Se-independent, identical to GSH-S-transferase) and inorganic peroxide for glutathione (GSH) oxidation, forming the corresponding disulfide, GSSG (reaction XXII). The function of glutathione reductases is to couple peroxide detoxification to intermediary redox metabolism utilizing NADPH (mostly derived from oxidative pentose phosphate cycle), thus re-reducing oxidized glutathione, GSSG (XXIII):

$$2 GSH + H_2O_2 \rightarrow GSSG + 2 H_2O \qquad \text{(XXII)}$$

$$GSSG + NADPH + H^+ \rightarrow 2 GSH + NADP^+ \qquad \text{(XXIII)}$$

In summary, superoxide and peroxides, as ubiquitous oxygen metabolites, are under control of efficient enzyme catalysis in which metabolic reductants (NADPH, GSH, ascorbate) serve as electron donors, cooperating with low molecular weight antioxidants specific for their corresponding compartments.

Antioxidants

Under stress conditions in which metabolic control is critical or lost (e.g., infections, partial loss of compartmentalization), more complex repair processes are required. In these cases, low molecular weight antioxidants are of great importance, serving as two-electron redox shuttles (o-diphenols → o-quinones), as free radical scavengers (phenol → phenoxy radical), or as transition metal chelators (phenolic acids, flavonoids, and others). In this case the critical determination of whether pro- or antioxidative properties are expressed largely depends on local concentrations and metabolic balances, such as the individual reduction charge in the compartment or the availability of free transition metals. This experimental field is especially subject to experimental artifacts. A "Handbook of Antioxidants" has been published recently (16).

ROS IN DIFFERENT COMPARTMENTS OF THE EYE

Oxyradicals are involved in various ophthalmic diseases such as ischemia–reperfusion injury, uveitis, diabetic retinopathy, cataract, and generally light damage (77). In the following section the different compartments of the eye are discussed with regard to the production and detoxification of ROS and their involvement in pathogenesis. However, it should be noted that ROS production in one compartment may have a dramatic impact on disease development at another place quite distant from the original ROS generation. Retinal lipid peroxidation initiated by uveitis is only one example (34,67,86). There is no detailed discussion of the basics of biochemistry in these compartments because this has recently been exhaustively dealt with by Berman (7) in a book that is a "must" for all interested researchers in this field.

Cornea

The cornea consists of three main layers, i.e., epithelium, stroma, and endothelium. Each layer comprises a more or less complex cellular and chemical structure.

Oxidative metabolism (glycolysis connected with mitochondrial tricarboxylic acid cycle and coupled oxidative phosphorylation) provides the energy requirements necessary for regenerative (healing) and metabolic (transport) functions. Oxygen penetration into the epithelium is calculated at a rate of 3–4 μl cm^{-2}/h (7). Production of ROS in this compartment is mostly due to photodynamic processes (see reactions I–VII) or as mitochondrial byproducts. Detoxification is caused by the presence of CAT, GSH-POD, and SOD (see reactions XI–XV and references in ref. 7). Cu–Zn–SOD is mainly localized in the basal and intermediate epithelial cells but not in the superficial ones. Unlike its function in the lens, corneal SOD is not continuously inactivated with age. A wealth of data concerning ROS production and detoxification in the endothelium has accumulated over the past 20 years. ROS, and therefore predominantly H_2O_2, are responsible for corneal swelling. Detoxification of peroxide appears to be mainly due to GSH-POD activity, and formation of H_2O_2 is mainly based on ascorbate oxidation in the immediate neighborhood (aqueous humor, AH) by a reaction that must be catalyzed by transition metals, for which Cu^{2+} is the most potent candidate. The balance between GSH and ascorbate–Cu^{2+} concentrations appears to govern the corresponding equilibrium. Photokeratitis caused by ultraviolet (UV-B) radiation results from necrosis of corneal epithelial cells. There appears to exist a threshold of acute exposure to this radiation. Even subthreshold exposure has recently been shown to produce hydrogen peroxide. Using dichlorofluorescein as a hydrogen peroxide–sensitive fluoroprobe and microfluorography equipment, Shimmura et al. (72) showed that low-dose UV-B (10 mJ cm^{-2} UV-B total) induced oxidative changes equivalent to 240 μM hydrogen peroxide. These changes were ameliorated by the iron chelators deferoxamine and lactoferrin, as well as by catalase. Lactoferrin is present in the tear fluids in concentrations of up to 2.2 mg/ml, suggesting a protective role against Fenton-type oxidations initiated by UV radiation.

Aqueous Humor

H_2O_2 in the AH of healthy subjects and patients with cataract has been measured by Spector and Garner (7) and amounts to 24 and 69 μM, respectively. Ascorbate, however, is present in $\sim$1-mM concentrations and glutathione in 1–10 μM. Several amino acids, urate, albumin, and transferrin may also contribute to ROS detoxification. There are reports of XOD reactions in AH that seem to be responsible for leukocyte infiltration and activation via production of chemotactic factors from XOD-derived ROS and corresponding precursors. ROS formation in AH appears to be partially responsible for induction and/or enhancement of cataract formation.

Iris, Ciliary Body, and Trabecular Meshwork

This compartment is responsible for AH formation and several regulatory functions (vessel tension) via prostaglandin and leukotriene production, cholinergic and adrenergic receptor functions, and drug metabolization. All of these processes produce ROS and can therefore also be strongly impaired by them. The ciliary body, in particular, appears to contain an inducible and very active P_{450} mono-oxygenase system (see above) and is therefore prone to ROS generation. The antioxidative capacity correspondingly is also very high in the ciliary body (SOD, CAT, and the Se-dependent GSH-POD-I). A second Se-independent GSH-POD-II is due to the activity of GSH-S-transferase and is particularly expressed in pigmented cells, whereas SOD, CAT, and GSH-POD-I are predominantly found in nonpigmented cells (references in ref. 7). Phagocytic activities of endothelial cells that line the TM appear to be of great importance, as well as ROS detoxification by TM via all mentioned enzymic pathways. Three SODs have been found in TM extracts: two Cu-Zn isoenzymes and Mn-SOD, which accounts for 10–20% of total SOD activity. The increase in methionine sulfoxide in TM proteins during aging is probably due to free radical processes, as has been shown for α_1-antiprotease in response to smoking and other protein-oxidizing processes. Oxidation of proteins also causes their aggregation, in which they form large complexes that might block their outflow into AH and thus (in the context of disturbed receptor properties as well as steroid and proteoglycan metabolism) can induce certain forms of glaucoma.

Primary open-angle glaucoma (POAG) was studied with enucleated pig eyes regarding the effects of elevated levels of H_2O_2 present in the AH (see above). Yan et al. (88) came to the conclusion that oxidative impacts facilitate volumetric washout (VW) and outflow facilities only under normal pressure but may increase the sensitivity of VW at elevated pressure. Peroxide exposure, in addition to directly affecting outflow properties, might also influence metabolic properties of trabecular cells in the context of hyaluronic acid metabolism and other components of connective tissues indirectly involved in VW (64). Likewise, destabilization of membranes by ROS and enhanced lipid peroxidation during acute attacks of glaucoma in cells of the drainage zone have been described by Kramorenko and Tsarevskii (44). This may become more important at advancing ages because SOD activity in TM cells significantly dropped with age, in contrast to that of CAT (21).

In epinephrine-induced glaucoma, lipid peroxidation and IOP can be regulated by "biologic antioxidants" (nature of the compound unclear) as mentioned by Alekseev et al. (1). In this context, it should be noted that TCDO (Ryoxon or Oxoferin), an inorganc chlorite complex, is able to attenuate epinephrine- and serotonin-induced blood vessel constriction by oxidizing these bioamines in a heme-catalyzed reaction (24,25,83). This may be of interest in association with the report of Pakalnis et al. (62), who investigated ocular oxygenation after vasoconstriction with phenylephrine, producing effects similar to those of epinephrine. The authors claim that hypoxia in neovascular glaucoma is induced by vasoconstriction. TCDO treatment therefore might possibly represent a new approach, not only in wound healing but also in glaucoma therapy. The report by Bojic et al. (10) addresses the possibility of hyperbaric oxygen treatment of glaucoma, indicating a positive effect especially for patients subjected to 30 sessions at 2 bars for 90 min each, after which the visual field was significantly increased. Because (cerebral?) oxygen deficiency appears to represent a general (causative) symptom in glaucoma (80), this situation might be at least partially overcome by topical treatment with oxygen-enriched water containing vitamine E and ubiquinone as antioxidants. Such an oxygen-enriched solvent (Aqua Nova; Aqua-Nova-Mannheim) has been shown to support oxygenation of solid tumors in the neck region, even when given orally (23).

Lens

Two types of cells are present in the lens: epithelial cells with high metabolic and transport activity and fiber cells with a high content of transparent cristallineproteins, which also appear to possess enzymic properties (dehydrogenases, proteases, lyases). High glutathione levels and active GSH metabolism protect against ROS toxicity and support detoxification of xenobiotics. ROS are either generated photodynamically by riboflavin or tryptophane (and its derivative, N-formyl kynurenine) or stem from ascorbate oxidation in AH, producing peroxide. Oxidation of essential SH groups in ATP-dependent ion translocator enzymes (pump-dependent K^+ fluxes) in epithelial cells (42) may initiate certain forms of cataract (references in refs. 7 and 26). Other types of cataract are induced by the hyperosmotic effects of sugars and sugar alcohols, such as sorbitol. Another mechanism may be seen in transition metal-catalyzed sugar oxidation, producing peroxides and modified proteins in analogy to ascorbate (diabetic situation). This process is also discussed in diabetic retinopathy, diabetic atherogenesis, diabetic neuropathy, and normal aging, in which the formation of AGEs (advanced glycation end products) is a characteristic phenomenon (14). Mechanisms of induction of cataract formation by different redox processes in the context of appropriate model reactions has recently been described by Schempp and Elstner (69).

As recently reviewed by Spector (76), irreversible protein modification in cataractous lenses is initiated in the epithelial layer by oxidative stress stemming both from peroxides (transition metal-dependent ascorbate oxidation) (31) in the AH and from photodynamic reactions. Initiation of cataract formation is extremely complex (23) and comprises a wealth of fields of influence ranging from genetic predisposition to environmental impacts such as smoking or exposure to smoky cooking fuel (71). There also appear to be correlations between cataract and atopic dermatitis, because in both diseases abnormalities in serum lipids (high levels) and decreased inducibility of leukocyte SOD are correlated. Most of these patients came from highly polluted environments (59). Lipid peroxidation under formation of diene conjugates, lipid hydroperoxides, and fluorescent products appears to be one dominating process in cataractogenesis (4).

Antioxidants play an important role in cataract development (74), although not visible at a nutritional (in serum plasma and red blood cells) level (49).

Vitreous

The main components of the vitreous are collagen, hyaluronic acid, and proteins, with little indication of active metabolism. Vitreous degeneration and therefore loss of its viscoelastic properties would result in loss of both mechanical and physiologic properties in surrounding tissues. Increased hydrogen peroxide, indicated by fluorophotometry using $2'$, $3'$-dichlorofluorescin has been studied in vivo (77) and was shown to be light-dependent. Increased hydrogen peroxide was detectable more than a week after light exposure of rabbit eyes at 1,800 lux for 24 h. Oxygen activation may occur through heme-catalyzed photodynamic reactions or through iron-catalyzed processes (Fenton chemistry) mediated by heme compounds and their degradation products derived from erythrocytes after blood influx after injury, or by blood vessel damage (hemorrhages in the retina) due to diabetes. Therefore, heme- or iron-mediated oxygen toxicity in vitro can be ameliorated by iron chelators, such as desferrioxamine, apo-transferrin, or the heme scavenger apo-hemopexin (38), for which protection of retinal pigment epithelial cells (RPEC) was reported.

Retina

The retina is an extremely complex structure. In its different structural elements, all of the above-mentioned mechanisms of oxygen activation and detoxification occur. Compared to other ocular compartments, lipid peroxidation in the retina due to the high concentrations of polyunsaturated fatty acids (PUFAs) in the photoreceptor membranes plays an outstanding role. Light-dependent retinal damage appears to be connected with duration, intensity, and wavelength of light exposure, where the accumulation of lipid peroxides can be measured (references in ref. 7). The photoreceptor rhodopsin itself may be the photodynamic agent that initiates ROS formation via the above-described mechanisms. Vitamin E (tocopherol) appears to play the dominant role in preventing lipid peroxidation, initiated either photodynamically or via transition metal catalysis (Haber–Weiss reaction). Ascorbic acid has been shown to quench the tocopheryl radical formed after tocopherol-mediated lipid protection (see above).

ROS produced via the cyclo-oxygenase pathway, on the other hand, may cause damage through oxidative stress-mediated vascular constriction and may initiate neovascularization in neonatal retinopathy (19). Prematurity is associated with well-known retinal problems resulting from lack of defenses against ROS (68). Part of this problem is undoubtedly due to accompanying lung disease and intraventricular hemorrhage requiring intense respiratory support, in which ischemia–reperfusion problems arise (41) and elevated levels of protoporphyrin IX add a high photodynamic risk (15). Although the neonatal CNS is relatively resistant to oxidative stress caused by physiologic responses such as cerebral vasoconstriction and reduction in ventilation (79), lack of selenium and therefore GSH-POD activity (together with vitamin E) may play an important role in neonatal retinopathy (63).

In addition to photodynamic- or iron-mediated initiation of retinal damage yet other mechanisms might be envisaged. Because it is known that in the retina both Müller glial cells and pigmented epithelial cells (RPECs) express NOS activity after corresponding stimulation by cytokines or lipopolysaccharide (LPS) (references in ref. 6), PON might work in such a way. Indeed, added synthetic PON in vitro induced concentration-dependent damage to RPECs (apoptosis), including tyrosine nitration. However, with RPECs expressing endogenous NO synthesis after stimulation, no nitration was observed, indicating that no PON was apparently formed under these conditions (6). In the case of retinal ischemia–reperfusion, however, NOS mRNA is expressed 12 h after reperfusion, especially in glial cells and in retina-infiltrating neutrophils (PMNs). Retinal damage, measured as electroretinogram (ERG) b-wave recovery, was ameliorated by N^G-1-iminoethyl)-L-ornithine (L-NIO), an inhibitor of NOS (36), indicating that under these conditions NO is involved in the formation of ROS. Therefore, one might speculate that only after PMN infiltration do superoxide and NO cooperate in HONOO production that initiates damage. Another condition that most likely initiates retinal damage by ROS is sustained activation of postsynaptic glutamate ionotropic receptors, such as the NMDA subtype, via Ca^{2+} influx, which causes LDH (lactate dehydrogenase) release from neuronal cells as an indicator of their impairment (22). In such retinal neurons, kainate-initiated ESR signals visualized in the presence of an appropriate spin-trap (DMPO) were abolished or ameliorated by the Ca chelator EGTA, the NOS antagonist nitro arginine, and the XOD antagonist oxopurinol.

Melanin, as the main "protective" pigment in the retinal pigmentary epithelium, appears to possess radical scavenging properties similar to those of synthetic 21-aminosteroids ("lazaroids" such as U74389G; Upjohn Co.), as shown for ischemia–reperfusion when pigmented and albino rabbit retinas were compared (58).

The synthesis in retina of endogenous antioxidants such as metallothionein and CAT appears to be initiated by H_2O_2 (or induced phagocytosis by RPECs) operating as a signal (78). Induction of CAT in retina of rats after ischemic periods has been recently reported by Lewden et al. (47). These inductive effects can be abrogated by addition of N-acetyl-cystein, a GSH precursor, indicating that GSH might be the dominating antioxidative principle. The efficiency of antioxidative systems in retinal tissues is well documented. It effectively protects mitochondrial DANN against oxidative damage (75) and appears to include novel proteins, counteracting neutrophil superoxide production without scavenging it or being cytotoxic. As reported by Wu et al. (86) and by Wu and Rao (84) a protein from retinal pigment epithelial cells with a protein doublet of 69/75 kDa exhibits some degree of similarity to the transferrin family. This protein blocks superoxide production by activated neutrophils, apparently acting directly on these white blood cells.

REFERENCES

1. Alekseev VN, Ketlinskii SA, Sharonov BP, Martynova EB, Lauta VF. Lipid peroxidation in experimental glaucoma and the possibilities for its correction (preliminary report). *Vestn Oftalmol* 1993;109:10–2.
2. Alexander RW. Hypertension and the pathogenesis of atherosclerosis—oxidative stress and the mediation of arterial inflammatory response: a new perspective. 1995;25:155–61.
3. Allen DR, Wallis GL, McCay PB. Catechol adrenergic agents enhance hydroxyl radical generation in xanthine oxidase systems containing ferritin: implications for ischemia/reperfusion. *Arch Biochem Biophys* 1994;315:235–43.

4. Babiszhayev MA, Costa EB. Lipid peroxide and reactive oxygen species generating systems of the crystalline lens. *Biochim Biophys Acta* 1994;1225:326–37.
5. Beckmann JS, Chen J, Crow JP, Ye YZ. Reactions of nitric oxide, superoxide and peroxynitrite with superoxide dismutase in neurodegeneration. In: Seil FJ, ed. *Progress in brain research.* Vol. 103. New York: Elsevier Science, 1994:371–80.
6. Behar-Cohen FF, Heydolph S, Faure V, Droy-Lefaix M-T, Courtois Y, Goureau O. Peroxynitrite cytotoxicity on bovine retinal pigmented epithelial cells in culture. *Biochem Biophys Res Commun* 1996;226:842–9.
7. Berman ER. *Biochemistry of the eye.* New York: Plenum Press, 1991.
8. Bing RJ. Introduction. *Int J Cardiol* 1995;50:203–5.
9. Böger RH, Bode-Böger SM, Mügge A, et al. Supplementation of hypercholesterolaemic rabbits with L-arginine reduces the vascular release of superoxide anions and restores NO production. *Artherosclerosis* 1995;117:273–84.
10. Bojic L, Kovacevic H, Andric D, Romanovic D, Petri NM. Hyperbaric oxygen dose of choice in the treatment of glaucoma. *Arh ööHig Rada Toksikol* 1993;44:239–47.
11. Bors W, Saran M, Elstner EF. Screening for plant antioxidants. In: Linskensd HF, Jackson JF, eds. *Plant toxin analysis.* Vol. 13. *Modern methods of plant analysis.* Berlin: Springer Verlag, 1992.
12. Bors W, Saran M, Tait D, eds. *Oxygen radicals in chemistry and biology.* Berlin: Walter de Gruyter Verlag, 1984.
13. Bratt J, Gyllenhammar H. The role of nitric oxide in lipoxin A₄-induced polymorphonuclear neutrophil-dependent cytotoxicity to human vascular endothelium in vitro. *Arthritis Rheum* 1995;38:768–76.
14. Brownlee M. Advanced protein glycosylation in diabetes and aging. *Annu Rev Med* 1995;46:223–34.
15. Bynoe LA, Gottsch JD, Sadda SR, Panton RW, Haller EM, Gleason CA. An elevated hematogenous photosensitizer in the preterm neonate. *Invest Ophthalmol Vis Sci* 1993;34:2878–80.
16. Cadenas E, Packer L, eds. *Handbook of antioxidants.* New York: Marcel Dekker, 1996.
17. Candeias LP, Patel KB, Stratford MRL, Wardman P. Free hydroxyl radicals are formed on reaction between the neutrophil-derived species superoxide anion and hypochlorous acid. *FEBS Lett* 1995;333:151–3.
18. Candeias LP, Stratford MRL, Wardman P. Formation of hydroxyl radicals on reaction of hypochlorous acid with ferrocyanide, a model iron (II) complex. *Free Rad Res* 1994;20:241–9.
19. Chemtob S, Hardy P, Abran D, et al. Peroxide-cyclooxygenase interactions in postasphyxial changes in retinal and choroidal hemodynamics. *J Appl Physiol* 1995;78:2039–46.
20. Davies KJA. Protein modification by oxidants and the role of proteolytic enzymes. *Biochem Soc Trans* 1993;21:346–53.
21. De La Paz MA, Epstein DL. Effect of age on superoxide dismutase activity of human trabecular meshwork. *Invest Ophthalmol Vis Sci* 1996;37:1849–53.
22. Dutrait N, Culcas M, Cazevieille Ch, et al. Calcium-dependent free radical generation in cultured retinal neurons injured by kainate. *Neurosci Lett* 1995;198:13–6.
23. Eble MJ, Lohr F, Wannenmacher M. Oxygen tension distribution in head and neck carcinomas after peroral oxygen therapy. *Onkologie* 1995;18:136–40.
24. Elstner EF. Hämaktivierte Oxidationen mit dem Chlorit-Sauerstoff-Komplex "TCDO" (OXOFERIN®)—eine Übersicht. *Z Naturforsch* 1988;43c:893–902.
25. Elstner EF. *Der Sauerstoff. Biochemie, Biologie, Medizin.* Mannheim, Wien, Zürich: BI Wissenschaftsverlag, 1990.
26. Elstner EF. *Sauerstoffabhängige Erkrankungen und Therapien.* Mannheim: BI Wissenschaftsverlag, 1993.
27. Elstner EF, Bors W, Wilmanns W, eds. *Reaktive Sauerstoffspezies in der Medizin. Grundlagen und Klinik.* Berlin: Springer-Verlag, 1987.
28. Elstner EF, Schempp H, Preibisch G, Hippeli S, Osswald W. Biological sources of free radicals. In: Nohl H, Esterbauer H, Rice-Evans C, eds. *Free radicals in the evironment. Medicine and toxicology.* London: Richelieu Press, 1994:13–45.
29. Euler DE. Role of oxygen-derived free radicals in canine reperfusion arrhythmias. *Am J Physiol* 1995;37:H295–300.
30. Folkes LK, Candeias LP, Wardman P. Kinetics and mechanisms of hypochlorous acid reactions. *Arch Biochem Biophy* 1995;323:120–6.

31. Garland D, Russell P, Zigler JS. Jr. The oxidative modification of lens proteins. *Basic Life Sci* 1988;49:347–52.
32. Gaziano JM, Manson JE, Hennekens CH. Natural antioxidants and cardiovascular disease: observational epidemiologic studies and randomized trials. In: *Natural antioxidants in human health and disease.* San Diego: Academic Press, 1994:387–409.
33. Ginsburg I, Kohen R. Cell damage in inflammatory and infectious sites might involve a coordinated "cross-talk" among oxidants, microbial haemolysins and ampiphiles, cationic proteins, phospholipases, fatty acids, proteinases and cytokines (an overview). *Free Rad Res* 1995;22:489–517.
34. Goto H, Wu GS, Chen F, et al. Lipid peroxidation in experimental uveitis: sequential studies. *Curr Eye Res* 1992;11:489–99.
35. Halliwell B, Gutteridge JMC. *Free radicals in biology and medicine.* 2nd ed. Oxford: Clarendon Press, 1989.
36. Hangai M, Yoshimura N, Hiroi K, Mandai M, Honda Y. Inducible nitric oxide synthase in retinal ischemia-reperfusion injury. *Exp Eye Res* 1996;63:501–9.
37. Hassoun PM, Yu FS, Zulueta JJ, White AC, Lanzillo JJ. Effect of nitric oxide and cell redox status on the regulation of endothelial cell xanthine dehydrogenase. *Am J Physiol* 1995;268:L809–17.
38. Hunt RC, Handy I, Smith A. Heme-mediated reactive oxygen species toxicity to retinal pigment epithelial cells is reduced by hemopexin. *J Cell Physiol* 1996;168:81–6.
39. Inoue S, Kawanishi S. Oxidative DNA damage induced by simultaneous generation of nitric oxide and superoxide. *FEBS Lett* 1995;371:86–8.
40. Kadiiska MB, Burkitt MJ, Xiang Q-H, Mason RP. Iron supplementation generates hydroxyl radical in vivo. An ESR spin-trapping investigation. *J Clin Invest* 1995;96:1653–7.
41. Kelly FJ. Free radical disorders of preterm infants. *Br Med Bull* 1993;49:668–78.
42. Kise K, Kosaka H, Nakabayashi M, Kishida K, Shiga T, Tano Y. Reactive oxygen species involved in phenazine-methosulfate-induced rat lens opacification. An experimental model of cataract. *Ophthal Res* 1994;26:41–50.
43. Kostka P. Free radicals (nitric oxide). *Anal Chem* 1995;67:411R–6R.
44. Kramorenko IuS, Tsarevskii LP. Chemiluminescence and activity of acid phosphatase in the drainage zone of the eye in *glaucoma* patients. *Vestn Oftalmol* 1992;108:32–4.
45. Lamarque D, Whittle BJR. Involvement of superoxide and xanthine oxidase in neutrophil-independent rat gastric damage induced by NO donors. *Br J Pharmacol* 1995;116:1843–8.
46. Lancelot E, Callebert J, Revaud M-L, Boulu RG, Plotkine M. Detection of hydroxyl radicals in rat striatum during transient focal cerebral ischemia: possible implication in tissue damage. *Neurosci Lett* 1995;197:85–8.
47. Lewden O, Garcher C, Morales C, Javouhey A, Rochette L, Bron AM. Changes of catalase activity after ischemia-reperfusion in rat retina. *Ophthal Res* 1996;28:331–5.
48. Li S, Nguyen TH, Schöneich C, Borchardt RT. Aggregation and precipitation of human relaxin induced by metal-catalyzed oxidation. *Biochemistry* 1995;34:5762–72.
49. Libondi R, Costagliola C, Della-Corte M, et al. Cataract risk factors: blood level of antioxidative vitamins, reduced glutathione and malondialdehyde in cataractous patients. *Metab Pediatr Syst Ophthalmol* 1991;14:31–6.
50. Marin J, Rodriguez-Martinez MA. Nitric oxide, oxygen-derived free radicals and vascular endothelium. *J Auton Pharmacol* 1995;15:279–307.
51. Martínez-Cayuela M. Oxygen free radicals and human disease: *Biochimie* 1995;77:147–61.
52. McCormick ML, Roeder TL, Railsback MA, Britigan BE. Eosinophil peroxidase-dependent hydroxyl radical generation by human eosinophils. *J Biol Chem* 1994;269:27914–9.
53. Miller RA, Britigan BE. Protease-cleaved iron-transferrin augments oxidant-mediated endothelial cell injury via hydroxyl radical formation. *J Clin Invest* 1995;95:2491–500.
54. Mira L, Maia L, Barreira L, Manso DV. Evidence for free radical generation due to NADH oxidation by aldehyde oxidase during ethanol metabolism. *Arch Biochem Biophys* 1995;318:53–8.
55. Mohsen M, Pinson A, Zhang R, Samuni A. Do nitroxides protect cardiomyocytes from hydrogen peroxide or superoxide? *Mol Cell Biochem* 1995;145:103–10.
56. Moore KP, Darley-Usmar V, Morrow J, Roberts LJ. II. Formation of F_2-isopropantes during oxidation of human low-density lipoprotein and plasma by peroxynitrite. *Circ Res* 1995;77:335–41.

57. Motterlini R, Foresti R, Vandegriff K, Intaglietta M, Winslow RM. Oxidative-stress response in vascular endothelial cells exposed to acellular hemoglobin solutions. *Am J Physiol* 1995; 269:H648–55.

58. Muller A, Villain M, Favreau B, Sandillon F, Privat A, Bonne C. Differential effect of ischemia/reperfusion on pigmented and albino rabbit retina. *J Ocul Pharmacol Ther* 1996;12:337–42.

59. Niwa Y, Iizawa O. Abnormalities in serum lipids and leukocyte superoxide dismutase and associated cataract formation in patients with atopic dermatitis. *Arch Dermatol* 1994;130:1387–92.

60. Nohl H, Esterbauer H, Ricce-Evans C, eds. *Free radicals in the environment, medicine and toxicology: Critical aspects and current highlights.* London: Richelieu Press, 1994.

61. Pagano PJ, Ito Y, Tornheim K, Gallop PM, Tauber AI, Cohen RC. An NADPH oxidase superoxide-generating system in the rabbit aorta. *Am J Physiol* 1995;268:H2274–80.

62. Pakalnis VA, Wolbarsht ML, Landers MB III. Ocular oxygenation: the effect of phenylephrine on anterior chamber oxygen tension. *Adv Exp Med Biol* 1986;200:233–41.

63. Papp A, Nemeth I, Pelle Z. Retrospective biochemical study of the preventive property of antioxidants in retinopathy of prematurity. *Orv Hetil* 1993;134:1021–6.

64. Polanski JR, Wood IS, Maglio MT, Alvarado JA. Trabecular meshwork cell culture in *glaucoma* research: evaluation of biological activity and structural properties of human trabecular cells in vitro. *Ophthalmology* 1984;91:580–95.

65. Pou S, Nguyen SY, Gladwell T, Rosen GM. Does peroxynitrite generate hydroxyl radical? *Biochim Biophys Acta* 1995;244:62–8.

66. Pryor WA, Squadrito GL. The chemistry of peroxynitrite: a product from the reaction of nitric oxide with superoxide. *Am J Physiol* 1995;268:L699–722.

67. Rao NA, Fernandez MA, Cid LL, Romero JL, Sevanian A. Retinal lipid peroxidation in experimental uveitis. *Arch Ophthalmol* 1987;105:1712–6.

68. Rao NA, Wu GS. Oxygen free radicals and retinopathy of prematurity [Editorial; comment]. *Br J Ophthalmol* 1996;80:387.

69. Schempp H, Elstner EF. Induction of cataract formation by redox processes. In: Eyer P, ed. *Metabolic aspects of cell toxicity.* Mannheim: BI Wissenschaftsverlag, 1994:31–50.

70. Schmidt HHHW, Hofmann H, Schindler U, Shutenko ZS, Cunningham DD, Feelisch M. No NO from No synthase. *Proc Natl Acad Sci USA* 1996;93:14492–7.

71. Shalini VK, Luthra M, Srinivas L, et al. Oxidative damage to the eye lens caused by cigarette smoke and fuel smoke condensates. *Indian J Biochem Biophys* 1994;31:261–6.

72. Shimmura S, Suematsu M, Shimoyama M, Tsubota K, Oguchi Y, Ishimura Y. Subthreshold UV radiation-induced peroxide formation in cultured corneal epithelial cells: the protective effects of lactoferrin. *Exp Eye Res* 1996;63:519–26.

73. Sies H. *Oxidative stress: oxidants and antioxidants.* London: Academic Press, 1991.

74. Sies H, Stahl W, Sundquist AR. Antioxidant functions of vitamins. Vitamins E and C, beta-carotene, and other carotenoids. *Ann NY Acad Sci* 1992;669:7–20.

75. Soong NW, Dang MH, Hinton DR, Arnheim N. Mitochondrial DNA deletions are rare in free radical-rich retinal environment. *Neurobiol Aging* 1996;17:827–31.

76. Spector A. Oxidative stress-induced cataract: mechanism of action. *FASEB J* 1995;9:1173–82.

77. Taguchi H, Ogura Y, Takanashi T, Hashizoe M, Honda Y. In vivo quantitation of peroxides in the vitreous humor by fluorophotometry. *Invest Ophthalmol Vis Sci* 1996;37:1444–50.

78. Tate DJ Jr, Miceli MV, Newsome DA. Phagocytosis and H_2O_2 induce catalase and metallothionein gene expression in human retinal pigment epithelial cells. *Invest Ophthalmol Vis Sci* 1995;36:1271–9.

79. Torbati D, Wafapoor H, Peyman GA. Hyperbaric oxygen tolerance in newborn mammals-hypothesis on mechanisms and outcome. *Free Rad Biol Med* 1993;14:695–703.

80. Troutneva KV, Zaretskaya RB. Cerebral cortex biopotential and blood oxygenation in glaucomatous patient. *J Fr Ophtalmol* 1979;2:629–31.

81. Volk T, Ioannidis I, Hensel M, deGroot H, Kox WJ. Endothelial damage induced by nitric oxide: synergism with reactive oxygen species. *Biochem Biophys Res Commun* 1995;213:196–203.

82. Weinbroum VG, Nielsen S, Tan S, et al. Liver ischemia-reperfusion increases pulmonary permeability in rat: role of circulating xanthine oxidase. *Am J Physiol* 1995;268:G988–96.

83. Wolin MS, Kleber E, Mohazzab KM, Elstner EF. Tetrachlorodecaoxygen, a wound healing

agent, produces vascular relaxation through hemoglobulin-dependent inactivation of serotonin and norepinephrine. *J Cardiovasc Pharmacol* 1994;23:664–8.

84. Wu GS, Rao NA. A novel retinal pigment epithelial protein suppresses neutrophil superoxide generation. I. Characterization of the suppressive factor. *Exp Eye Res* 1996;63:713–25.

85. Wu GS, Swiderik KM, Rao NA. A novel retinal pigment epithelial protein suppresses neutrophil superoxide generation. II. Purification and microsequencing analysis. *Exp Eye Res* 1996;63:727–37.

86. Wu GS, Walker J, Rao NA. Effect of deferoxamine on retinal lipid peroxidation in experimental uveitis. *Invest Ophthalmol Vis Sci* 1993;34:3084–9.

87. Xia Y, Dawson VL, Dawson TM, Snyder SH, Zweier JL. Nitric oxide synthase generates superoxide and nitric oxide in arginine-depleted cells leading to peroxynitrite-mediated cellular injury. *Proc Natl Acad Sci USA* 1996;93:6770–4.

88. Yan DB, Trope GE, Ethier CR, Menon IA, Wakeham A. Effects of hydrogen peroxide-induced oxidative damage on outflow facility and washout in pig eyes. *Invest Ophthalmol Vis Sci* 1991;32:2515–20.

89. Youngman RJ, Elstner EF. Oxygen species in paraquat toxicity: the crypto-OH radical. *FEBS Lett* 1981;129:265–8.

Nitric Oxide and Endothelin in the Pathogenesis of Glaucoma, edited by I. O. Haefliger and J. Flammer.
Lippincott–Raven Publishers, Philadelphia © 1998.

12

Distribution and Regulation of Optic Nerve Head Tissue PO$_2$

*Constantin J. Pournaras, †Evrydiki A. Bouzas, and *Guy Donati

*Department of Clinical Neurosciences, University Eye Department,
Geneva University Hospital, Geneva, Switzerland; and †Neuro-ophthalmology Unit,
Neurology Department, Athens University, Athens, Greece*

Glaucomatous optic neuropathy is a multifactorial disease. It is well known that, among others, vascular factors play a major role in its pathogenesis (1,2). Blood flow modifications and disturbances of the optic nerve head (ONH) autoregulatory mechanisms have been incriminated (3–5). Basic knowledge regarding the blood supply to the ONH and the various factors that control ONH blood flow contribute to the understanding of the vascular etiology of glaucomatous optic neuropathy (5).

The optic nerve, as part of the nervous system, has high oxygen consumption and high metabolic activity, both of which are required for the process of neuronal transport. Nutrition and oxygenation of the optic nerve depend on its blood flow. Blood flow can be calculated by the equation: blood flow = perfusion pressure/resistance to flow. At the ONH, the value of the perfusion pressure is given by the mean blood pressure minus the intraocular pressure (IOP). The resistance to the flow depends on the contractile state of the smooth muscle of the arterioles irrigating the ONH and, potentially, of the pericytes of the ONH capillary network (6). This contraction is regulated by multiple factors, including neurotransmitters, circulating vasoactive substances, local metabolic factors (partial pressure of O$_2$ and CO$_2$, pH, metabolic products), and endothelium-derived substances such as endothelin, nitric oxide (NO), and proteoglycans (PGs) (6,7). Autoregulatory mechanisms may ensure the constant supplementation of the ONH with oxygen and nutritional elements, despite the variation in parameters that influence the ONH blood flow.

Tissue partial pressure of O$_2$ (PO$_2$) measurements with microelectrodes represent a precise technique for the study of ONH oxygenation which, according to Fick's diffusion law, is closely related to the local ONH blood flow (8). Studies on oxygenation of the ONH include measurements made, using PO$_2$-sensitive microelectrodes, from the vitreous close to the ONH in cats (9,10) and monkeys (11), and in ONH tissue in cats (12) and minipigs (13,14). In addition, intravascular oxygen measurements from the ONH in cats were obtained using a phosphorescence method (15).

The autoregulatory capacities of the ONH circulation and the modifications of ONH tissue PO_2 during variation of local metabolic parameters, modifications of the perfusion pressure, and inhibition of endothelial NO release are discussed in this article.

TISSUE ONH PO₂ DISTRIBUTION

Systemic Normoxia

Measurements of the ONH tissue PO_2 were performed in anesthetized miniature pigs with double-barreled, recess-type, O_2-sensitive microelectrodes (16) mounted on an electronic micromanipulator (17) that allows smooth radial and angular movements within the eye, in front of the surface of the optic disc or at the desired depth for PO_2 recordings within the prelaminar region of the optic nerve head (18) (Fig. 1).

The PO_2 values in front of the optic disk were significantly higher close to the arterioles ($PO_2 = 33.1 \pm 3.9$ mm Hg; $PaO_2 = 106.9 \pm 4.4$ mm Hg; $n = 8$) than at intervascular locations ($PO_2 = 16.6 \pm 1.4$ mm Hg; $PaO_2 = 104.0 \pm 4.3$ mm

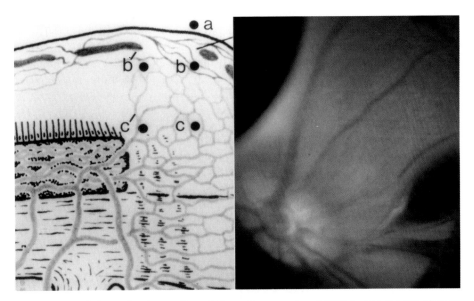

FIG. 1. Left: Schematic of a section of the optic nerve head (ONH) showing the sites at which the PO_2 measurements were performed: near the center, in front of the optic disk (*a*), at 50-μm depth within the ONH (*b*), and at 200-μm depth within the ONH (*c*), and at the rim of the ONH, at 50 μm (*b′*) and 200-μm (*c′*) depth within the ONH. **Right:** Oxygen-sensitive microelectrode placed within the ONH of the miniature pig.

TABLE 1. *Distribution of tissue PO$_2$ (mm Hg ± SEM) at the optic nerve head (ONH) during systemic normoxia and hyperoxia*

	Normoxia	Hyperoxia	*n*
PO$_2$ in front of the ONH			
Juxta-arteriolar	33.1 ± 3.9	81.1 ± 8.8	8
Intervascular	16.6 ± 1.4	17.4 ± 1.4	8
Intervascular PO$_2$ within the ONH tissue at 50-μm depth			
Central area	9.6 ± 1.2	10.0 ± 1.4	7
Rim	10.8 ± 1.9	10.6 ± 1.4	8
Intervascular PO$_2$ within the ONH tissue at 200-μm depth			
Central area	9.4 ± 0.8	8.7 ± 1.1	12
Rim	8.2 ± 1.8	46.8 ± 7.5	6

Hg; $n = 8$) ($p<0.05$) during systemic normoxia (13). This heterogeneous oxygen distribution was first discussed by Ernest, who compared the tissue PO$_2$ in the vicinity of the central retinal artery and away from it at the surface of the ONH of monkeys and concluded that this may be due to the diffusion of O$_2$ from the central retinal artery (11). In miniature pigs, PO$_2$ values were found to be elevated in areas adjacent to arterioles both in front of the optic disk and within the ONH tissue (19). A similar heterogeneous distribution was found in the inner retina (18,20).

At a depth of 50 μm within the ONH, the intervascular PO$_2$ values at both the central area (PO$_2$ = 9.6 ± 1.2 mm Hg; PaO$_2$ = 98.8 ± 4.21 mm Hg; $n =$ 7) and the rim (PO$_2$ = 10.8 ± 1.9 mm Hg; PaO$_2$ = 104.4 ± 4.2 mm Hg; $n =$ 8) were significantly lower than those measured at intervascular locations in front of the optic disk. Similarly, at a depth of 200 μm within the ONH, the intervascular PO$_2$ values at both the central area (PO$_2$ = 9.4 ± 0.8 mm Hg; PaO$_2$ = 97.7 ± 2.1 mm Hg; $n = 12$) and the rim (PO$_2$ = 8.2 ± 1.8 mm Hg; PaO$_2$ = 101.0 ± 5.1 mm Hg; $n = 6$) were lower than those measured at intervascular locations in front of the optic disk. The PO$_2$ values at a depth of 200 μm did not significantly differ from those obtained at a depth of 50 μm ($p>0.05$) (Table 1). Similar homogeneous oxygen distribution in intervascular tissue areas within the ONH was also found in cats (12).

The lower tissue PO$_2$ values within rather than in front of the ONH are probably due to oxygen consumption by the neuronal tissue. Tissue PO$_2$ values were constant in intervascular areas at various depths within the ONH, although the vascular supply of the ONH is not uniform because it is dependent on the retinal arterioles at the more superficial part of the ONH and on the choroidal arterioles at the prelaminar ONH area (21), and the tissue PO$_2$ at the juxtapapillary choroid is much higher than in the inner retina (18).

TISSUE ONH PO$_2$ REGULATION DURING MODIFICATION OF SYSTEMIC PaO$_2$

Systemic Hyperoxia

Measurements of local ONH PO$_2$ during hyperoxia induced by 100% O$_2$ breathing, performed at the same areas as during normoxia, showed that in front of the optic disk systemic hyperoxia induced a significant increase in juxta-arteriolar PO_2 values (PO_2 = 81.1 ± 8.8 mm Hg; PaO_2 = 373.2 ± 22.2 mm Hg; n = 8), whereas it did not significantly change ($p>0.05$) intervascular PO_2 values (PO_2 = 17.4 ± 1.4 mm Hg; PaO_2 = 331.1 ± 42.5 mm Hg; n = 8) (Table 1, Fig. 2).

At a depth of 50 μm within the ONH, systemic hyperoxia did not induce a significant change in the intervascular PO_2, either at the central area (PO_2 = 10.0 ± 1.4 mm Hg; PaO_2 = 318.8 ± 29.4 mm Hg; n = 7) or at the rim (PO_2 = 10.6 ± 1.4 mm Hg; PaO_2 = 318.9 ± 28.1 mm Hg; n = 8) of the ONH. However, at this depth, juxta-arteriolar recordings showed an increase of the local PO_2 (Fig. 2). At a depth of 200 μm within the ONH, systemic hyperoxia did not significantly change the PO_2 values at intervascular locations at the central area of the ONH (PO_2 = 8.7 ± 1.1 mm Hg; PaO_2 = 287 ± 24.9 mm Hg; n = 12), whereas it induced an enormous rise in local PO_2 (PO_2 = 46.8 ± 7.5 mm Hg; PaO_2 = 381.5 ± 24.4 mm Hg; n = 6) at the ONH rim, because the PO_2 at the choroid increases tremendously during hyperoxia (18).

During hyperoxia, O_2 diffuses from the arterioles, accounting for the increase in PO_2 observed at the juxta-arteriolar areas. Interestingly, during hyperoxia the PO_2 values in intervascular areas in front of the ONH and at different depths are maintained constant and similar to those recorded during normoxia, despite the important PaO_2 increase in the retinal and choroidal circulation.

ONH blood flow measurements by laser Doppler flowmetry showed an ONH blood flow decrease of 34.2 ± 6.5%, n = 8, during hyperoxia (14). In miniature pigs a similar autoregulation during hyperoxia has been demonstrated in the inner retina (18), whose oxygenation depends on the retinal vessels. In contrast to miniature pigs, a PO_2 increase at different depths within the ONH has been reported during 100% oxygen breathing in cats, indicating that in these animals tissue PO_2 regulation during hyperoxia is not efficient (12). It should be noted that in cats 100% oxygen breathing induces a sharp rise in PO_2 in the inner retina as well (22). In miniature pigs, a statistically significant PO_2 increase was found during hyperoxia only at the rim of the ONH at a depth of 200 μm, close to the choroid. This PO_2 increase is probably caused by diffusion of O_2 from the choroidal vessels lying close to the rim of the ONH. Indeed, during hyperoxia

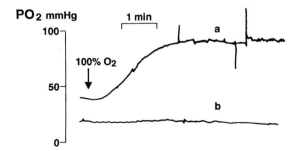

FIG. 2. Tissue PO_2 measurements, recorded after 100% O_2 breathing, in front of the optic nerve head at a juxta-arteriolar (**a**) and an intervascular area (**b**). Hyperoxia induces a significant increase in juxta-arteriolar tissue PO_2, whereas measurements at the intervascular area remain stable.

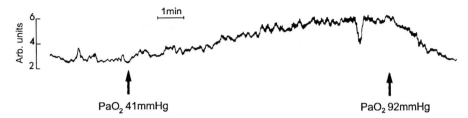

FIG. 3. Typical recording of modifications of optic nerve head (ONH) blood flow during systemic hypoxia. Systemic PaO$_2$ of 41 mm Hg induces a progressive increase in ONH blood flow of approximately 40%. Normoxia induces a decrease in ONH blood flow to previous hypoxic values.

choroidal PO$_2$ increases (18,22), and it may diffuse toward the surrounding tissues.

Systemic Hypoxia

Because an identical regulation at intervascular areas close to the center of the ONH at 50- and 200-μm depth was observed, the 200-μm location was selected for the subsequent experiments. Hypoxia was obtained by decreasing the O$_2$ in the inspired gas mixture by 10–20%. PO$_2$ values at a depth of 200 μm within the ONH during hypoxia (PO$_2$ = 11.28 ± 0.5 mm Hg; PaO$_2$ = 51.5 ± 6.85 mm Hg; n = 10) were not significantly different from those measured during normoxia (PO$_2$ = 11.23 ± 0.49 mm Hg; PaO$_2$ = 102.4 ± 8.38 mm Hg; n = 10).

Figure 3 shows a typical ONH blood flow recording by laser Doppler flowmetry during systemic hypoxia. The ONH blood flow progressively increases as systemic PaO$_2$ drops to hypoxic values. Recovery to systemic normoxia induces a ONH blood flow decrease. During hypoxia, in the same way as during hyperoxia, tissue PO$_2$ autoregulation was demonstrated in the inner retinal layers, whereas no autoregulation was found near the choroid (23,24). However, the absence of choroidal blood flow autoregulation does not affect tissue ONH PO$_2$ in miniature pigs, in which it is maintained at constant values by ONH blood flow modifications.

TISSUE ONH PO$_2$ DURING VARIATIONS OF PERFUSION PRESSURE

The retinal and choroidal circulations have a different response to variations of the perfusion pressure. The retinal blood flow is regulated and remains stable during increases and decreases in the perfusion pressure (25,26). In contrast, a decrease in the perfusion pressure induces choroidal blood flow changes in a linear fashion with a decrease in perfusion pressure (27). However, it has been suggested (28) that during variation of the perfusion pressure even the choroidal circulation may have some autoregulatory capacity.

Local ONH PO₂ Measurements After Acute Increases in Blood Pressure

Local ONH PO_2 measurements were performed after acute increases in blood pressure at intervascular areas close to the center of the ONH at a depth of 200 μm. Increase of the arterial pressure was induced by i.v. injection of 0.3 mg epinephrine, which rapidly elevates both diastolic and systolic blood pressure. The mean systolic blood pressure before injection was 107.5 ± 3.7 mm Hg and increased to 177.5 ± 5.2 mm Hg ($n = 14$) after injection. ONH PO_2 values at intervascular areas and at a depth of 200 μm did not differ before ($PO_2 = 9.18 \pm 1.68$ mm Hg; $n = 14$) and after ($PO_2 = 9.66 \pm 1.28$ mm Hg; $n = 14$) the acute increase of the blood pressure induced by epinephrine.

Local ONH PO₂ Measurements After Acute Decrease in Blood Pressure

Local ONH PO_2 measurements were performed after acute decrease in blood pressure at intervascular areas close to the center of the ONH at a depth of 200 μm. Hypotension was induced by i.v. injection of 10 mg of trinitrine, which induced a decrease in systolic arterial pressure from 98.75 ± 3.09 mm Hg to 53.75 ± 2.54 mm Hg ($n = 6$). During the rapid initial phase of blood pressure modifications, transient changes in ONH PO_2 were recorded. However, once the systemic blood pressure was stabilized at hypotensive values, PO_2 measurements ($PO_2 = 10.95 \pm 1.23$ mm Hg; $n = 6$) were not significantly different from those recorded during steady state ($PO_2 = 11.85 \pm 1.01$ mm Hg; $n = 6$).

Previous PO_2 measurements have demonstrated an autoregulation in front of the ONH when the perfusion pressure was lowered in the eyes of cats by an increase in IOP (9,10) and in eyes of monkeys (11) by a decrease in blood pressure. The PO_2 measurements shown here demonstrate that, even within the ONH tissue at a depth of 200 μm, PO_2 is maintained stable during important increases or decreases in systemic arterial pressure, suggesting autoregulation of the ONH blood flow during variations of the perfusion pressure (29–31).

LOCAL ONH PO₂ MEASUREMENTS AFTER INHIBITION OF ENDOTHELIAL NO RELEASE

NO which is released mainly by endothelial cells, plays an important role in the regulation of the vascular tone in several tissues (7,32). NO is a powerful vasodilator because it inhibits vascular contraction. In the eye, NO has a different role in the retinal and choroidal circulations. Injection of the NO synthase inhibi-

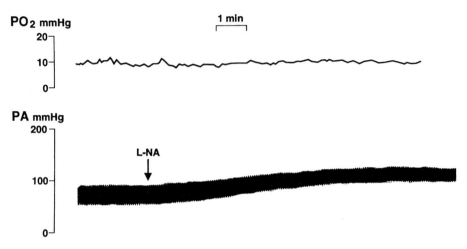

FIG. 4. Simultaneous recording of optic nerve head tissue PO_2 and systemic arterial pressure after i.v. injection of 20 mg/kg nitro-L-arginine. Nitro-L-arginine induces a subtle increase in systemic blood pressure, but the tissue PO_2 remains unchanged.

tor nitro-L-arginine (L-NA) in isolated, perfused porcine eye induced a decrease in choroidal blood flow (33). Intravenous injection of L-NA caused a 40% decrease of choroidal blood flow, without any modification of the retinal blood flow, in anesthetized dogs (34). In addition, in vivo experiments in the miniature pig demonstrated that i.v. infusion of L-NA has no measurable effect on the diameter of the retinal arterioles (35). PO_2 measurements in intervascular areas at a depth of 200 μm were also performed after i.v. perfusion of 20 mg/kg of the NO synthase inhibitor L-NA. Intravenous infusion of nitro-L-arginine had no effect on tissue PO_2. The PO_2 values were 12.16 ± 0.79 mm Hg ($n = 10$) before and 11.97 ± 0.78 mm Hg ($n = 10$) after the infusion. The postinfusion measurements were obtained 10 min after administration of L-NA. Its systemic effect was evident by an increase in systolic blood pressure from 90 ± 2.2 to 115 ± 2.1 mm Hg, $n = 10$ (Fig. 4).

DISCUSSION

In vivo microelectrode PO_2 measurements in the intact eye provide information concerning the ONH oxygenation and, indirectly, concerning ONH blood flow. During normoxia, PO_2 values are elevated in areas adjacent to arterioles both in front of the optic disk and within the ONH tissue, a PO_2 distribution similar to that of the inner retina (18,20). Furthermore, tissue PO_2 values are lower within than in front of the ONH, probably owing to oxygen consumption by the neuronal tissue. Tissue PO_2 values are constant in intervascular areas at various depths within the ONH. During hyperoxia, O_2 diffuses from the arterioles, accounting for the observed increase in PO$_2$ in the juxta-arteriolar areas. However, by autoregulatory modifications of the ONH blood flow, PO$_2$ values in intervascular areas in front of the ONH and at different depths in the prelaminar area are maintained constant and are similar to those recorded during normoxia, despite an important PaO$_2$ increase in the retinal and choroidal circulation. Similar autoregulation during hyperoxia has been demonstrated in the inner retina, although in the external retinal layers, whose oxygenation depends on the choroidal circulation, tissue PO$_2$ increases (18). Autoregulation at the level of the inner retina is achieved by a decrease in blood flow (20) and, probably, by an increase in O$_2$ consumption (18). A similar mechanism of regulation of ONH tissue PO$_2$ during hyperoxia, by decrease in ONH blood flow, was shown. The PO$_2$ increase during hyperoxia at the rim of the ONH at a depth of 200 μm, close to the choroid, is probably due to diffusion of O$_2$ from the choroidal vessels lying close to the rim of the ONH. During hypoxia, as during hyperoxia, tissue PO$_2$ autoregulation was demonstrated in the inner retinal layers, whereas no autoregulation was found near the choroid (23,24). However, as during hyperoxia, the tissue ONH PO$_2$ is maintained at constant values by ONH blood flow modification.

The PO$_2$ measurements performed in miniature pigs (19) demonstrate that within the ONH tissue PO$_2$ is maintained stable during decreases or increases in systemic arterial pressure, suggesting autoregulation of the ONH blood flow during variations in perfusion pressure. In addition, blood flow autoregulation within the ONH during increased IOP, which induces a simultaneous decrease in ONH perfusion pressure, was shown using radioactively labeled microspheres (29) or a tracer, iodoantipyrine I-125 (30,31). The ONH blood flow autoregulation is also confirmed by findings showing that intravascular ONH PaO$_2$ was remarkably stable during similar experimental conditions (15).

Perfusion of L-NA did not change tissue PO$_2$ in the ONH. These results point to the fact that, as in the retina, the endothelium-derived NO probably does not play an important role in the control of the vascular tone in the ONH under physiologic conditions. However, in the CNS the endothelial cell is not the sole site of NO production. Both neurons (35) and astrocytes (36) are involved in NO production and release and, in the retina, it has been shown that NO released during neuronal activity plays a role in regulation of vascular tone (37). A similar role for neuronal but not endothelium-derived NO, which would not have been significately inhibited by systemic administration of L-NA, may also exist in the ONH. In addition, the role of other vasodilatory or vasoconstricting factors, such as PGs or endothelin, remains to be investigated.

Despite the double anatomic origin of the ONH vascularization, both retinal and choroidal, our findings indicate that the regulatory mechanisms of ONH circulation responding to metabolic stimuli and perfusion pressure variations are similar to those of the retina rather than to those of the choroid. It therefore appears that tissue ONH PO$_2$ remains stable during variations in perfusion pressure. However, a role for such variations in the pathogenesis of glaucomatous optic neuropathy is still possible. First, autoregulation may be efficient only within certain limits of variations in perfusion pressure. Second, the experiments described above give no information on the long-term effect of perfusion pressure variations. Finally, the autoregulatory mechanisms themselves may be impaired in glaucomatous optic neuropathy.

REFERENCES

1. Ernest JT, Potts AM. Pathophysiology of the distal portion of the optic nerve. 2. Vascular relationships. *Am J Ophthalmol* 1968;66:380–7.
2. Fechtner RD, Weinreb RN. Mechanisms of optic nerve damage in primary open angle glaucoma. *Surv Ophthalmol* 1994;39:23–42.
3. Hayreh SS, Zimmerman MB, Podhajsky P, Alward WL. The role of nocturnal hypotension in ocular and optic nerve ischemic disorders. *Invest Ophthalmol Vis Sci* 1993;34:994–9.
4. Robert Y, Steiner D, Hendrickson P. Papillary circulation dynamics in glaucoma. *Graefes Arch Clin Exp Ophthalmol* 1989;227:436–9.
5. Hayreh SS. Progress in the understanding of the vascular etiology of glaucoma. *Curr Opin Ophthalmol* 1994;5:26–35.
6. Haefliger IO, Zschauer A, Anderson DR. Relaxation of retinal pericyte contractile tone through the nitric oxide-cyclic guanosine monophosphate pathway. *Invest Ophthalmol Vis Sci* 1994;35:991–7.
7. Haefliger IO, Meyer P, Flammer J, Lüscher TF. The vascular endothelium as a regulator of the ocular circulation: a new concept in ophthalmology? *Surv Ophthalmol* 1994;39:123–32.
8. Tsacopoulos M. Quelques aspects des relations existant entre le fonctionnement neuronal et rétinien, le metabolisme oxydatif et l'apport constant d'O₂ par la microcirculation. *Klin Mbl Augenheilk* 1985;186:477–9.
9. Ernest JT. In vivo measurements of optic-disk oxygen tension. *Invest Ophthalmol Vis Sci* 1973;12:927–31.
10. Ernest JT. Optic disk oxygen tension. *Exp Eye Res* 1977;24:271–8.
11. Ernest JT. Autoregulation of optic-disk PO₂. *Invest Ophthalmol Vis Sci* 1974;13:101–6.
12. Ahmed J, Linsenmeier RA, Dumm R Jr. The oxygen distribution in the prelaminar optic nerve head of the cat. *Exp Eye Res* 1994;59:457–66.
13. Pournaras CJ, Munoz JL, Abdesselem R. Regulation de la PO₂ au niveau de la papille en hyperoxie. *Klin Mbl Augenheilk* 1991;198:404–5.
14. Pournaras CJ, Munoz J-L, Riva CE, Brazitikos PD. Local PO₂ in the optic nerve of miniature pigs during systemic hyperoxia [Abstract]. *Invest Ophthalmol Vis Sci* 1991;32(suppl):786.
15. Shonat RD, Wilson DF, Riva CE, Cranstoun SD. Effect of acute increases in intraocular pressure on intravascular optic nerve head oxygen tension in cats. *Invest Ophthalmol Vis Sci* 1992;33:3174–80.
16. Tsacopoulos M, Lehmenkuhler A. A double-barreled Pt microelectrode for simultaneous measurements of PO₂ and bioelectrical activity in excitable tissue. *Experientia* 1977;33:1337–8.
17. Pournaras CJ, Shonat RD, Munoz JL, Petrig BL. New ocular micromanipulator for measurements of retinal and vitreous physiologic parameters in the mammalian eye. *Exp Eye Res* 1991;53:723–7.
18. Pournaras CJ, Riva CE, Tsacopoulos M, Strommer K. Diffusion of O₂ in the retina of anesthetized pigs in normoxia and hyperoxia. *Exp Eye Res* 1989;49:347–60.
19. Bouzas EA, Pournaras CJ, Donati G. Distribution and regulation of the optic nerve head tissue PO₂. *Surv Ophthalmol* 1997 (in press).
20. Riva CE, Pournaras CJ, Tsacopoulos M. Regulation of local oxygen tension and blood flow in the inner retina during hyperoxia. *J Appl Physiol* 1986;61:592–8.
21. Hayreh SS. Blood supply of the optic nerve head in health and disease. In: Ed Lambrou GN, Greve EL, eds. *Ocular blood flow in glaucoma: means, methods, measurements.* Amstelveen: Kugler & Ghedini, 1989:3–54.
22. Linsenmeier RA, Yancey CM. Effects of hyperoxia in the oxygen distribution in the intact cat eye. *Invest Ophthalmol Vis Sci* 1989;30:612–8.

23. Linsenmeier RA, Braun RD. Oxygen distribution and consumption in the cat retina during normoxia and hypoxemia. *J Gen Physiol* 1992;99:177–97.

24. Moret Ph, Pournaras CJ, Munoz J-L. Profils de la PO₂ distribution and regulation of the optic nerve head tissue PO₂: I. Profils de la PO₂ transrétinienne en hypoxie. *Klin Mbl Augenheilk* 1992;200:498–501.

25. Riva CE, Sinclair SH, Grunwald JE. Autoregulation of retinal circulation in response to decrease of perfusion pressure. *Invest Ophthalmol Vis Sci* 1981;21:34–8.

26. Riva CE, Grunwald JE, Petrig BL. Autoregulation of human retinal blood flow: an investigation with laser Doppler velocimetry. *Invest Ophthalmol Vis Sci* 1986;27:1706–12.

27. Alm A, Bill A. Ocular and optic nerve blood flow at normal and increased intraocular pressures in monkeys (Cacaca irus): a study with radioactively labeled microspheres including flow determinations in brain and some other tissues. *Exp Eye Res* 1973;15:15–29.

28. Kiel JW, Shepherd AP. Autoregulation of choroidal blood flow in the rabbit. *Invest Ophthalmol Vis Sci* 1992;33:2399–410.

29. Geijer C, Bill A. Effects of raised intraocular pressure on retinal, prelaminar, laminar, and retrolaminar optic nerve blood flow in monkeys. *Invest Ophthalmol Vis Sci* 1979;18:1030–42.

30. Sossi N, Anderson DR. Effect of elevated intraocular pressure on blood flow. Occurrence in cat optic nerve head studied with iodoantipyrine I 125. *Arch Ophthalmol* 1983;101:98–101.

31. Quigley HA, Hohman RM, Sanchez R, Addicks EA. Optic nerve head blood flow in chronic experimental glaucoma. *Arch Ophthalmol* 1985;103:956–62.

32. Moncada S. Nitric oxide: physiology, pathophysiology and pharmacology. *Pharmacol Rev* 1991;43:109–42.

33. Meyer P, Flammer J, Luscher TF. Endothelium-dependent regulation of the ophthalmic microcirculation in the perfused porcine eye: role of nitric oxide and endothelins. *Invest Ophthalmol Vis Sci* 1993;34:3614–21.

34. Deussen A, Sontag M, Vogel R. L-arginine-derived nitric oxide: a major determinant of uveal blood flow. *Exp Eye Res* 1993;57:129–34.

35. Gally JA, Montagne PR, Recke GN, Edelman GM. The NO hypothesis: possible effects of a short-lived, rapidly diffusible signal in the development and the function of the nervous system. *Proc Natl Acad Sci USA* 1990;87:3547–51.

36. Murphy S, Minor RL, Welk G, Harrison DJ. Evidence for an astrocyte-derived releasing factor with properties similar to nitric oxide. *J Neurochem* 1990;55:349–51.

37. Donati G, Pournaras CJ, Munoz JL, Poitry S, Poitry-Yamate CL, Tsacopoulos M. Nitric oxide controls arteriolar tone in the retina of the miniature pig. *Invest Ophthalmol Vis Sci* 1995;36:2228–37.

Nitric Oxide and Endothelin in the Pathogenesis of
Glaucoma, edited by I. O. Haefliger and J. Flammer.
Lippincott–Raven Publishers, Philadelphia © 1998.

13

Oxygenation in the Ocular Fundus by Phosphorescence Quenching

Charles E. Riva

*Institut de Recherche en Ophtalmologie, Sion, and University of Lausanne,
Medical School, Lausanne, Switzerland*

Compromised oxygenation of the fundus has been implicated in a variety of ocular diseases, such as diabetic retinopathy (1), vascular occlusive diseases, and possibly glaucoma (2,3). This oxygenation is dependent on local blood flow, tissue consumption of oxygen, and on oxygen partial pressure (pO_2) in the blood and the tissue. Measurements of tissue pO_2 have been limited to animal studies using microelectrodes (4–7). This method requires insertion of the microelectrode into the eye. Furthermore, it provides information only on changes in pO_2 in locally defined regions a few micrometers in diameter. The results are assumed to hold for the entire tissue.

This article reviews the application of a recently developed method that allows the measurement of intravascular pO_2 by the oxygen-dependent quenching of phosphorescence (PQ). Two modes of this technique have been applied: the imaging mode (IPQ) and the focal mode (FPQ). The description of these techniques is extensively borrowed from the original investigations of Shonat et al. (8,9) and Cranstoun et al. (10), with permission of the respective publishers.

BACKGROUND

Phosphorescence is the emission of light during an energy transition from a long-lived, spin-forbidden, excited triplet state to the ground state (11). When a molecule that is capable of phosphorescence, such as a metalloporphyrin derivative, is excited into the triplet state, it may emit phosphorescence or, alternatively, transfer its energy to another molecule without light emission (quenching). In the blood, oxygen is the only significant quenching agent (12), with the degree of quenching dependent on the concentration of oxygen in the vicinity of the phosphorescent molecule. By measuring the quenching effect, the intravascular pO_2 can be determined.

Previous studies investigating phosphorescence emission have demonstrated that the intensity decay conforms to a single exponential with a characteristic lifetime τ that is dependent on the oxygen concentration (11,13). In a zero oxygen environment, the lifetime is maximal ($\tau = \tau_0$), but when oxygen is present, quenching becomes important and the lifetime is shortened. The relationship between τ and pO_2 surrounding the probe is given by the Stern–Volmer equation:

$$\tau_0/\tau = 1 + (k_q)(\tau_0)(pO_2)$$

where k_q is the quenching constant (Torr-1 s^{-1}) for the particular triplet-state probe (11).

In the study of Shonat et al. (8) a palladium (Pd) complex of *meso-tetra* (4-carboxyphenyl) porphine was used as the oxygen probe for the following reasons: its sensitivity to oxygen over the range of pO_2 values typically found in vivo; its excitation spectrum within the visible range; and its phosphorescence emission in the near infrared, where the retinal tissue absorbs minimally. Figure 1 shows the excitation and emission spectra for this probe.

For both in vitro calibration and in vivo measurements, the probe was bound to albumin. The reason for that has been discussed by Shonat et al. (8). In particular, because of this binding in vitro and in vivo, no additional calibration of τ_0 and k_q was necessary, so that absolute pO_2 values could be obtained in vivo.

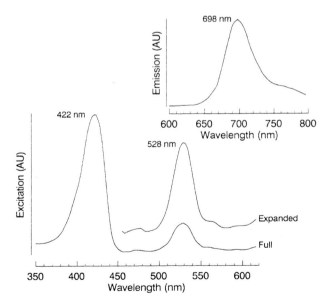

FIG. 1. Excitation and emission spectra for Pd-*meso-tetra* (4-carboxyphenyl) porphin bound to albumin (8). See this reference for detailed information on the preparation of the probe and measurements of the spectra. From ref. 8.

pO₂ IN THE IMAGING MODE

In this imaging mode (IPQ), the probe was excited and the phosphorescence was collected through a Wild Macrozoom microscope with an epifluorescence attachment (Wild-Leitz USA, Malvern, PA), as shown in Fig. 2 (8). A 45-W xenon flash lamp generated the excitation flash ($\approx$5 μs width at half maximum) and the resulting phosphorescence was observed with an intensified CCD camera (Xybion Electronic Systems, San Diego, CA) placed in the image plane of the microscope. The timing of the flash and the gating of the CCD intensifier were under the control of an 80386 microcomputer. A hardware and software video image processing system (Image 1/AT; Universal Imaging, Malvern, PA) generated all the timing signals and digitized (512 $\times$ 480 pixels) the video images. The excitation was centered at a wavelength of 528 nm, using a bandpass filter. Emission was filtered through a longpass cutoff filter with 50% transmission at 630 nm. The energy levels delivered to the eye were well below the maximal permissible limit for the retina.

The phosphorescence lifetime was calculated from images collected at different delay times after a flash at time zero, with the number of delay times large enough to characterize the exponential decay. One measurement required about 10 different delay times and 80 separate images, and generated 10 stored images on disk, with the entire procedure taking about 20 s. Calculation of the lifetime and pO₂ was done off-line.

A color map of the pO₂ obtained from a cat is shown in Fig. 3A. Full-scale pO₂ is 0–150 Torr, with the optic nerve tissue regions and venules showing

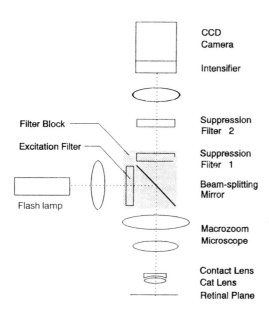

FIG. 2. Phosphorescence imaging microscope. A filter block (*shaded*) inside the epifluorescence attachment holds the primary excitation filter, beam-splitter mirror, and the first suppression filter. The negative power contact lens is used to view the fundus with the microscope optics. From ref. 8.

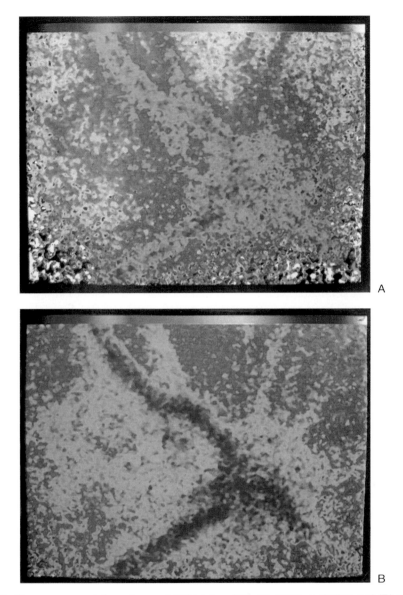

FIG. 3. Oxygen maps of the retina and ONH taken (**A**) with green excitation and (**B**) with blue excitation. The color scale band across the top designates full-scale pO$_2$ from 0–150 Torr (left to right). ×20.

lower pO_2 than the retinal regions around the disk. The average pO_2 in three different regions of this map is shown in Table 1 (8). The most striking feature is the high pO_2 in the capillary region ($\approx$69 Torr), which is much higher than the previously measured values using microelectrodes in the cat. The explanation provided by Shonat et al. (8) is that this map was generated with a green excitation flash (bandwidth 515–560 nm), with a range of wavelengths to which the retina is mostly transparent. A map obtained with an excitation in the blue (center wavelength 422 nm) from the same region of the fundus in the same cat, under identical physiologic conditions as in Fig. 3B, indeed shows lower pO_2 values everywhere, as shown in Table 1 (8).

Using this technique, Shonat et al. (9) investigated the effect of acute increases in intraocular pressure (IOP) on ONH and retinal pO_2 in anesthetized cats. Five adult cats weighing 2.0–3.5 kg were used and prepared as previously described (14). Each cat was premedicated with atropine (0.04 mg/kg s.c.) and anesthetized with i.m. ketamine HCl (22 mg/kg) and acepromazine maleate (2 mg/kg). Catheters were placed in a femoral artery and vein and a tracheostomy was performed. A loading dose of pancuronium bromide (0.2 mg/kg) was given i.v. and the animal was ventilated with 21% O_2 and 79% N_2. Arterial blood pressure, end-tidal CO_2, and heart rate (HR) were monitored continuously. Arterial pH, pCO_2, and pO_2 were monitored intermittently using a blood gas analyzer, and adjustments of the inspired gas mixture, end-tidal volume, and respiration rate were made to keep pH $\approx$7.4, pCO_2 $\approx$31 mm Hg, pO_2 $\geq$90 mm Hg. Rectal temperature was maintained at $\approx$38°C. Enflurane (1.7–2.5%) was administered and pancuronium bromide (0.10 mg/kg/h) infused continuously. The pupils were dilated with 1% tropicamide and 10% phenylephrine, and the cat was placed prone on a table with the head secured in a stereotactic head holder. A ring was sutured to the eye with three stitches at the limbus and was held in a fixed position to prevent eye motion. A zero-diopter contact lens was placed on the cornea protected with Healon. All experimental procedures conformed to the ARVO Resolution on the Use of Animals in Research.

Two 18-gauge needles were inserted into the vitreous, one connected to a reservoir containing a balanced salt solution to raise the IOP, the other to measure it. After generating a pO_2 map at an IOP of 15–20 mm Hg, assumed to be the normal IOP, the IOP was raised in increasing increments and the pO_2 was mapped again after a few minutes of equilibration at each level. The IOP was

TABLE 1. *Average pO_2 (mm Hg) in different regions from Figs. 3a and b*

	pO$_2$ (Torr)	
Region	Fig. 3a	Fig. 3b
Optic nerve head center	33	27
Superior venule	30	25
Nasal capillary region	69	41

raised until the blood flow stopped or the reservoir reached the ceiling. Figure 4A–C shows pO_2 maps obtained at normal IOP, IOP = 60, and IOP = 79 mm Hg, where flow was practically stopped. We observe very little difference between Fig. 4A and B. However, when the flow is stopped, the pO_2 is close to zero at the nerve and slightly above it at the retina and choroid.

On the basis of such maps, Shonat et al. (9) evaluated the pO_2 in various regions of the fundus and determined the effect of acute increases in IOP on ONH and retinal capillary pO_2 (Fig. 5A and B), plotted as function of mean perfusion pressure (PP_m = mean blood pressure minus IOP). In both figures, the pO_2 values found before insertion of the needles appear above the abscissa region, labeled "control." These figures demonstrate that the pO_2 is well regulated in the ONH and nasal capillary region, even at low PP_ms. The decline in pO_2 is shallow until the blood flow stops. At this point, the pO_2 falls rapidly to zero, as expected. However, because the excitation light was centered at 530 nm, a wavelength that penetrates deep into the ONH and retina, the data actually represent an integration of pO_2 from the vitreal surface to an unspecified depth. It is probable that the results reflect a choroidal influence, especially in the choroidal region. Although a perfect oxygen-regulatory capacity would require that the slope of the pO_2 vs. PP_m be zero, the shallowness of the slope we found suggests that regulation is good and fails only when the IOP is raised above ophthalmic arterial pressure.

These results may have important implications for the understanding of glaucomatous damage and the role of oxygen. ONH hypoxia was observed only at very low PP_m. However, because the study was done in cats and because it involves an acute elevation of IOP, the effect of chronically elevated IOP on the ONH pO_2 in humans remains to be investigated.

pO_2 IN THE FOCAL MODE

Imaging in the focal mode (FPQ) is too slow for determination of the time course of the pO_2 in response to rapid changes in the physiologic conditions. For this reason, Cranstoun et al. (10) developed a technique that allows local measurement of the intravascular pO_2 with a time constant of approximately 1 s. In addition, the instrument developed for this purpose also allows the quasi-simultaneous measurement from the same location of blood flow by laser Doppler flowmetry (LDF). Furthermore, the FPQ technique can be used simultaneously with measurements of tissue pO_2 using oxygen microelectrodes.

Using these techniques, Cranstoun et al. (10) investigated the relationship between tissue blood flow and intra- and extravascular pO_2 in the ONH, with the aim of obtaining a better understanding of metabolic demand and delivery of oxygen. Measurements were performed under different well-controlled conditions, such as hyperoxia, hypoxia, hypercapnia, dark adaptation, and euthanasia.

The FPQ system was implemented in a Zeiss fundus camera. It measures the

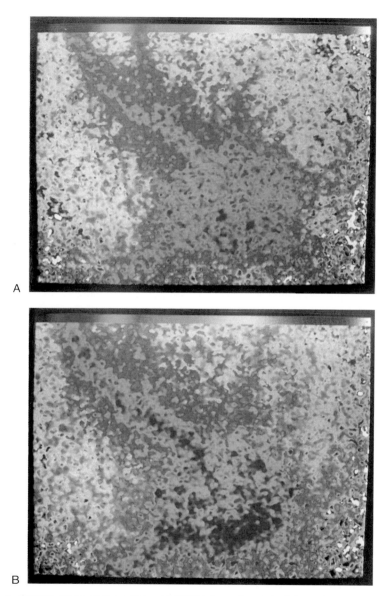

FIG. 4. Oxygen maps of the retina and ONH taken at various intraocular pressures (IOP) with a green flash for the excitation. **A:** IOP = 24 mm Hg; **B:** IOP = 60 mm Hg; and **C:** IOP = 79 mm Hg (almost no flow).

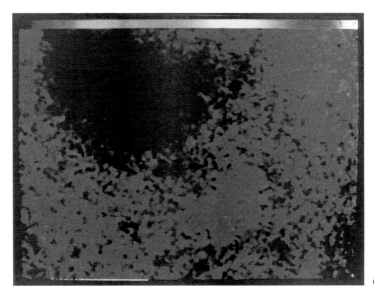

C

FIG. 4. *Continued.*

phosphorescence emission with a photomultiplier tube (PMT) from an area with a diameter of $\approx$300 μm at the fundus. The PMT photocurrent is amplified and digitized by an 80486 computer, which calculates the pO_2 and displays the results on the monitor. A typical measurement from the ONH tissue can be made in less than 1 s, allowing measurement of rapid changes in pO_2. LDF is continuously monitored between PQ measurements, using the same instrument and computer program. Because the LDF laser line (670 nm) is close to the phosphorescence emission (698 $\pm$ 30 nm), both measurements are not performed simultaneously. Instead, the program turns the laser off when a FPQ measurement is being made, and turns it back on to continue LDF.

LDF, as applied to measurement of blood flow in the ONH, has been described in more detail in a previous publication (14,15). In short, a diode laser (λ = 670 nm), delivered to the eye through a modified fundus camera, is focused on the ONH tissue away from visible vessels. Laser light scattered by the red blood cells is collected in the image plane of the camera by an optical fiber and is detected by a photomultiplier tube. The photocurrent is amplified and digitized by a personal computer which calculates, from the photocurrent power spectrum, the flux of these red blood cells through the sampled volume.

Experiments were performed in adult miniature pigs (10–13 kg). These animals have a retina that anatomically resembles that of the human. All procedures conformed to the ARVO Statement for the Use of Animals in Ophthalmic and Vision Research. Animals were anesthetized with metomidate hydrochloride (HCl). Arterial and venous catheters were inserted and the animal was paralyzed

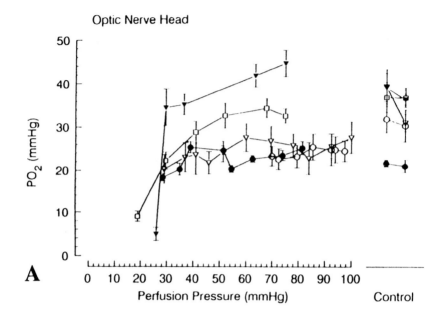

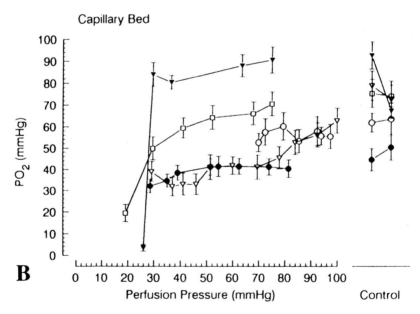

FIG. 5. pO$_2$ in the central region of the ONH (**A**) and in the nasal capillary bed (**B**) in five cats. For each cat, the pO$_2$ distribution was mapped before the pressure-controlling needles were inserted. They are shown as control. The two pO$_2$ values below 10 mm Hg at low perfusion pressure in two cats were taken shortly after the blood flow stopped. From ref. 9.

with curare and artificially ventilated. Anesthesia was maintained by continuous infusion of Hypnodil. For preparation of the porphyrin probe, blood was drawn from the animal ($\sim$4 ml/kg) and the serum extracted. The probe (20 mg/kg) was mixed with the serum, the pH was adjusted to 7.4, and the serum/probe solution was filtered with a 0.2-mm sterile filter. The solution was infused and allowed to equilibrate with the blood before measurements proceeded. Various physiologic stimuli were applied and the pO_2 response to these stimuli was documented (10).

Hyperoxia

The animal was ventilated with 100% O_2. Arterial blood gases were taken during normoxia and after 5 min of increased oxygen breathing. Arterial pO_2 increased from 130 to 356 mm Hg after 5 min. Figure 6a shows only a small increase in intravascular pO_2 (7.5%) after 7 min of hyperoxia. Blood flow was reduced by 22%.

Hypoxia and Euthanasia

The animal was ventilated with 0% O_2 until death (at approximately 11.5 min). Blood flow increased 75%, and intravascular pO_2 remained relatively constant (Fig. 6b).

Hypercapnia

The animal was ventilated with a gas mixture containing CO_2. Arterial blood gases were taken during normoxia and after 5 min of CO_2 breathing. Arterial pO_2 increased from 99 to 120 mm Hg and pCO_2 from 38 to 99 mm Hg. Tissue pO_2 remained constant, but intravascular pO_2 increased by $\sim$33% (Fig. 6c).

Dark Adaptation

The pO_2 was measured by FPQ and an oxygen microelectrode with the animal in a state of light adaptation and then after various periods of total darkness. Figure 6d shows the results of such an experiment. Intravascular pO_2 increased by 100% after only 2 min of adaptation. It then decreased as the result of light adaptation by the PQ excitation flash. There was no change in tissue pO_2. The hatched boxes in the figure represent time in the dark. Although not shown in the figure, changes in blood flow during dark adaptation were not significant.

These new methods for obtaining intravascular pO_2 in the ocular fundus, which are noninvasive to the eye and require only a small bolus injection of phosphorescent dye, should find important applications in the study of ocular

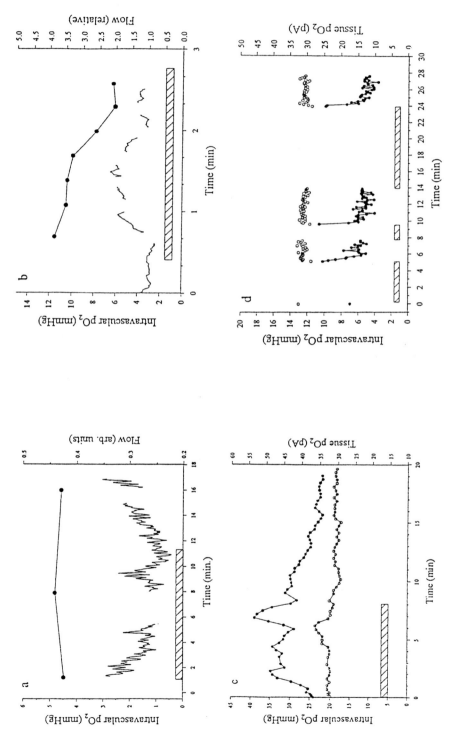

FIG. 6. Effect of hyperoxia (**a**), euthanasia (**b**), hypercapnia (**c**), and dark adaptation on intravascular (●) and tissue pO₂ (○), and blood flow (– –) (**d**). The application of the stimuli are indicated by a hatched rectangle. From ref. 10.

vascular diseases in experimental animals. Furthermore, coupled with oxygen-sensitive microelectrodes, a measure of extravascular oxygen, a more complete model of blood flow and oxygenation to the ocular fundus should be gained.

ACKNOWLEDGMENTS

Supported by a research grant no. 3200-043157.95 from Fonds National Suisse de la Recherche Scientifique and by Loterie Suisse Romande.

REFERENCES

1. Stefansson E. Oxygen and diabetic eye disease. *Graefes Arch Clin Exp Ophthalmol* 1990;228:120–3.
2. Hayreh SS. Pathogenesis of optic nerve lesion in glaucoma. *Trans Am Acad Ophthalmol Otolaryngol* 1976;81:197–213.
3. Schwartz B, Rieser J, Fishbein S. Fluorescein angiographic defects of the optic disk in glaucoma. *Arch Ophthalmol* 1977;95:1961–74.
4. Alder VA, Cringle SJ. Vitreal and retinal oxygenation. *Graefes Arch Clin Exp Ophthalmol* 1990;228:151–7.
5. Linsenmeier RA. Effect of light and darkness on oxygen distribution and consumption in the cat retina. *J Gen Physiol* 1986;88:521–42.
6. Pournaras CJ, Tsacopoulos M, Riva CE, Roth A. Diffusion of O_2 in normal and ischemic retinas of anesthetized miniature pigs in normoxia and hyperoxia. *Graefes Arch Clin Exp Ophthalmol* 1990;228:138–42.
7. Riva CE, Pournaras CJ, Tsacopoulos M. Regulation of local oxygen and blood flow in the inner retina during hyperoxia. *J Appl Physiol* 1986;61:592–8.
8. Shonat RD, Wilson DF, Riva CE, Pawlowski M. Oxygen distribution in the retinal and choroidal vessels of the cat as measured by a new phosphorescence imaging method. *Appl Opt* 1992;231:3711–8.
9. Shonat RD, Wilson DF, Riva CE, Cranstoun SD. Effect of acute increases in intraocular pressure on intravascular optic nerve head oxygen tension in cats. *Invest Ophthalmol Vis Sci* 1992;33:3174–80.
10. Cranstoun SD, Riva CE, Munoz J-L, Pournaras CJ. Measurements of intra and extra vascular pO_2 and blood flow in the optic nerve head of the minipig. *Proc 6th World Congr Microcirc* 1996:249–53.
11. Vanderkooi J, Mainara G, Green TJ, Wilson DF. An optical method for measurement of dioxygen concentration based upon quenching of phosphorescence. *J Biol Chem* 1987;252:5476–82.
12. Wilson D, Vanderkoi JM, Green G, et al. A versatile and sensitive method for measuring oxygen. *Adv Exp Med Biol* 1987;215:71–7.
13. Rumsy W, Vanderkooi J, Wilson D. Imaging of phosphorescence: a novel method for measuring oxygen distribution in perfused tissue. *Science* 1988;241:1649–51.
14. Riva CE, Harino S, Petrig BL, Shonat RD. Laser Doppler flowmetry in the optic nerve. *Exp Eye Res* 1992;55:499–506.
15. Petrig B, Riva CE. New continuous real-time analysis system for laser-Doppler flowmetry and velocimetry in the ocular fundus using a digital signal processor. *Vis Sci Appl* 1994;2:238–41.

Nitric Oxide and Endothelin in the Pathogenesis of Glaucoma, edited by I. O. Haefliger and J. Flammer. Lippincott–Raven Publishers, Philadelphia © 1998.

14

Nitric Oxide in the Outflow Pathways of the Aqueous Humor

Ernst R. Tamm and *Elke Lütjen-Drecoll

*Laboratory of Molecular and Developmental Biology, National Eye Institute, National Institutes of Health, Bethesda, Maryland; and *Department of Anatomy, University of Erlangen-Nürnberg, Erlangen, Germany*

Normal human eyes have an intraocular pressure (IOP) of 17–19 mm Hg, which is maintained because most of the aqueous humor leaves the eye by flowing against a certain resistance. The resistance is provided by the trabecular meshwork that is located between anterior chamber and Schlemm's canal (Fig. 1). The trabecular meshwork consists of three different portions: the uveal meshwork, the corneoscleral meshwork, and the cribriform or juxtacanalicular layer, which is located directly underneath the endothelial lining of Schlemm's canal (1). Recent experimental studies strongly indicate that the cribriform layer accounts for most of trabecular meshwork's resistance to aqueous outflow in the primate eye (2). Unlike the other two layers of the meshwork, the cribriform layer is less ordered and does not form trabecular beams. In contrast, it can be regarded as some sort of loose connective tissue composed of relatively free cells that are attached to each other and to the endothelial cells lining Schlemm's canal. In addition, the cribriform cells form contacts with fine collagen fibrils and a network of elastic fibers in the cribriform layer, the cribriform plexus (Fig. 2) (3). This elastic cribriform plexus is also connected with smaller fibrils to the endothelial cells of Schlemm's canal and, at its posterior aspect, with the elastic fibers in the scleral spur and the anterior elastic tendons of the ciliary muscle. A combined physiologic and morphometric study in monkeys showed a positive correlation between outflow facility and the area of optically empty spaces in the cribriform region (4). On the other hand, theoretical calculations about the pressure gradient in the cribriform area have shown that the area of these optically empty spaces is too large to provide a significant resistance to aqueous outflow (5,6). Therefore, it must be assumed that the spaces between cribriform cells and extracellular fibers are at least partly filled with some sort of ground substance, which probably consists of a variety of different glycosaminoglycans or proteoglycans. Some of the individual components of this ground substance, e.g., hyaluronic acid (7),

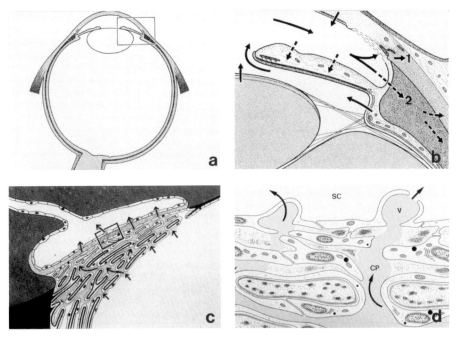

FIG. 1. Schematic drawing of the aqueous humor outflow pathways. **b:** Inset from **a.** Aqueous humor is secreted by the ciliary epithelium into the posterior chamber and flows through the pupil into the anterior chamber (*arrows*). Most of the aqueous humor leaves the eye by passing through the trabecular meshwork into Schlemm's canal (*1*). A minor part of the aqueous humor leaves the eye via the uveoscleral outflow pathways (*2*). **c:** Outflow pathways of aqueous humor (yellow) within the trabecular meshwork. **d:** Inset from c. Outflow pathways of the aqueous humor (yellow) within the cribriform area of the trabecular meshwork. SC, Schlemm's canal; V, vacuole.

have been identified. Others are still unknown. In addition, it remains unclear which of the components in the cribriform layer is finally responsible for the normal resistance to aqueous outflow.

Glaucoma is characterized by an IOP that is too high for the health of the eye and causes cupping and atrophy of the optic disk. In primary open-angle glaucoma (POAG), the reason for elevated IOP is an unusually high aqueous outflow resistance in the trabecular meshwork. In trabeculectomy specimens from patients with later stages of POAG, Rohen and Wittmer (8) found large amounts of extracellular material in the cribriform layer, which they called "plaque material." This observation was later confirmed by quantitative studies showing that the area of plaque material in eyes with POAG is significantly higher than in normal eyes of the same age group (9). A similar increase in plaque material was seen in trabeculectomy specimens from patients without prior treatment with antiglaucomatous drugs, indicating that the accumulation of plaque material is not due to secondary effects caused by therapy (10). The

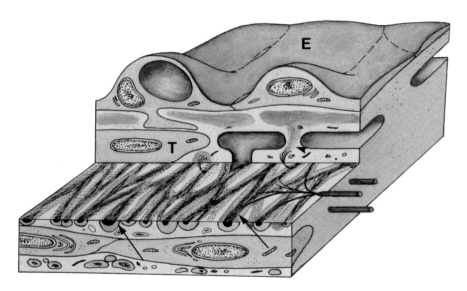

FIG. 2. Schematic drawing of the cribriform area of the trabecular meshwork. The extracellular fibrils in the cribriform region form a network, the so-called cribriform plexus (*arrows*). The fibers of the cribriform plexus are connected with trabecular cells (T) and, via connecting fibrils (*arrowhead*) with the endothelium (E) of Schlemm's canal.

nature of the plaque material is still not understood. Tangential sections through the inner wall of Schlemm's canal indicate that the plaques consist of thickenings of the elastic fibers in the cribriform region (11). Recently, we investigated donor eyes from patients with POAG in different stages of the disease, including early stages, and showed that the increase in IOP can occur before an increase in the amount of extracellular plaque material and/or before optic nerve damage (12). Even in eyes with advanced POAG, not all pathways for aqueous humor in the cribriform area are filled with plaque material, indicating that additional unknown structural or functional events have to contribute to the increase in outflow resistance in POAG. A possible candidate might be the "trabecular meshwork-induced glucocorticoid response protein" (TIGR), a reportedly secreted glycoprotein produced in large amounts by cultured human trabecular meshwork cells after long-term treatment with dexamethasone (13,14). Stone and co-workers (15) recently described mutations in the TIGR gene in families with juvenile glaucoma as well as in some patients with adult-onset POAG.

NITRERGIC NERVES AND INTRAOCULAR PRESSURE

In both normal and glaucomatous eyes, contraction of the ciliary muscle reduces IOP by decreasing trabecular meshwork resistance (4,16). The reason for this influence of ciliary muscle contraction on aqueous outflow resistance is the connection of the anterior tendons of the ciliary muscle with the connective tissue elements in the trabecular meshwork, especially with the elastic fiber plexus in the cribriform layer (3). Contraction of the muscle appears to change the architecture of the fibrillar extracellular components in the cribriform area, causing an increase in outflow pathways. Experimental studies in monkeys showed that by disinserting the ciliary muscle from the trabecular meshwork, the increase in outflow facility after ciliary muscle contraction induced by muscarinic agents could be abolished (17).

Recent studies indicate that there are other contractile cells in the chamber angle that might influence outflow resistance independently of ciliary muscle contraction. These cells reside in the scleral spur, a wedge-shaped ridge that projects from the inner side of the anterior sclera and provides the posterior attachment for the connective tissue elements of the corneoscleral and cribriform parts of the trabecular meshwork. The scleral spur cells (SSC) show structural characteristics of contractile myofibroblasts (18). They stain for α-smooth-muscle actin (Fig. 3a) and smooth-muscle myosin but not for desmin, which is the characteristic intermediate filament of ciliary muscle cells (19). In contrast to the adjacent longitudinal ciliary muscle bundles, the SSC form no bundles and are circumferentially oriented. The SSC form tendon-like contacts with the elastic fibers of the scleral spur, which are continuous with those of the adjacent trabecular meshwork (Fig. 3b). It is reasonable to assume that changes in SSC tone cause changes in trabecular meshwork architecture, thereby modulating the size of the outflow pathways for aqueous humor. Individual SSC are innervated by autonomic nerve endings that closely contact their cell membrane (Fig. 3d) (18). We characterized the nature of this innervation and found that a considerable number of terminal varicose axons contacting SSC stained for the neuronal isoform of nitric oxide synthase (NOS 1) (20), the enzyme that synthesizes nitric oxide (NO) in neuronal tissue (Fig. 3c) (21). In addition, the varicose axons in the scleral spur stain for NADPH-diaphorase (NADPH-D), a histochemical reaction that is considerably specific in visualizing neuronal NOS (22). It is extremely likely that NOS- and NADPH-D–positive scleral spur axons use NO as a neurotransmitter. Other scleral spur nerve fibers were immunoreactive for substance P, calcitonin gene-related peptide, vasoactive intestinal polypeptide, and neuropeptide Y (20). The NOS-positive or ''nitrergic'' axons in the scleral spur derive from nerve fiber bundles that run in the supraciliary space and appear to come from the posterior eye segment. They probably originate from the pterygopalatine ganglion, or perhaps from choroidal ganglion cells. Thus far, the physiologic role of the nitrergic SSC innervation remains the subject of speculation because no experimental data on the action of SSC in human eyes are available. A reasonable hypothesis is that a nitrergic innervation causes a decrease in SSC tone. In isolated bovine trabecular meshwork strips, relaxation was induced by application of organic nitrovasodilators (23). The posterior part of the bovine trabecular meshwork consists of many myofibroblast-like cells and appears to

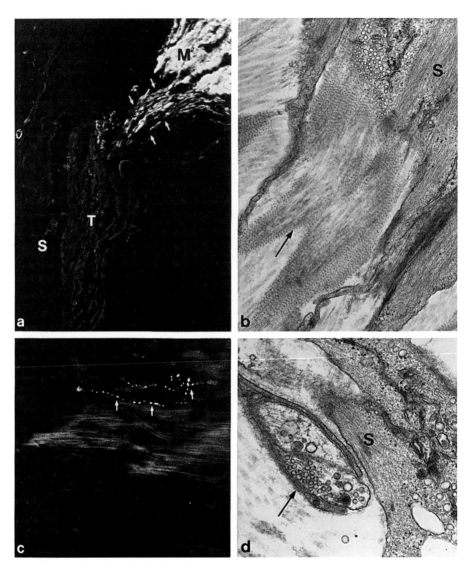

FIG. 3. Morphology of scleral spur cells and their innervation in the human eye. **a:** Chamber angle of a human eye after immunostaining for α-smooth-muscle actin. In addition to the cells of the ciliary muscle (M), many cells in the scleral spur (*arrows*) are positively labeled (×320. S, Schlemm's canal; T, trabecular meshwork. **b:** Tangential sections show that the cytoplasmic processes of the scleral spur cells (S) form tendon-like structures with the elastic fibers in the scleral spur (*arrow*) (×32,400). **c:** Tangential section through the scleral spur region in a human eye. Immunostaining with antibodies against neuronal NOS visualized many varicose, circumferentially oriented axons (*arrows*) in the scleral spur (×300). **d:** Electron micrograph of a nerve ending (*arrow*) contacting a scleral spur cell (S). The terminal contains both small (30−60-nm) agranular and large (65−100-nm) granular vesicles (×30,000). From ref. 46.

be equivalent to the scleral spur region in the human eye (24). Agents that cause relaxation of isolated bovine meshwork increase outflow facility in organ cultures of bovine anterior segments (25). In human and monkey eyes, application of organic nitrovasodilators decreases IOP (26,27), an effect that is caused in monkeys by a decrease in resistance to aqueous humor outflow. Taking these points together, it appears not to be unlikely that NO released from nitrergic scleral spur nerves decreases outflow resistance in the human eye.

No nitrergic nerves are found in the longitudinal or meridional portion of the ciliary muscle, which is responsible for the effects of the ciliary muscle on outflow facility. There is, however, a population of NOS-positive nerve cells in the inner, circular, and reticular portions, those parts of the human ciliary muscle that are crucial for accommodation (28). Because of this localization, NOS-positive ciliary muscle nerve cells are very probably not involved in modulating outflow facility but rather contribute to the processes of accommodation and disaccommodation.

The NADPH-D reaction stains not only the nerve cells in the ciliary muscle, but also, albeit with weaker intensity, ciliary muscle cells proper (28,29). It is very likely that this staining does not reflect the presence of neuronal NOS, because antibodies against this isoform do not react with ciliary muscle cells (28,29). Immunohistochemical findings by Nathanson and McKee (29) indicate that endothelial nitric oxide synthase (eNOS or NOS 3) in ciliary muscle cells might be responsible for the positive NADPH-D staining, although some nonspecific activity of the antibodies used to detect eNOS was noted by the authors. eNOS immunoreactivity has been found in mitochondria isolated from most mammalian tissues (30) and is especially abundant in oxidative, mitochondria-rich skeletal muscle fibers (31). Mitochondria may also contribute to positive eNOS and NADPH-D staining in ciliary muscle cells, because primate ciliary muscle cells are extremely rich in mitochondria (32,33). In addition, many structural details of ciliary muscle cells, such as the almost parallel myofibrils, the Z-band–like extensions of the dense bands, the rich innervation, and the absence of gap junctions all resemble those of striated skeletal muscle (33–35), as does the ciliary muscle's ability to contract and relax very rapidly (17). The role of mitochondrial NOS has yet to be determined. Two possibilities are involvement in oxidative phosphorylation or inactivation of mitochondrion-derived oxygen free radicals (30,31). Nathanson and McKee (36) reported that NADPH-D staining in the ciliary muscle of eyes with POAG was less intense than in controls. Although it should be emphasized that the NADPH-D reaction is a qualitative rather than a quantitative method, a decrease in muscle NADPH-D staining could indicate that structural changes in ciliary muscle cells are associated with POAG. Such changes have been reported earlier (37) but they probably reflect symptoms rather than the causative events of POAG, because they are also found in eyes with secondary glaucoma (38). Nathanson and McKee (36) also reported that in eyes with POAG the anterior insertion of the ciliary muscle to the scleral spur and trabecular meshwork was more posterior than in controls, and suggested a glaucoma-associated loss of anterior ciliary muscle cells. These findings are difficult to interpret, because large interindividual variations exist regarding the position of the anterior insertion of the ciliary muscle in the normal human eye (39).

Positive NADPH-D reactivity was also observed in the human trabecular meshwork by Nathanson and McKee (29), a finding that was not observed in our studies, at least not with incubation times that were sufficient to stain nerve cells, ciliary muscle, and ciliary epithelial cells. This indicates that NADPH-D

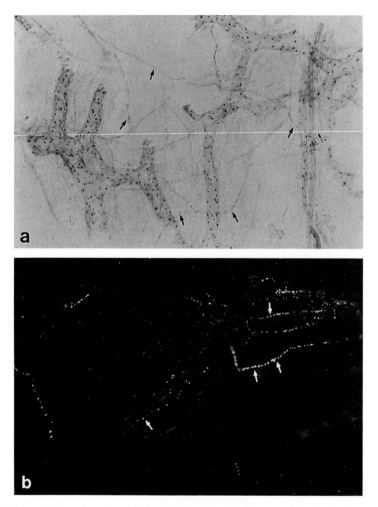

FIG. 4. Tangential sections through the episcleral region in a human eye. A dense network of NADPH-D–positive (**a**) and NOS-immunoreactive (**b**) axons (*arrows*) is observed in close contact with the vessels forming the episcleral venous plexus. In addition, there is markedly positive NADPH-D staining in the endothelial cells of the episcleral vessels (×200).

(and presumably NOS) activity in the human trabecular meshwork is considerably weaker than in other cell types of the human anterior eye segment.

After passing through the trabecular meshwork into Schlemm's canal, aqueous humor leaves the eye via flat collector channels that lead into the episcleral venous plexus (40). Resistance to aqueous humor outflow depends on the difference between IOP and episcleral venous pressure. There is some evidence that nitrergic nerves might influence outflow resistance, not only by modulating resistance in the trabecular meshwork but also by changing the diameter of the episcleral vessels, thus influencing episcleral venous pressure. In the human eye, the individual vessels of the episcleral venous plexus are in contact with a dense network of NADPH-D/NOS–positive axons (Fig. 4a,b). In addition, their endothelial cells stain intensely for NADPH-D, suggesting the presence of eNOS (NOS 3). In rabbit, dog, monkey, and human, the episcleral venous plexus forms arteriovenous anastomoses with arterioles that derive from branches of the anterior ciliary arteries (41–43). There is some evidence in the rabbit that the diameter of the anastomoses and the amount of blood shunted may influence episcleral venous pressure and, indirectly, outflow resistance (44). The arteriolar part of the arteriovenous anastomoses in rat, rabbit, and dog expresses a dense nitrergic innervation (45).

In summary, there appear to be two mechanisms by which nitrergic nerves might modulate IOP: by changing the tone of scleral spur cells, thereby modulating the architecture of the trabecular meshwork and in turn its outflow resistance, and by dilating episcleral vessels, thereby lowering episcleral venous pressure.

ACKNOWLEDGMENTS

Supported by grants from the Ria Freifrau von Fritsch-Stiftung of the University Erlangen-Nürnberg, Germany (ERT) and the Deutsche Forschungsgemeinschaft (ELD, Dr 124/6-3). ERT is the recipient of a Heisenberg Award from the Deutsche Forschungsgemeinschaft (Ta 115/8-1).

REFERENCES

1. Lütjen-Drecoll E, Rohen JW. Morphology of the aqueous outflow pathways in normal and glaucomatous eyes. In: Ritch R, Shields MB, Krupin T, eds. *The glaucomas, basic sciences,* 2nd ed. St. Louis: Mosby, 1996:89–123.
2. Maepea O, Bill A. Pressures in the juxtacanalicular tissue and Schlemm's canal in monkeys. *Exp Eye Res* 1992;54:879–83.
3. Rohen JW, Futa R, Lütjen-Drecoll E. The fine structure of the cribriform meshwork in normal and glaucomatous eyes as seen in tangential sections. *Invest Ophthalmol Vis Sci* 1981;21:574–85.
4. Lütjen-Drecoll E. Structural factors influencing outflow facility and its changeability under drugs. *Invest Ophthalmol Vis Sci* 1973;12:280–94.
5. Seiler T, Wollensak J. The resistance of the trabecular meshwork to aqueous humor outflow. *Graefes Arch Clin Exp Ophthalmol* 1985;223:88–91.

6. Ethier CR, Kamm RD, Palaszewski BA, Johnson MC, Richardson TM. Calculations of flow resistance in the juxtacanalicular meshwork. *Invest Ophthalmol Vis Sci* 1986;27:1741–50.
7. Lütjen-Drecoll E, Schenholm M, Tamm E, Tengblad A. Visualization of hyaluronic acid in the anterior segment of rabbit and monkey eyes. *Exp Eye Res* 1990;51:55–63.
8. Rohen JW, Witmer R. Electron microscopic studies on the trabecular meshwork in glaucoma simplex. *Graefes Arch Clin Exp Ophthalmol* 1972;183:251–66.
9. Lütjen-Drecoll E, Shimizu T, Rohrbach M, Rohen JW. Quantitative analysis of "plaque material" in the inner and outer wall of Schlemm's canal in normal and glaucomatous eyes. *Exp Eye Res* 1986;42:443–55.
10. Rohen JW, Lütjen-Drecoll E, Flügel C, Meyer M, Grierson I. Ultrastructure of the trabecular meshwork in untreated cases of primary open-angle glaucoma (POAG). *Exp Eye Res* 1993;56:683–92.
11. Lütjen-Drecoll E, Futa R, Rohen JW. Ultrahistochemical studies on tangential sections of the trabecular meshwork in normal and glaucomatous eyes. *Invest Ophthalmol Vis Sci* 1981;21:563–73.
12. Gottanka J, Johnson DH, Martus P, Lütjen-Drecoll E. Severity of optic nerve damage in eyes with POAG is correlated with changes in the trabecular meshwork. *J Glaucoma* 1997;6:123–32.
13. Fauss DJ, Bloom E, Lui GM, Kurtz RM, Polansky JR. Glucocorticoid (GC) effects on HTM cells: biochemical approaches and growth factor responses. In: Lütjen-Drecoll E, ed. *Basic aspects of glaucoma research III.* Stuttgart, New York: Schattauer-Verlag, 1993:319–30.
14. Polansky JR, Fauss DJ, Chen P, et al. Cellular pharmacology and molecular biology of the trabecular meshwork inducible glucocorticoid response (TIGR) gene product. *Ophthalmologica* 1997;211:126–39.
15. Stone EM, Fingert JH, Alward WLM, et al. Identification of a gene that causes primary open angle glaucoma. *Science* 1997;275:668–70.
16. Kaufman PL. Pressure-dependent outflow. In: Ritch R, Shields MB, Krupin T, eds. *The glaucomas.* St. Louis: CV Mosby, 1989:219–40.
17. Kaufman PL. Accommodation and presbyopia. In: Hart WMJ, ed. *Adler's physiology of the eye.* 9th ed. St. Louis: Mosby–Year Book, 1992:391–411.
18. Tamm E, Flügel C, Stefani FH, Rohen JW. Contractile cells in the human scleral spur. *Exp Eye Res* 1992;54:531–43.
19. Tamm E, Flügel C, Baur A, Lütjen-Drecoll E. Cell cultures of human ciliary muscle: growth, ultrastructural and immunocytochemical characteristics. *Exp Eye Res* 1991;53:375–87.
20. Tamm ER, Koch TA, Mayer B, Stefani FH, Lütjen-Drecoll E. Innervation of myofibroblast-like scleral spur cells in human and monkey eyes. *Invest Ophthalmol Vis Sci* 1995;36:1633–44.
21. Förstermann U, Kleinert H. Nitric oxide synthase: expression and expressional control of the three isoforms. *Naunyn Schmiedebergs Arch Pharmacol* 1995;352:351–64.
22. Blottner D, Grozdanovic Z, Gossrau R. Histochemistry of nitric oxide synthase in the nervous system. *Histochem J* 1995;27:785–811.
23. Wiederholt M, Sturm A, Lepple-Wienhues A. Relaxation of trabecular meshwork and ciliary muscle by release of nitric oxide. *Invest Ophthalmol Vis Sci* 1994;35:2515–20.
24. Flügel C, Tamm E, Lütjen-Drecoll E. Different cell populations in bovine trabecular meshwork: an ultrastructural and immunohistochemical study. *Exp Eye Res* 1991;52:681–90.
25. Wiederholt M, Bielka S, Schweig F, Lütjen-Drecoll E, Lepple-Wienhues A. Regulation of outflow rate and resistance in the perfused anterior segment of the bovine eye. *Exp Eye Res* 1996;61:223–34.
26. Wizemann A, Wizemann V. Untersuchungen zur ambulanten und perioperativen Augendrucksenkung mit organischen Nitraten. *Klin Mbl Augenheilk* 1980;177:292–5.
27. Schuman JS, Erickson K, Nathanson JA. Nitrovasodilator effects on intraocular pressure and outflow facility in monkeys. *Exp Eye Res* 1994;58:99–105.
28. Tamm ER, Flügel-Koch C, Mayer B, Lütjen-Drecoll E. Nerve cells in the human ciliary muscle. Ultrastructural and immunocytochemical characterization. *Invest Ophthalmol Vis Sci* 1995;36:414–26.
29. Nathanson JA, McKee M. Identification of an extensive system of nitric oxide-producing cells in the ciliary muscle and outflow pathway of the human eye. *Invest Ophthalmol Vis Sci* 1995;36:1765–73.

30. Bates TE, Loesch A, Burnstock G, Clark JB. Mitochondrial nitric oxide synthase: a ubiquitous regulator of oxidative phosphorylation? *Biochem Biophys Res Commun* 1996;218:40–4.
31. Kobzik L, Stringer B, Balligand J-L, Reid MB, Stamler JS. Endothelial type nitric oxide synthase in skeletal muscle fibers: mitochondrial relationships. *Biochem Biophys Res Commun* 1995;211:375–81.
32. Rohen JW, Kaufman PL, Eichhorn M, Goeckner PA, Bito LZ. Functional morphology of accommodation in the raccoon. *Exp Eye Res* 1989;48:523–37.
33. Tamm ER, Lütjen-Drecoll E. Ciliary body. *Microsc Res Tech* 1996;33:390–439.
34. van der Zypen E. Licht- und elektronenmikroskopische Untersuchungen über den Bau und die Innervation des Ziliarmuskels bei Mensch und Affe (*Cercopithecus ethiops*). *Graefes Arch Clin Exp Ophthalmol* 1967;174:143–68.
35. Samuel U, Lütjen-Drecoll E, Tamm ER. Gap junctions are found between iris sphincter smooth muscle cells but not in the ciliary muscle of human and monkey eyes. *Exp Eye Res* 1996;63:187–92.
36. Nathanson JA, McKee M. Alterations of ocular nitric oxide synthase in human glaucoma. *Invest Ophthalmol Vis Sci* 1995;36:1774–84.
37. Fine BS, Yanoff M, Stone RA. A clinicopathologic study of four cases of primary open-angle glaucoma compared to normal eyes. *Am J Ophthalmol* 1981;91:88–105.
38. Ueno M, Naumann GOH. Uveal damage in secondary glaucoma. *Graefes Arch Clin Exp Ophthalmol* 1989;227:380–3.
39. Fischer F. Entwicklungsgeschichtliche und anatomische Studien über den Skleralsporn im menschlichen Auge. *Graefes Arch Ophthalmol* 1933;133:318–58.
40. Ashton N. Anatomical study of Schlemm's canal and aqueous veins by means of neoprene casts: II Aqueous veins. *Br J Ophthalmol* 1952;36:265–77.
41. Rohen J. Arteriovenöse Anastomosen im Limbusbereich des Hundes. *Graefes Arch Ophthalmol* 1956;157:361–7.
42. Meighan SS. Blood vessels of the bulbar conjunctiva in man. *Br J Ophthalmol* 1956;40:513–26.
43. Funk RHW, Rohen JW. Scanning electron microscopic study of episcleral arteriovenous anastomoses in the owl and cynomolgus monkey. *Curr Eye Res* 1995;15:321–7.
44. Funk RHW, Gehr J, Rohen JW. Short-term hemodynamic changes in episcleral arteriovenous anastomoses correlate with venous pressure and IOP changes in the albino rabbit. *Curr Eye Res* 1996;15:87–93.
45. Funk RHW, Mayer B, Wörl J. Nitrergic innervation and nitrergic cells in arteriovenous anastomoses. *Cell Tissue Res* 1994;277:477–84.
46. Tamm E, Flügel C, Stefani FH, Rohen JW. Immunzytochemische und ultrastrukturelle Untersuchungen am menschlichen Skleralsporn. *Ophthalmologe* 1993;90:66–72.

Nitric Oxide and Endothelin in the Pathogenesis of Glaucoma, edited by I. O. Haefliger and J. Flammer. Lippincott–Raven Publishers, Philadelphia © 1998.

15

Nitric Oxide and Endothelin in Aqueous Humor Outflow Regulation

Michael Wiederholt

Institut für Klinische Physiologie, Universitätsklinikum Benjamin Franklin, Freie Universität Berlin, Berlin, Germany

FUNCTIONAL ANTAGONISM BETWEEN CILIARY MUSCLE AND TRABECULAR MESHWORK

The exact mechanism of outflow regulation is not fully understood. It has been generally accepted that contraction of the ciliary muscle (CM) via its insertion at the scleral spur and its tendons expands and spreads the trabecular lamellae and thus increases the filtration area of the cribriform meshwork (7,15,24,25). The experimental model of disinsertion of the CM in monkey eyes supported the concept that pilocarpine increased aqueous humor (AH) outflow by inducing contraction of the CM (8). The trabecular meshwork (TM) was considered to have no direct effect on AH outflow.

Recently, we presented evidence for contractile properties of the TM and postulated a direct contribution of the TM to the regulation of outflow in addition to the effect of the CM (31). In Table 1, the arguments for contractile properties of the TM are summarized. (a) It has been demonstrated that TM tissue and cultured meshwork cells of the eye of humans and various animals contain contractile filaments (α-actin) that are consistent with a smooth-muscle–like function of the meshwork. (b) In electrophysiologic experiments, we could show that cultured bovine and human TM cells showed voltage spikes typical of smooth-muscle cells, which could be inhibited by nifedipine but were insensitive to tetrodotoxin. The excitability of TM cells indicates that they function as contractile smooth-muscle cells. There is no principal difference between human and bovine TM cells concerning K^+ and Ca^{2+} channels. Using patch-clamp techniques, a Ca^{2+}-dependent maxi-K^+ channel could be described in bovine and human TM cells. This channel is of major importance for regulation of balance between contraction and relax-

TABLE 1. *Evidence for contractile properties of the trabecular meshwork (TM)*

Morphology
  Smooth-muscle–specific α-actin
Electrophysiology
  Membrane voltage measurements
    Voltage spikes typical for smooth-muscle cells
  Patch-clamp techniques
    Ca^{2+}-dependent maxi-K^+ channel involved in balance contraction/relaxation
Direct measurement of contractility of isolated TM
  Contraction induced by
    Cholinergic agonists
    α-Adrenergic agonists
    Endothelin
    Thromboxane
  Relaxation induced by
    Cholinergic antagonists
    β-Adrenergic agonists
    Ca^{2+}-channel blockers
    Nitric oxide
Perfused anterior segment (only TM)
  Substances that induce contraction of isolated TM
    → decrease of outflow
  Substances that induce relaxation of isolated TM
    → increase of outflow

ation of smooth-muscle cells (27). (c) Direct measurements of contractility of isolated meshwork strips could be performed for the first time (12,31). These measurements revealed muscarinic (mainly of the M_3 subtype), α- and β-adrenergic and endothelin receptors in TM and CM cells. Cholinergic and α-adrenergic (mainly α_2-agonists) induced contractions, whereas β-agonists produced relaxations. Relaxation was induced by release of nitric oxide (NO) (32). Most important, the contractile properties of TM and CM are differently modulated by various drugs. (d) In perfused anterior segments of the eye with only remaining functional TM, it could be demonstrated that substances that produced contraction in isolated TM strips induced a decrease in the outflow rate of the anterior segment. Relaxing substances induced an increase of the outflow rate (29).

From these experiments, a functional antagonism between CM and TM in regulation of AH outflow was postulated (31). This functional antagonism is illustrated in Fig. 1. Pilocarpine has a dual effect on CM and TM. In accordance with the conventional model of outflow regulation, contraction of the CM induced by pilocarpine leads to a functional relaxation of the TM and may decrease intraocular pressure (IOP) via an increase in the outflow. The concept that the CM is the exclusive modulator of AH regulation must be extended, because pilocarpine has an additional direct effect on the TM. The direct contraction of the TM induced by pilocarpine may lead to an increase in IOP via decrease of outflow. In this functional antagonism, the effect of

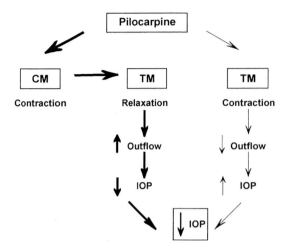

FIG. 1. Schematic representation of the effect of pilocarpine on aqueous humor outflow and regulation of intraocular pressure.

pilocarpine on CM is dominant. Therefore, the overall effect of pilocarpine might be a decrease in IOP.

This dual effect of pilocarpine can be exemplified by malignant glaucoma, in which a ciliary block quite often exists (23). It has been shown that miotics such as pilocarpine further increase the IOP in malignant glaucoma. This can be explained by our model (Fig. 2). Because of the ciliary block, pilocarpine may lead only to contraction of the TM and thus increase IOP.

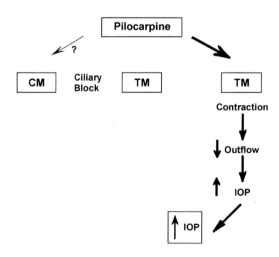

FIG. 2. Possible mechanism of increase in intraocular pressure induced by pilocarpine in malignant glaucoma.

MECHANISMS OF ACTION OF NO IN OUTFLOW REGULATION

The NO/cGMP system functions as an important intracellular mechanism for signal transduction (16). Nitric oxide synthase (NOS)-specific activity could be detected in ciliary processes and TM of the bovine eye (5). Recently, NOS has been described in the human outflow system and adjacent CM (17). The reactivity of NOS decreased in patients with primary open-angle glaucoma (POAG) (18). In various animal models, it has been shown that activation of the NO/cGMP system increases AH outflow and decreases IOP (2). Therefore, NO may be an important intracellular messenger in regulation of AH dynamics by modulating the contractile properties of the trabecular meshwork.

The NO/cGMP system is shown in Fig. 3. The entire cascade was tested in isolated TM and CM strips (32). The membrane-permeable 8-bromo-cGMP relaxed TM and CM strips precontracted by carbachol. As an inhibitor of NOS, L-arginine was used, which further contracted tissues stimulated by carbachol. The data indicate that in both TM and CM there is a constant release of NO, the TM system being more sensitive. As organic nitrates we used isosorbide dinitrate (ISDN) and isosorbide-5-mononitrate (ISMN). Both organic nitrates relaxed TM and CM strips precontracted by carbachol. Whereas organic nitrates are known to activate the soluble guanylate cyclase indirectly (via interaction with a thiol), non-nitrate vasodilators, such as sodium nitroprusside (SNP) and S-nitroso-N-acetyl penicillamine (SNAP), are known to be direct stimulators of

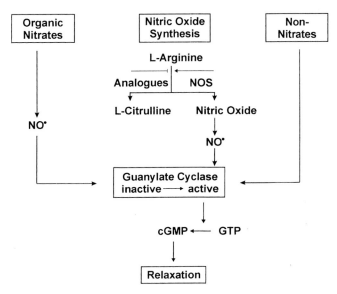

FIG. 3. Modulation of the guanylate cyclase/cGMP-system by three different pathways.

the cyclase (16). Both non-nitrates had the most effective relaxant activity on TM and CM. The powerful relaxing effect of the vasodilators demonstrates the presence of NOS in TM and CM. In general, the relaxant effects were stronger in TM compared to CM. Four different isoforms of NOS have been characterized and the enzyme may exist in soluble or particulate fractions of cells and may be constitutive or inducible (16). To test for the presence of the constitutive isoforms, ISDN and SNP were tested in tissues that were neither stretched nor stimulated by carbachol. Because both substances significantly relaxed resting TM and CM (32), there is evidence for the constitutive and inducible isoforms in TM and CM cells. In a recent article, a direct effect of NO on ion channels without requiring cGMP has been postulated (1,3). Among the various channels, a nonselective cation channel that is permeable to Na^+, K^+, and Ca^{2+} might be involved. Such a channel regulated by carbachol probably exists in TM and CM (30,33). From our experiments on direct measurements of contractility, however, it can be concluded that there is no interaction between the NO/cGMP system and the carbachol-regulated nonselective cation-channel pathway in inducing relaxation of TM and CM tissue. In smooth-muscle cells, a calcium-dependent maxi-K channel is receiving increasing attention (19). This channel appears to be most important for the regulation of smooth-muscle tone and is a target protein mediating the effect of various relaxant substances. By using patch-clamp techniques, we concentrated on the function of the maxi-K channel in TM cells (27). In single-channel recordings performed on bovine and human TM cells, we were able to demonstrate a high density of maxi-K channels. In whole-cell experiments, application of the membrane-permeable 8-bromo-cGMP

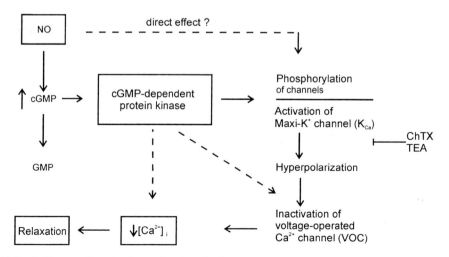

FIG. 4. Proposed mechanisms of action of NO/cGMP on relaxation of smooth muscle tissues such as trabecular meshwork and ciliary muscle. Modified from refs. 1 and 3.

to the external bathing solution led to a large increase in outward current. A specific blocker of the maxi-K channel, charybdotoxin, led to a reduction in the current induced by cGMP. The importance of the NO/cGMP system was recently documented in transformed human TM cells by an increase of intracellular cGMP by application of sodium nitroprusside (21).

The proposed mechanism of the NO/cGMP system on TM cells is summarized in Fig. 4. After activation of this channel by intracellular cGMP/NO, potassium leaves the cell through this channel, inducing hyperpolarization. This hyperpolarization then leads to inactivation of voltage-operated calcium channels and finally decreases intracellular calcium, inducing relaxation of the trabecular meshwork. As described for other smooth-muscle cells (19), the maxi-K channel also appears to serve as a negative-feedback mechanism in TM cells. This channel thus regulates the membrane voltage and intracellular calcium and hence the balance between contraction and relaxation. In TM, NO may modulate contractility and thus AH outflow by modulation of this channel.

ENDOTHELIN IN CONTRACTION OF TM AND CM

As summarized in Table 2 endothelin depolarized membrane voltage and increased intracellular calcium in TM and CM muscle cells. These are typical data in smooth-muscle cells indicating that endothelin might induce contraction. Contraction was directly measured in isolated strips of TM and CM (Table 2). Both tissues were contracted by 10^{-6} mol/L carbachol, which was the reference contractility in our measurements (100%). Compared to the contraction induced by carbachol, endothelin was much more effective on TM contraction (157%) compared to CM (54%). Furthermore, the endothelin-induced contractions were sensitive to intracellular calcium (13). Because the effect of endothelin on the TM is the dominating force, endothelin in high concentrations should increase IOP (Fig. 5).

Our data are in line with the present model of the effect of endothelin on contractility (19,22,26,28). Endothelin-induced contractions are partly dependent

TABLE 2. *Effects of endothelin-1*

	Trabecular meshwork	Ciliary muscle	References
Membrane voltage	Depolarization	Depolarization	9,11,13,14
Intracellular calcium	Increase	Increase	9,14
Contractility			13,30
Carbachol (10^{-6} mol/L)	100%	100%	
Endothelin (10^{-8} mol/L)	157%	54%	
Endothelin + flufenamic acid			
(10^{-4} mol/L)	32%	28%	

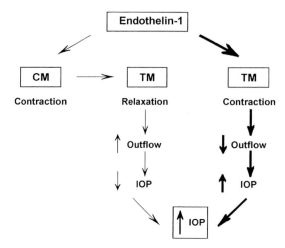

FIG. 5. The dominating effect of endothelin-1–induced contraction of the trabecular meshwork leads to an increase in intraocular pressure.

on extracellular calcium and L-type Ca^{2+} channels. In addition, outward Ca^{2+}-activated K^+ currents are involved. Furthermore, activation of nonspecific cation channels (which are permeable to Na^+, K^+, and Ca^{2+}) by endothelin has been postulated (13,28). To test this hypothesis, we applied the currently most sensitive blocker of nonselective cation channels, flufenamic acid (30). Most of the endothelin-induced contractions could be inhibited by the blocker of nonspecific cation channels (Table 2). The data support the assumption that a main effect of endothelin on contraction of TM (and CM) is by modulation of nonselective cation channels. A blocker of this channel can reduce the opening probability of the channel and thus decreases the influx of calcium from the extracellular compartment. This decrease in intracellular calcium induces relaxation, which is much more pronounced in TM as compared with the CM.

ENDOTHELIN IN AQUEOUS HUMOR

We demonstrated for the first time (Table 3) that endothelin-like immunoreactivity in AH of human and bovine eyes is two- to threefold higher than the

TABLE 3. *Endothelin-1 (ET-1) in aqueous humor*

Nonpigmented ciliary epithelial cells (10)
Release of ET-1 into aqueous humor
Immunocytochemical staining with antibodies against ET-1
Concentration of ET-1
Aqueous humor > Plasma (10)
Aqueous humor > Aqueous humor (20)
(POAG)   (Control)

corresponding plasma level (10,31). Furthermore, we showed that human nonpigmented ciliary epithelial cells express a high potential for releasing endothelin-like immunoreactivity. Immunocytochemically, intense staining for endothelin was found in cultured human nonpigmented ciliary epithelial cells and in ciliary epithelial cells of donor eyes (10). This suggests an important role of endothelin in regulation of AH secretion and outflow.

In perfused anterior segments of the bovine eye with only remaining TM, endothelin was a powerful substance to reduce AH outflow (29). These measurements are in contrast to data obtained in the perfused human eye, in which endothelin induced an increase in outflow (4). However, in this preparation the fraction of remaining TM and CM cells was not measured. The authors postulate an effect of endothelin on the CM (4). Indeed, according to our model (Fig. 5) this would lead to an increase in AH outflow.

In addition to being an important circulating vasoregulatory hormone, endothelin may represent a local humoral factor involved in regulation of AH dynamics (31). The constant secretion of endothelin by nonpigmented ciliary epithelial cells into the AH probably defines the basic contractility of contractile elements in the anterior part of the eye (TM, CM, iris). It is important to note that release of endothelin may be increased by stretch and by stimulation of fluid flow (26). Endothelin release into the aqueous humor may thus be changed by AH flow and/or IOP. Endothelin could be an intraocular factor partially responsible for the interaction between AH secretion and outflow. It can be speculated that dysfunction of such a feedback system may be involved in POAG. Recently, we found that endothelin-like immunoreactivity in AH of patients with POAG was significantly higher than in age-matched controls (patients with cataract) with normal IOP (Table 3) (20). There is no indication from our data whether the increase in endothelin in AH of patients with POAG is the cause or the consequence of glaucoma. It is interesting to note that plasma endothelin concentrations in normal-tension glaucoma are abnormal (6).

ACKNOWLEDGMENT

Supported by the Deutsche Forschungsgemeinschaft (DFG Wi 328/11 and Wi 328/19).

REFERENCES

1. Archer SL, Huang JMC, Hampl V, Nelson DP, Shultz PJ, Weir EK. Nitric oxide and cGMP cause vasorelaxation by activation of a charybdotoxin-sensitive K channel by cGMP-dependent protein kinase. *Proc Natl Acad Sci USA* 1994;91:7583–7.
2. Behar-Cohen FF, Goureau O, D'Hermies F, Courtois Y. Decreased intraocular pressure induced by nitric oxide donors is correlated to nitrite production in the rabbit eye. *Invest Ophthalmol Vis Sci* 1996;37:1711–5.

3. Bolotina VM, Najibi S, Palacino JJ, Pagano PJ, Cohen RA. Nitric oxide directly activates calcium-dependent potassium channels in vascular smooth muscle. *Nature* 1994;368:850–3.
4. Erickson-Lamy KA, Korbmacher C, Schuman JS, Nathanson JA. Effect of endothelin on outflow facility and accommodation in the monkey eye in vivo. *Invest Ophthalmol Vis Sci* 1991;32: 492–5.
5. Geyer O, Podos SM, Mittag TW. Nitric oxide synthase: distribution and biochemical properties of the enzyme in the bovine eye [Abstract]. *Invest Ophthalmol Vis Sci* 1993;34:826.
6. Kaiser HJ, Flammer J, Wenk M, Lüscher T. Endothelin-1 plasma levels in normal-tension glaucoma: abnormal response to postural changes. *Graefes Arch Clin Exp Ophthalmol* 1995; 233:484–8.
7. Kaufman P. Aqueous humor outflow. *Curr Top Eye Res* 1984;4:97–138.
8. Kaufman P, Bárány E. Loss of acute pilocarpine effect on outflow facility following surgical disinsertion and retrodisplacement of the ciliary muscle from the scleral spur in the cynomolgus monkey. *Invest Ophthalmol Vis Sci* 1976;15:793–807.
9. Korbmacher C, Helbig H, Haller H, Erickson-Lamy KA, Wiederholt M. Endothelin depolarizes membrane voltage and increases intracellular calcium concentration in human ciliary muscle cells. *Biochem Biophys Res Commun* 1989;164:1031–9.
10. Lepple-Wienhues A, Becker M, Stahl F, et al. Endothelin-like immunoreactivity in the aqueous humour and in conditioned medium from cultured ciliary epithelial cells. *Curr Eye Res* 1992;11:1041–6.
11. Lepple-Wienhues A, Rauch R, Clark AF, Grässmann A, Berweck S, Wiederholt M. Electrophysiological properties of cultured human trabecular meshwork cells. *Exp Eye Res* 1994;59:305–11.
12. Lepple-Wienhues A, Stahl F, Wiederholt M. Differential smooth muscle-like contractile properties of trabecular meshwork and ciliary muscle. *Exp Eye Res* 1991;53:33–8.
13. Lepple-Wienhues A, Stahl F, Willner U, Schäfer R, Wiederholt M. Endothelin-evoked contractions in bovine ciliary muscle and trabecular meshwork: interaction with calcium, nifedipine and nickel. *Curr Eye Res* 1991;10:983–9.
14. Lepple-Wienhues A, Stahl F, Wunderling D, Wiederholt M. Effects of endothelin and calcium channel blockers on membrane voltage and intracellular calcium in cultured bovine trabecular meshwork. *Germ J Ophthalmol* 1992;1:159–63.
15. Lütjen-Drecoll E, Rohen JW. Morphology of aqueous outflow pathways in normal and glaucomatous eyes. In: Klein EA, ed. *The glaucomas.* St. Louis: CV Mosby, 1989;89–123.
16. Moncada S, Palmer RMJ, Higgs EA. Nitric oxide: physiology, pathophysiology, and pharmacology. *Pharmacol Rev* 1991;43:109–42.
17. Nathanson JA, McKee M. Identification of an extensive system of nitric oxide-producing cells in the ciliary muscle and outflow pathway of the human eye. *Invest Ophthalmol Vis Sci* 1995;36:1765–73.
18. Nathanson JA, McKee M. Alterations of ocular nitric oxide synthase in human glaucoma. *Invest Ophthalmol Vis Sci* 1995;36:1774–84.
19. Nelson MT, Quayle JM. Physiological roles and properties of potassium channels in arterial smooth muscle. *Am J Physiol* 1995;268:C799–822.
20. Noske W, Hensen J, Wiederholt M. Endothelin-like immunoreactivity in aqueous humor of primary open angle glaucoma and cataract patients. *Graefes Arch Clin Exp Ophthalmol* 1997;235:551–2.
21. Pang IH, Shade DL, Clark AF, Steely HT, DeSantis L. Preliminary characterization of a transformed cell strain derived from human trabecular meshwork. *Curr Eye Res* 1994;13:51–63.
22. Pollock DM, Keith TL, Highsmith RF. Endothelin receptors and calcium signaling. *FASEB J* 1995;9:1196–204.
23. Rieser JC, Schwartz B. Miotic-induced malignant glaucoma. *Arch Ophthalmol* 1972;87:706–12.
24. Rohen J. Das Auge und seine Hilfsorgane. In: v. Möllendorff W, Bargmann W, eds. *Handbuch der mikroskopischen Anatomie des Menschen.* Bd. III/2 *Haut und Sinnesorgane.* Berlin: Springer-Verlag, 1964:189–328.
25. Rohen J, Futa R, Lütjen-Drecoll E. The fine structure of the cribriform meshwork in normal and glaucomatous eyes. *Invest Ophthalmol Vis Sci* 1981;21:574–85.

26. Rubanyi GM, Polokoff MA. Endothelins: molecular biology, biochemistry, pharmacology, physiology, and pathophysiology. *Pharmacol Rev* 1994;46:325–415.
27. Stumpff F, Strauss O, Boxberger M, Wiederholt M. Characterization of maxi-K-channels in trabecular meshwork and their regulation by cGMP. *Invest Ophthalmol Vis Sci* 1997;38 (in press).
28. van Renterghem C, Vigne P, Barhanin J, Schmid Alliana A, Frelin C, Lazdunski M. Molecular mechanism of action of the vasoconstrictor peptide endothelin. *Biochem Biophys Res Commun* 1989;157:977–85.
29. Wiederholt M, Bielka S, Schweig F, Lütjen-Drecoll E, Lepple-Wienhues A. Regulation of outflow rate and resistance in the perfused anterior segment of the bovine eye. *Exp Eye Res* 1995;61:223–34.
30. Wiederholt M, Dörschner N, Groth J. Effect of diuretics, channel modulators, and signal interceptors on contractility of the trabecular meshwork. *Ophthalmologica* 1997;211:153–61.
31. Wiederholt M, Lepple-Wienhues A, Stahl F. Contractile properties of trabecular meshwork and ciliary muscle. In: Lütjen-Drecoll, ed. *Basic aspects of glaucoma research, III.* Stuttgart: Schattauer, 1993:287–306.
32. Wiederholt M, Sturm A, Lepple-Wienhues A. Relaxation of trabecular meshwork and ciliary muscle by release of nitric oxide. *Invest Ophthalmol Vis Sci* 1994;35:2515–20.
33. Wiederholt M, Stumpff F. The trabecular meshwork and aqueous humor reabsorption. In: Civan MM, ed. *Current topics in membranes.* Vol. 45. *The eye's aqueous humor: from secretion to glaucoma.* San Diego: Academic Press, 1998;163–202 (in press).

Nitric Oxide and Endothelin in the Pathogenesis of Glaucoma, edited by I. O. Haefliger and J. Flammer. Lippincott–Raven Publishers, Philadelphia © 1998.

16

Nitric Oxide in the Human Eye: Sites of Synthesis and Physiologic Actions on Intraocular Pressure, Blood Flow, Sodium Transport, and Neuronal Viability

Dorette Ellis and James Nathanson

Department of Neurology, Harvard Medical School, and Neuropharmacology Research Laboratory, Massachusetts General Hospital, Charlestown, Massachusetts

This article investigates the tissue and cellular distribution of nitric oxide (NO) synthesis in the human anterior segment. Because this part of the eye contains a variety of tissues and cell types, which perform a variety of physiologic functions, it is not surprising that physiologic responses to NO and NO agonists are varied and complex. In part, this explains reported variability in the response of anterior segment tissues to exogenous agents but, at the same time, such complexity will eventually result in greater flexibility in using NO agonists and antagonists therapeutically. Particular areas of complexity and variability have involved the following: (a) changes in ocular blood flow in response to the same NO agonist in different parts of the ocular circulation; (b) differences in intraocular pressure (IOP) in response to different doses of the same agent or of the same agent evaluated in different species; (c) differences in whether inflow or outflow predominates in the effects of seemingly similar NO agents; and (d) varied reports of the actions of different NO agonists in either helping or hindering neuronal survival. Table 1 summaries some of the physiologic actions and pathophysiologic effects of NO in the human eye. Rather than being a hindrance to understanding, the rich and complex distribution of the NOS system creates possibilities for the use of NO-related agents, not only in the control of IOP in primary open-angle glaucoma (POAG) but also in the reduction of vasospasm in normotensive glaucoma (NTG), and possible prevention or ameliorations of the optic neuropathy in all of the glaucomas. (This same complexity has resulted in a large number of recent publications which, due to space limitations, can not all be noted here. For reviews and a more complete list of citations, see references.)

TABLE 1. *Nitric oxide in glaucoma: evidence for diverse physiologic and pathologic functions and a variety of therapeutic approaches[a]*

Effects on AH production
  NOS in secretory epithelium, likely inhibition
Effects on AH outflow
  NOS in TM spindle cells, probably decreasing resistance
  NOS in collecting channels and distal veins, decreasing resistance
  NOS in CM, increasing resistance in normal eye but less effect in POAG
  NOS in TM endothelium and Schlemm's canal endothelium; regulation of outflow at
    membrane level via effects on Na,K,Cl co-transporter; water channels
Limiting NO-mediated glutamate excitotoxicity (ganglion cells and optic nerve)
  Blocks NMDA receptors; channels or NOS
  Activate NTG/redox downregulation of NMDA receptor
Blocking NOS-initiated apoptosis of ganglion cells
  Blocks downstream cell death
Preventing NOS-mediated damage to optic nerve
  NOS in unmyelinated portion of optic nerve head (45)
  Induction of NOS isoforms in POAG (Hernandez et al., personal communication)
Optimizing ganglion cell energy metabolism
  NO alters ATP levels via Na pump regulation
Effects on ocular blood flow [optimize flow in POAG and eliminate vasospasm in
    normotensive glaucoma (NTG)]
  Use of NO agonists and endothelin antagonists to reverse evidence of altered choroidal,
    retinal, and ONH blood flow
  Interfere with hormone or flow-mediated NO mechanisms in arterial endothelium
  Interfere with NO mechanisms in vascular smooth muscle
Limiting action of oxygen free radicals
  Remove or reduce generation of free radicals by NO to block free radical toxicity
  Reverse modulating effects of free radicals on cell energy metabolism by blocking
    cGMP/PKG pathway
Alter primary disease process
  Recent evidence for defect of NOS-containing cells in long CM
  Possible additional alterations in ONH and retrochoroidal NOS; primary? secondary?
    implications for function?

[a] Above data are from experiments in this and other laboratories. See text for references.

HISTORICAL BACKGROUND

NO is a key inter- and intracellular regulator in a number of organs and tissues, including blood vessels, immune cells, smooth muscle, nervous system, and some endothelia. Historically, our interest in wanting to establish the existence of a NO synthase (NOS) system in the anterior segment began before the original discovery that NO can serve as a physiologic regulator in cells. The reason for this early recognition of NO's potential role provides an interesting scientific sidelight on NO action, and begins with work of this and other laboratories on the systemic, fluid-regulating natriuretic peptides (NPs). It was an understanding of how NPs act, especially their use of cGMP as a second messenger, that led to investigation of nitrovasodilators (NTVs) as IOP-lowering agents and eventually to speculation (1) that NTVs mimic some natural nonpeptide, cGMP-stimulating substance in the eye. Because of this conceptual connection with NPs and cGMP, it is of interest to describe briefly some of these earlier findings.

ATRIOPEPTIN-ACTIVATED MEMBRANE GUANYLYL CYCLASE: ROLE IN AQUEOUS HUMOR AND CEREBROSPINAL FLUID PRODUCTION

About a decade ago, we proposed that the then newly discovered atrial natriuretic factor (or peptide; ANF; ANP), a salt-losing, diuretic regulatory factor present in the circulation, also acts on the choroid plexus (CP) and ciliary process (Cil. Proc.) to decrease cerebrospinal fluid (CSF) secretion, inhibit aqueous humor (AH) production, lower IOP, and cause large increases in membrane guanylyl cyclase (mGC) activity (for reviews see refs. 1–8). Of related interest was the puzzling discovery in CP (1) and Cil. Proc (8) of DARPP-32, a dopamine- and cAMP-regulated phosphoprotein (DARPP-32). The discovery of DARPP-32 in the CP epithelium (Fig. 1a,b) was rather puzzling because the CP lacks D-1 dopaminergic receptors [which, when activated, increase cAMP production and stimulate cAMP-dependent protein kinase (PKA) and the phosphorylation of substrate proteins including DARPP-32] (Fig. 2).

The discovery that CP contains high concentrations of NP receptors and PKG raised the question of whether CP DARPP might be phosphorylated, not in response to dopamine (DA)-activating cAMP and PKA but in response to ANP-stimulating cGMP. Using antibodies that distinguish between phosphorylated and dephosphorylated forms of DARPP, it was demonstrated that when ANP stimulates cGMP it also phosphorylates DARPP-32 (9) at the same site phosphorylated by DA-activated PKA, an effect mimicked by the cell-permeable analogue of cGMP, 8-bromo-cGMP. Phosphorylated DARPP-32 is a potent inhibitor of protein phosphatase type 1 (PP type 1), a major protein phosphatase inhibitor present in many cell types. Because of this, DARPP-32 is a functional enhancer of the phosphorylation of other substrates, phosphorylated by either the cAMP- or cGMP-dependent pathway. It was therefore of interest to determine the biochemical mechanism by which ANP (NPs) regulate fluid homeostasis in these tissues.

$\longrightarrow$

FIG. 1. A: Shown by immunostaining, the phosphoprotein DARPP-32 (bright yellow) is highly enriched in secretory epithelium of Cil. Proc. and CP (shown here) and is largely absent from vascular and other cell types, visible as a faint green color (the streak is an autofluorescent artifact). In this experiment, the CP was subjected to a procedure that removed most of the epithelium but left the seven cells shown (15–20 μm in diameter). A similar localization has been observed in Cil. Proc and appears to be involved in secretion of AH. DARPP-32 regulates the activity of Na,K-ATPase through dephosphorylation. DARPP-32 itself is regulated by certain hormones and cellular messengers, including ANF and NO, which alter cellular cGMP levels (see text). **B:** Secretory epithelial cells of the type found in CP and Cil. Proc. (NPE), whose fluid production is regulated by both NO and NPs. Stained here with an antibody to DARPP-32, such isolated cells accumulate large amounts of cGMP when stimulated with NO agonists or NPs, and are highly enriched in PKG and Na,K-ATPase.

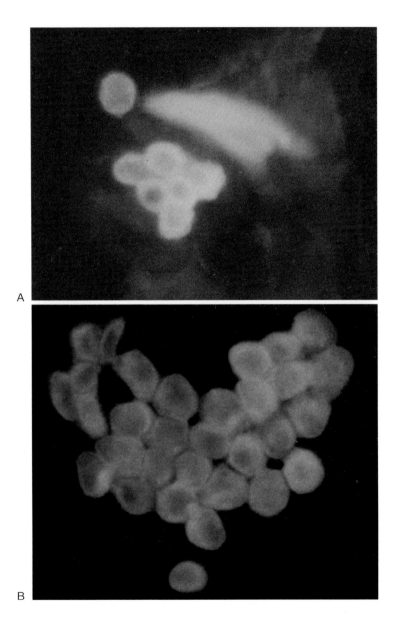

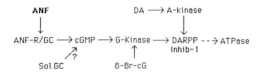

FIG. 2. Proposed pathway by which NPs such as ANF regulate active sodium transport in secretory epithelium and certain other cell types. Previous research had restricted activation of the pathway to hormones, such as dopamine, that stimulate synthesis of cAMP which, in turn, activated PKA. Studies of ANF action in the kidney and eye indicate that hormones and messengers that function through cGMP synthesis can stimulate PKG to phosphorylate the same sites as PKA. This observation laid the groundwork for the discovery that other cGMP-generating hormones and messengers, such as NO, also use this regulatory pathway.

FUNCTIONAL ASPECTS OF ANP AND mGC: REGULATION OF THE Na,K-ATPase

The Na,K-ATPase (sodium pump) is a plasma membrane protein composed of two different polypeptides, the catalytic α-subunit and the β-subunit. There are four known isoforms of Na,K-ATPase, $\alpha1$, $\alpha2$, $\alpha3$, and $\alpha4$, which are inhibitable by the cardiac glycosides digitalis and ouabain. The Na,K-ATPase catalyzes transfer of $2K^+$ (from the extracellular space into the cell) and the extrusion from the cell of $3Na^+$, while hydrolyzing ATP to ADP and P_i. This creates an electrochemical gradient, necessary for ion movement through passive channels and needed for the function of certain other ion transporters and co-transporters. The expression of different Na,K-ATPase isoforms is highly tissue- and species-dependent. However, the functional significance of this diversity is not clear. For example, three isoforms have been identified in the Cil. Proc. (10). The $\alpha1$ isoform is the major form in the kidney, and $\alpha2$ and $\alpha3$ isoforms are enriched in the brain (11).

ANP inhibits sodium and water reabsorption in tubule epithelial cells of the CP-like kidney via a cGMP-dependent process. Although this effect is due in part to the passive regulation of a cation channel, there is also evidence of active Na^+ reabsorption by ANP. Because DA can regulate active Na^+ transport via a mechanism involving cAMP-dependent phosphorylation of DARPP-32, and because of ANP's ability to phosphorylate DARPP-32 in the CP, we investigated the possibility that the Na,K-ATPase might be regulated by hormones and messengers using cGMP. The small amount of tissue available in CP made kidney a more practical initial target of investigation.

Studies in the kidney did indeed demonstrate that ANP causes long-term modulation of the Na,K-ATPase, concomitant with increases in cGMP levels (12). cGMP-dependent protein phosphorylation is involved, because inhibitors of PKG completely obliterated ANP inhibition of the sodium pump, whereas PKA inhibitors had no effect on ANP-induced modulation of the sodium pump (12). Various controls showed that the effect of ANP occurs as a result of hormone activation, and not in response to alterations of intracellular sodium concentrations or to indirect effects of cAMP-dependent alterations in phosphodiesterase activity. These findings were the first to supply strong evidence that regulation of the Na,K-ATPase is not limited to cAMP [and perhaps the protein kinase C (PKC) pathway as well] but is also regulated by cGMP and hormones, such as ANP, that use this second messenger (Fig. 2). Inhibition of Na,K-ATPase reduces the driving force for sodium reabsorption and is an important mechanism for altering the rate of Na$^+$ and water movement across certain epithelia.

Although therapeutic use of ANP for lowering IOP is limited because of poor absorption of topically applied peptide, the above findings raised an important question. Because local cGMP synthesis in the eye appears to be involved in the ocular hypotensive effect of ANP, might exogenous lipophilic activators of other GCs, such as soluble GC (sGC), mimic the action of ANP and bring about ocular hypotension when applied topically to the eye? [It should be noted that recent studies indicate that NP action is more complex than described, due in part to the presence of NP receptor subtypes, some more responsive to BNP or CNP than to ANP. These receptors are present not only in CP but also in the TM and possibly in other outflow areas.]

NITROVASODILATORS: SOLUBLE GUANYLYL CYCLASE REGULATION OF IOP

Nitrovasodilators (NTVs) are a group of nitrogen-containing compounds, including nitroglycerin, amyl nitrite, sodium nitroprusside (SNP), and hydralazine, that have been used for many years to relax blood vessels and treat systemic hypertension and coronary vasospasm. Because NTVs stimulate sGC (13) and increase cGMP levels, it was of interest to test the effects of NTVs on IOP. Topical application of nitroglycerin, hydralazine, and a number of other NTVs to normal or ocular hypertensive rabbits, caused a decrease in IOP (Fig. 3)

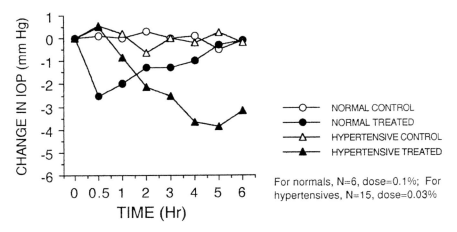

FIG. 3. Ocular hypotensive effect of topical hydralazine on IOP in normal and ocular hypertensive rabbits. The hypotensive effect of this NTV was greater in animals that had an elevated IOP. In humans, POAG patients may also show an increased sensitivity relative to normal patients due to an observed atrophy of the anterior longitudinal portion of the ciliary muscle.

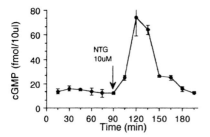

FIG. 4. Direct evidence for the presence of an endogenous NO-synthesizing system in the human outflow pathway is shown in this experiment, in which an isolated anterior segment containing TM, Schlemm's canal, collecting channels, and draining veins is examined in organ culture. Addition of a bolus of nitroglycerine to the entering superfusion fluid results in a marked increase in cGMP levels in the exiting fluid (average facility increase was 35% to 10 μM NTG and 69% to 100 μM) (Nathanson and Erickson, unpublished studies).

without any observable alterations in systemic blood pressure. Of interest, over the past 70 years there have been several anecdotal reports of the ocular effects of systemic NTVs, and results have been varied. In one well-controlled study, however, administration of nitroglycerin lowered IOP at doses that did not change systemic blood pressure (14). These findings take on significance now that it is known that NTVs mimic NO, and therefore suggest a role for NO in the regulation of IOP and other physiologic processes in the anterior segment. Consistent with a mechanism involving cGMP, perfusion of the isolated, organ-cultured human anterior segment is associated with a marked increase in cGMP in AH exiting the eye (Fig. 4).

Of considerable interest, and somewhat surprising, was the fact that, although NTVs do cause a small decrease in AH secretion, they have a larger effect on outflow facility. In contrast, NPs cause a large decrease in AH secretion and a rather modest decrease in outflow facility. In addition, whereas the small effect of NPs on outflow is to increase resistance, NTVs cause a a decrease in outflow resistance. This difference in physiology suggested that NTVs act independently of NPs and affect a different set of target tissues. These results also suggested that NO may have a normal physiologic role in regulating IOP in the eye.

Earlier immunohistochemical studies using an antibody to the nNOS (bNOS) looking for endogenous NO production in rat anterior segment demonstrated a modest but not extensive array of NO-synthesizing nerve terminals (15). This was surprising because of the assumption that the action of NTVs on AH regulation was due to the fact that NTVs mimic some endogenous NO-like substance in the anterior segment of the eye. The failure to identify much in the way of endogenous NOS raised the possibility (later disproved) that NTVs lack an endogenous NO counterpart and might be working through an entirely different mechanism, one not involving cGMP.

MECHANISM OF ACTION OF NTVs IN THE EYE

One way of supplying evidence of whether or not NTVs are working, at the cellular level, through cGMP was to determine their ability to modulate the cGMP/PKG-initiated modulation of the sodium pump. A positive result would also supply important information, in general, about the mechanisms that NO

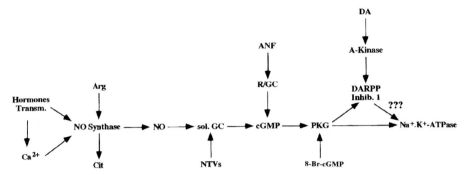

FIG. 5. Experiments in CP, kidney, eye, and brain indicate that stimulation of NO synthesis by a variety of hormones causes major alterations in activity of the key enzyme, Na,K-ATPase. Such regulation has relevance to water and ion transport as well as cell viability (see text). Hormones often activate NOS by mobilizing calcium. NO, produced from the conversion of arginine (arg) to citrulline (cit), stimulates GC and the synthesis of cGMP which, through PKG and other proteins (e.g., DARPP, inhibitor-1), eventually alters activity of the sodium pump. This same pathway is shared, in part, by NPs such as ANF and hormones acting through PKA (A-kinase) or PKC (not shown). Because of the complexity of the pathway, there exist a number of sites that can be targeted by drugs (e.g., NTVs, 8-Br-cGMP) aimed at altering sodium pump activity.

uses in various cell types. Because of its relative tissue abundance and uniformity and because of our prior work showing NP regulation of Na,K-ATPase, rat and calf kidney were used to investigate the actions of NTVs on the sodium pump. In this organ, acetylcholine and bradykinin have been implicated in activating NO synthesis, and by use of procedures similar to those used for the NPs it was demonstrated that NTVs mediate the action of these hormones to exert a potent regulation of Na,K-ATPase (16). This regulation was blocked by hemoglobin and by inhibitors of PKG, indicating a pathway similar to that used by the NPs. However, distinct from NP action, the effects of hormones capable of stimulating NO synthesis differed from that of NPs in being blockable by inhibitors of NOS, such as nitro-arginine. This result, supported by similar studies in brain (17), provides a new mechanism to help explain some of the observed physiological actions of NO in a variety of tissues (see Fig. 5). [NO also acts through other mechanisms. In smooth muscle, e.g., it appears that NO causes deactivation of myosin light-chain kinase, opposing the pathway by which acetylcholine initiates calcium-mediated smooth-muscle contraction.]

NOS ISOZYMES AND FACTORS AFFECTING THE DISCOVERY OF ENDOGENOUS NO IN THE HUMAN ANTERIOR SEGMENT

The eventual discovery of isozymes of NOS in human ocular anterior segment resulted from studies in the kidney, where, as was the case for the eye, NO distribution had been believed to be limited to a very small part of the kidney, the juxtaglomerular apparatus. This localization had been based on studies of bNOS, one of the three genetically distinct isoform of NOS (18,19). Another isoform is endothelial NOS (eNOS), originally discovered in blood vessels and previously known as endothelium-derived relaxing factor (EDRF), mediating the action of blood-borne hormones and shear stress on vasodilation. The third isoform is inducible or macrophage NOS (iNOS or mNOS), made in macrophages during certain inflammatory responses and capable of producing NO at concentrations high enough to induce formation of oxygen free radicals and to be toxic to invading organisms (18,20).

As noted above, the substantial effects of NTVs on sodium pump regulation were not consistent with the small amount of NOS reported in the juxtaglomerular apparatus. This suggested a more extensive source of NO. When other isozymes were evaluated using isozyme-specific antisera, an extensive system of eNOS-containing tubule cells was discovered both in the thick ascending medullary limb (TAL) and in the cortical portion of the distal convoluted nephron (16). In studies using porcine LLC-PK1 tubule epithelial cells, eNOS makes a marked appearance as cell monolayers differentiate into renal tubule-like structures (Fig. 6). Although undifferentiated monolayers showed very low levels of

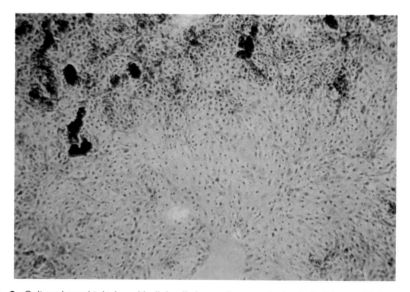

FIG. 6. Cultured renal tubule epithelial cells have pharmacologic similarities to Cil. Proc NPE and have been developed by the authors as a model for studying NO action in the eye. This low-power photomicrograph demonstrates how the cellular monolayer (top) differentiates into tubule-like structures that stain intensely for the NOS marker NADPH-d and appear almost black. A method has been developed for harvesting and purifying the tubules, which demonstrate NO synthesis and cGMP accumulation in response to acetylcholine and certain other hormones (16). Tubule NOS can be further induced with application of certain cytokines, suggesting that such epithelial cells may also contain an inducible isoform of NOS. This latter observation, if present in ciliary epithelium, is relevant to studies showing increased NO synthesis in experimental uveitis.

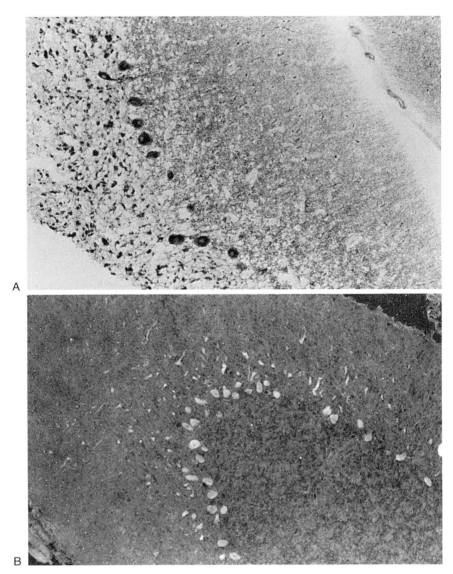

FIG. 7. Use of current nomenclature for NOS isoforms can be restrictive and misleading. Thus, the endothelial isoform (eNOS) is present also in epithelial cells (Fig. 6) and smooth muscle (Fig. 8). Furthermore, as shown here, cerebellar Purkinje neurons of the cerebellum contain a macrophage isoform of NOS. Photomicrographs show diaphorase reactivity of these large cells (**A**), and another section (**B**) shows immunoreactivity specific for mNOS (Nathanson and McKee, unpublished observations). Earlier schemes explaining NO function in the cerebellum assumed that NO was absent in these cells, but were formulated incorrectly, using data for localization of the neural isoform.

NOS immunoreactivity, at 3–5 days the cells assembled into tubule-like structures, with a selective increase in eNOS immunoreactivity.

MISLEADING NOMENCLATURE: eNOS IN EPITHELIAL CELLS AND mNOS IN NERVE CELLS

The fact that the presence of an entire renal tubule system could be overlooked emphasizes the importance of examining all isoforms of NOS when a tissue is evaluated for NO function. It also points out that current terminology of NOS isoforms may inadvertently restrict thinking about the true extent of NO function. As noted above, eNOS is not found solely in endothelia but also in some epithelial cell layers and in smooth muscle (see below). Another example, noted several years ago (Nathanson and McKee, unpublished observations), is the incorrect notion, derived from immunochemical studies using anti-bNOS, that Purkinje neurons of the cerebellum do not produce NO. However, as shown in Fig. 7A, diaphorase reactions show extensive reactivity of these cells, and immunochemical studies (Fig. 7B) reveal that this is due to the presence of the macrophage isoform of NOS in these large-output neurons. This finding has implications for physiologic studies of NO function in the brain, yet went undetected for some time, in part because of restrictive notions of the distribution of NOS isoforms based on nomenclature.

NO SYNTHASE: DISTRIBUTION IN ANTERIOR SEGMENT

Results in the kidney suggested that all NOS isoforms needed to be evaluated in the search for endogenous NO-generating cells in human anterior segment. Using NADPH-diaphorase (NADPH-d), a technique that identifies all three isoforms of NOS, the human anterior segment was found to be markedly enriched in NOS. This was confirmed in immunohistochemical studies using isozyme-specific antisera (Fig. 8), which show dramatically that most NOS in the human anterior segment is of the eNOS isoform, thus explaining why localization of bNOS apparently showed relatively few sites of NO synthesis.

→

FIG. 8. Distribution of the three isoforms of NOS in the human anterior segment, showing dramatically, using immunocytochemistry, that most NO synthesis is from the endothelial isoform (**a**), explaining why prior studies localizing the neural isoform (**b**) concluded incorrectly that NO is confined primarily to NPE and a small number of nerve fibers. Actually, extensive NO synthesis occurs in the ciliary muscle and smooth muscle of the iris as well as in TM and in endothelia and smooth-muscle cells throughout the AH outflow pathway. A few mNOS-containing macrophage-like cells are seen in (**c**) although cytokine stimulation studies by the authors suggest that some epithelia also demonstrate an inducible form of NOS. From Nathanson et al. (22).

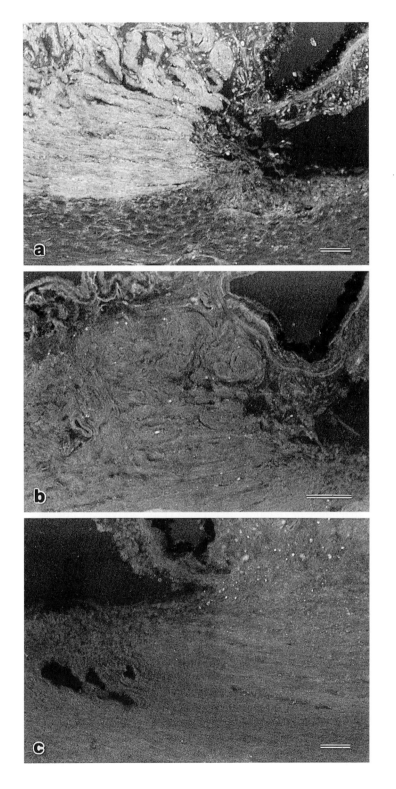

Ciliary Process

In addition to its presence in the ciliary vascular endothelium, NOS activity is highly enriched in the nonpigmented ciliary epithelium, with very little in the pigmented epithelium. Interestingly, it appears that both bNOS and eNOS are present (note, however, that immunochemical studies of ciliary epithelium need careful interpretation because of the presence of many immunoglobulin receptors, which can create false localization). The presence of NOS in ciliary epithelium suggests the possibility of regulation of AH secretion. In fact, a small degree of regulation has been observed (21), but the intensity of NOS labeling and the apparent presence of two isoforms suggest that additional functions for NO may exist in this tissue. NOS is also present in a small number of nerve fibers, both in the stroma and near blood vessels, in the Cil. Proc, as well as in other parts of the anterior segment, suggesting the existence of neural regulation of uveal blood flow (see below).

Ciliary Muscle

The human ciliary muscle (CM) contains high concentrations of NADPH-d and immunostaining for eNOS isoform. The CM consists of two morphologically distinct muscles, each with its own unique function: the longitudinal CM with its tendonous connections to the TM (implicated in the regulation of AH outflow and IOP), and the inner, circular, and reticular portion of the CM (connected to the lens and regulating accommodation) are both markedly enriched in eNOS (22). NADPH-d activity is present in muscle fibers, some NO-containing nerve fibers within the muscle (Fig. 9), and a small number of CM neuronal cell bodies. The presence of eNOS in the CM has been substantiated by biochemical demonstration of NO production (22). Other laboratories have independently confirmed NO production in the CM (23) and in other smooth muscles such as the trachea (24). Biochemical studies have also demonstrated that NTVs cause a cGMP-dependent modulation of Na,K-ATPase activity in bovine CM slices (25). Other studies (26) have shown that NTVs raise cGMP levels not only in CM culture cells line but also in TM endothelial cells and in TM actin-containing muscle-like cells.

TM and Schlemm's Canal

TM cells are heterogeneous in nature, consisting of TM endothelial cells, actin-containing muscle-like cells, nerve fibers, and phagocytic cells. eNOS is localized to a subset of cells present in the outer, intermediate, and juxtacanalicular areas of the TM (Fig. 10). The deepest innermost layers of the TM, which traditionally have been believed to be the areas of greatest resistance to AH outflow, are especially enriched in NOS, as visualized by NADPH-d staining (Fig. 11). In Schlemm's canal, NOS is present in the endothelium of both the

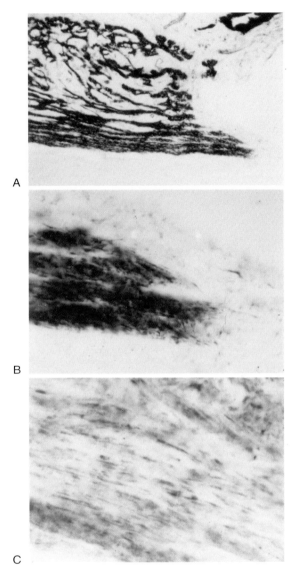

FIG. 9. Diaphorase reactivity in human CM, showing the presence of NOS marker throughout the muscle, but most intensely (blue-black) in the anterior portion of the longitudinal portion (**B**; higher magnification of **A**). When under-reacted, the CM reveals, at high power (**C**) that activity is present in both smooth muscle and nerve fibers and (see later figures) in a small number of nerve cell bodies.

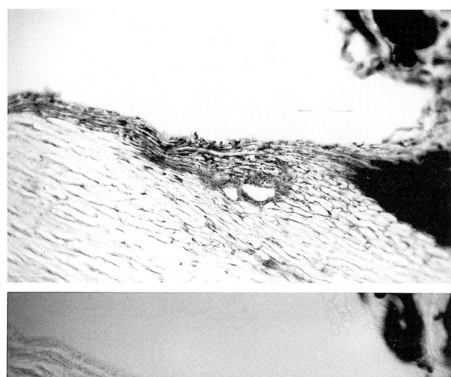

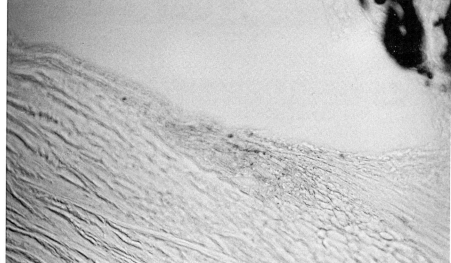

FIG. 10. A: Medium power view of human outflow pathway stained for diaphorase. Note presence of NOS reactivity in TM and endothelium of Schlemm's canal. At right is the intensely-stained anterior portion of longitudinal CM. Upper right is pigment. **B:** When NADPH co-factor is omitted, diaphorase reaction fails to stain, revealing a small amount of pigment in the TM as well.

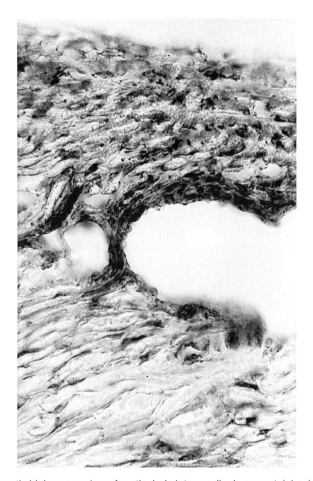

FIG. 11. Dramatic high-power view of particularly intense diaphorase staining in subcanicular cells of TM just below endothelia of Schlemm's canal, which is also reactive. Also positive are many of the giant vacuoles budding from Schlemm's endothelium. TM also shows many positive spindle-like cells as well as more typical endothelia and amorphous (possibly phago-cytic) cells. Heavy reactivity in area of TM near canal coincides with area of TM known to contain tighter packing of cells and much of the known resistance of the TM. This new finding further supports a possible regulatory role for NO in outflow resistance.

inner and the outer wall. Of particular interest, NOS is co-localized with Na,K-ATPase in the walls of giant vesicles budding from the inner wall, raising the possibility of active regulation of transport in the area.

Collecting Channels and Draining Veins

eNOS is also present in the endothelium of collecting channels as well as in vascular endothelium of draining veins.

Vasculature

eNOS is present in arteriolar endothelial and smooth-muscle cells throughout the anterior segment. Like blood vessels in other organs, NO agonists have been shown by a number of laboratories to induce vasodilatation of smooth muscle and large vessels and to increase blood flow to the choroid and anterior segment of the eye. These agonists may mimic certain blood-borne hormones that stimulate synthesis of NO in the endothelium, which diffuses and subsequently causes the relaxation of vascular smooth muscle. It is not yet clear which hormones may be most important in ocular vessels. Blood flow may also act as a mechanical trigger for endothelial NO production and subsequent vasodilatation. A third trigger may come from bNOS-containing nerve endings which surround many ocular vessels. Such nerves are presumably autonomic motor nerves called nonadrenergic, noncholinergic (NANC). The origins of such nerves are primarily from the ciliary and pterygopalatine ganglia.

Intrinsic NO-Containing Neurons in the Choroid and CM: Evidence for Intrinsic Autonomic Ganglia Within the Eye

Although nerves from parasympathetic ganglia located outside the eye are thought to supply much of the ocular NO input, diaphorase-reacted human eye sections also reveal intrinsic nerve cell bodies with processes scattered in a layer in the external part of the choroid. These neurons appear heterogeneous, some unipolar (pseudounipolar), many bipolar, and some multipolar (see Fig. 12C). Sections of human CM also reveal diaphorase-positive cell bodies. In our studies, these appear in groups of 5–25 cells, usually in the posterior half of the longitudinal CM, well into the substance of the muscle and not at its border (see Fig. 13). Both choroid and CM NO neurons have also been reported by other investigators

---

→

FIG. 12. A,B: First demonstration of the presence of NOS in human optic nerve head and apparent existence of a transition zone for NO production (**A,** low power; **B,** high power). Unmyelinated ganglion cell nerve bundles show intense diaphorase reactivity (left), which is lost as the bundles pass through the cribiform plate and become myelinated (to right). Reactivity can also be seen in thinner fibers scattered at right angles, which may be vascular or neural structures. This same transition area for myelination is also a transition area for blood flow; both facts support a possible functional role for NO in the optic nerve head. **C:** Diaphorase in retina and choroid, showing existence of diaphorase neurons (cell bodies) present throughout the choroid below the retinal pigment epithelium (to the left of arrowhead). The function of these intrinsic NO neurons is as yet unknown. Other intrinsic diaphorase neurons exist in the CM (see Fig. 13). The neural retina shows reactivity in ganglion cells and their axons (*top layer*). Additional reactivity is present in other retinal cells and, particularly, in the inner segment of cones and, to a lesser extent, rods. NO in inner segments could play a role in regenerating cGMP degraded by light-activated phosphodiesterase or play a slower metabolic role in regulating photoreceptor Na,K-ATPase activity.

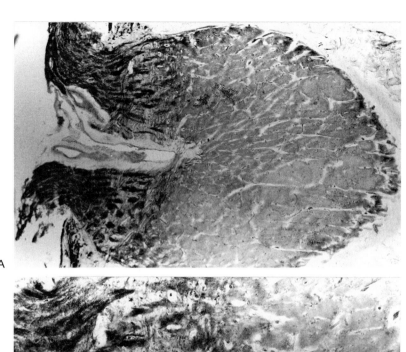

A

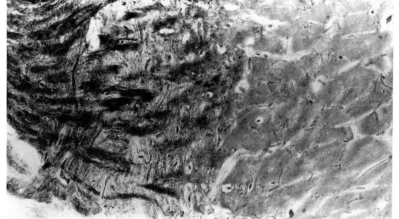

B

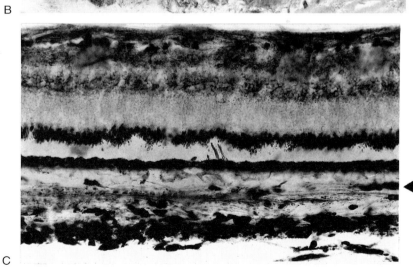

C

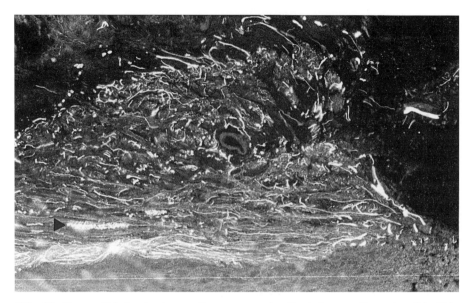

FIG. 13. Human CM showing immunofluorescence of antibody to neurofilament protein. This marker visualizes most nerve fibers in the muscle, showing extremely dense innervation of this muscle. Two types of fibers (thin and thick) are readily visualized, as is the particularly dense innervation of the longitudinal portion of the CM. Of particular interest is the elongated patch of neuron-like cell bodies to the left and just above the area of most intense innervation of the longitudinal CM (to right of arrowhead). In double-labeling experiments with NADPH-d, many of these cells appear to contain NOS, suggesting the existence of intrinsic ganglion-like cells within the muscle. Studies by this and other investigators also reveal the existence of extrinsic NOS neurons in parasympathetic ganglia outside the eye.

(27,28). These intrinsic NO cell bodies in the CM and choroid may be analogous to the small autonomic ganglia found in intestinal smooth muscle, such as Auerbach's myenteric plexus. If so, this finding indicates that local regulation of blood flow as well as smooth muscle in other tissues of the eye could be subject to local feedback loops, the existence of which has somehow gone unnoticed for years.

ALTERATIONS OF OCULAR NOS IN POAG

In a study involving 15 postmortem eyes from patients with POAG (vs. 14 control eyes), there was reported to be a significant reduction in the amount of NADPH-d staining in the longitudinal. CM, as well as in the TM and Schlemm's canal. Associated with the decrease in diaphorase staining were substantial structural alterations in the longitudinal CM, suggesting, although not proving, that the loss of the NOS marker was associated with, or possibly resulted from, a loss of muscle mass (Fig. 14). Eyes in this study were matched for age and postmortem delay, and statistical analysis revealed that prior surgery or treatment by drugs could not explain the differences observed. It will be important in

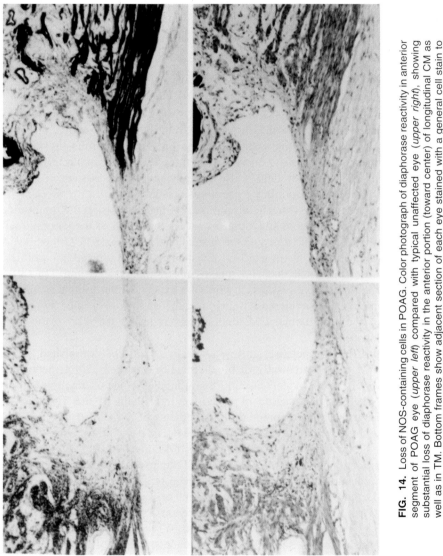

FIG. 14. Loss of NOS-containing cells in POAG. Color photograph of diaphorase reactivity in anterior segment of POAG eye (*upper left*) compared with typical unaffected eye (*upper right*), showing substantial loss of diaphorase reactivity in the anterior portion (toward center) of longitudinal CM as well as in TM. Bottom frames show adjacent section of each eye stained with a general cell stain to show that many cells still remain in areas of diaphorase loss in POAG eye.

future studies to see if this alteration in diaphorase or NOS can be confirmed. It is not yet possible to say whether such alterations are causally related to POAG or are merely secondary manifestations resulting from glaucoma. Nevertheless, even in the latter case, a loss of integrity of the anterior portion of the longitudinal CM would tend to increase AH outflow resistance due to reduction or loss of the CM connections to the TM that normally act to decrease resistance (see below).

FUNCTIONAL ACTIONS OF NO IN THE ANTERIOR SEGMENT: EFFECTS ON OUTFLOW FACILITY

In the normal human eye, the distribution of NOS in the ocular anterior segment is complex, which makes it difficult to predict the overall physiologic effects of NO and NO agonists on AH dynamics. Prediction of the effects of NO through use of animal models is also complicated by the existence of morphologic variations among outflow systems of various species.

In higher primates, the existence of tendinous connections from the longitudinal CM to TM (29) leads to a situation in which contraction of the longitudinal CM by cholinergic agonists causes, in the normal eye, an increase in TM extracellular spaces and a lowering of outflow resistance. Electrophysiologic studies have recently demonstrated that NO relaxes precontracted CM and TM (30). Keeping in mind the above caveats, it would be expected that drugs that mimic NO would tend to cause an increase in precanicular outflow resistance by reducing tension of the longitudinal CM tendons and reducing the size of the TM extracellular spaces.

This action of NO to increase outflow resistance would be diminished if the longitudinal CM were structurally or biochemically impaired, as has been observed in cases of POAG. A decrease in longitudinal CM size or function would also tend to decrease the degree of repetitive movement of the TM that is believed to occur during accommodative movements of the CM. If, in fact, this movement of the TM by the longitudinal CM tends to "flush" the TM of accumulated debris from filtered AH, as has been postulated (31), then the observed dysfunction of the muscle in POAG might tend to contribute to the accumulation of plaque-like material, as has been reported in POAG.

The TM, like the CM, also contains muscle-like cells and, because NO agonists can affect TM contractility, any loss of endogenous NO-producing cells in the TM could directly influence outflow resistance. NO tends to oppose contractile responses in vitro but, because of our poor understanding of the role of the intrinsic smooth-muscle–like cells in the TM, it is not clear what the directionality of the effects of NO might be in vivo. Distal to the TM, NO would also have a tendency to induce relaxation of any smooth muscle present in collecting channels or draining veins. By lowering such "postcanicular" resistance, the action of NO at this level would contribute to an increase in overall outflow facility.

On the basis of information from non-ocular tissues, it appears that the bio-chemical mechanism mediating the relaxation induced by NO in smooth-muscle cells, described above, involves the ability of NO to oppose the action of contractile agents to regulate phosphorylation of myosin light-chain kinase, which ultimately leads to ATP-dependent contraction of the muscle fiber.

FUNCTIONAL ASPECTS OF NO: REGULATION OF OCULAR VASCULAR BEDS

Another important action of ocular NOS has been revealed by a number of recent studies indicating that the blood flow to several areas of the eye—choroid, uvea, retina, and optic nerve head—is regulated by endogenously secreted NO, and that the nature of the regulation is often specific for a particular microcirculation. This is of great importance, not only in normotensive glaucoma but also as an ancillary factor in POAG, and must be considered during the overall evaluation of NO agents and their potential therapeutic use in glaucoma. The diversity of response seen among various vascular beds results from differences in cell types involved [e.g., smooth muscle vs. pericyte (or both) vs. additional flow-related regulation of endothelium] and from the fact that circulating hormones can have markedly different effects, depending on whether the endothelial layer of the vessels being affected forms a barrier to penetration as opposed to endothelium, which has fenestrations that allow hormones to regulate additional cells (e.g., muscle cells, pericytes) as well. Because other investigators in this volume deal with NO regulation of blood flow, it will not be further discussed.

FUNCTIONAL ASPECTS OF NO: REGULATION OF Na,K-ATPase

In addition to altering the contractile response of the muscle light-chain kinase pathway in smooth muscle, NO can also influence regulation of membrane Na,K-ATPase. On the basis of studies of NO action in the kidney and brain (12,16,17), NO, like the NPs, is able to initiate long term alterations in the activity of the sodium pump via a soluble GC, cGMP-dependent mechanism. NO-stimulated cGMP causes PKG to phosphorylate DARPP-32 at the same site phosphorylated by ANP (through cGMP) and DA (through cAMP) (32). The directionality of the NO-induced alteration in Na,K-ATPase activity varies according to species and tissue, causing, e.g., stimulation of Na,K-ATPase in rat brain but inhibition in rat kidney. Although not fully understood, it appears that such differences may be associated with the particular distribution of Na,K-ATPase isoforms present in a given tissue.

Because the sodium pump acts to establish the primary *trans*-membrane electrical and ion gradient, regulation of the Na,K-ATPase by NO has far-reaching effects, from alteration of active fluid secretion in the Cil. Proc NPE (NO causes a small inhibition of secretion here) to effects on other transport mechanisms dependent on the primary sodium/potassium gradient.

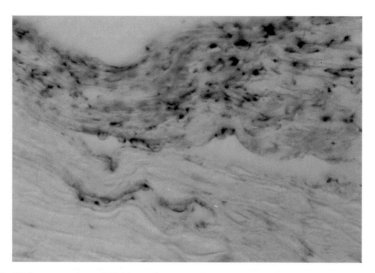

FIG. 15. High-power view of Schlemm's canal showing intense diaphorase activity in giant vacuoles budding from endothelial cells. Other experiments showed that these cells are enriched in Na,K-ATPase, raising the possibility that movement of AH across Schlemm's endothelium may not be an entirely passive process, as had been thought, and may be subject to regulation, perhaps through NO modulation of the sodium pump, as the authors have shown. Regulation may also occur through other channels or co-transporters that are dependent on presence of a *trans*-membrane sodium gradient.

Although outflow resistance has traditionally been considered to be a passive process, there is increasing evidence that specific transporters may be involved. Therefore, it is of interest, relative to NO's action on Na,K-ATPase, that application of ouabain to the outflow system has resulted in marked decrease in outflow facility. In immunohistochemical studies, we have found that the endothelium of Schlemm's canal is enriched in Na,K-ATPase activity and that NOS is present in giant vacuoles budding from this endothelium (Fig. 15). If NO were to stimulate sodium transport in the endothelium of the TM or Schlemm's canal, then, in POAG, a decrease in NO might act to cause a decrease in AH facility.

A change in the primary sodium gradient may also affect secondary transport mechanisms. In the eye, these may include one or more of several potassium channels that are known, in other tissues, to be regulated by cGMP-dependent mechanisms. Another possible cGMP-regulated mechanism is the Na,K,Cl co-transporter, a protein highly enriched in the TM, which has recently been suggested to be a site of action of NPs and could provide, in part, an explanation for reports of NP effects on outflow facility (33). cGMP-regulation of the co-transporter has previously been noted in some other cell types containing NP receptors (34), and recent studies show an abundance of NP receptors in cultured human TM (35). Whether the Na,K,Cl co-transporter is also regulated by NO remains to be determined.

NO/GLU/cGMP: POSSIBLE NEUROPROTECTIVE ROLE?

Recent studies have demonstrated that there is a selective loss of retinal ganglion cells in glaucomatous compared to normal eyes (36,37). Although the relationship between ocular hypertension and retinal degeneration in glaucoma is unclear, several studies have suggested that increased IOP is a risk factor for visual dysfunction of this disease (38).

From investigations of the brain, it is known that NO plays a role in modulating the neurotoxic response of excitatory amino acid neurotransmitters such as glutamate (39), and affects the survival of injured and metabolically stressed cells (40), including retinal neurons. Recent studies (41) have demonstrated an increase in glutamate levels in vitreous humor of glaucomatous humans and monkeys and in induced rats. Furthermore, in several species, retinal ganglion cells contain glutamate receptors. These observations suggest that excitotoxicity may be another important mechanism through which NO can influence the pathophysiology and treatment of POAG.

Although the biochemical mechanisms mediating glutamate- and NO-initiated excitotoxicity are complex, one line of research has shown that NOS inhibitors influence ganglion neuronal survival after ischemia-induced excitotoxic injury (42). Furthermore, a number of other studies have shown the presence of mitochondrial defects in certain chronic neurodegenerative diseases (43). Therefore, physiologic or pathophysiologic mechanisms that alter cell energy metabolism may be of considerable relevance to the course and treatment of excitotoxic nerve damage and neurodegenerative disease, including that in the optic neuropathy of glaucoma.

NO can alter the usage of high-energy metabolites in secretory cells through modulating the activity ATP-requiring sodium pump (16) and, in nerve tissue, NO modulation of the sodium pump may serve as a normal mechanism for the brain to regulate neuronal energy metabolism (17). Through this mechanism, NO, glutamate, and certain other intercellular messengers bring about a marked and prolonged alteration in Na,K-ATPase activity through a multistep biochemical pathway involving, in part, synthesis of carbon monoxide, stimulation of sGC, and activation of PKG. This pathway is also regulated by NO and certain oxygen free radicals, and therefore, by serving as a possible physiologic feedback system for modulating cell energy usage, forms a focal point for the action of several cellular messengers that have been implicated in neuronal viability in certain neurodegenerative diseases and under conditions of stress.

Physiologic experiments indicate that the maintenance of the *trans*-membrane Na/K gradient by Na,K-ATPase in actively firing nerve cells, or in cells with tonically open ion channels, requires up to 50% of the cell's ATP and other high-energy phosphates (44). In fact, if photoreceptors are kept in the dark for too long (cation channels open), ATP stores are insufficient to sustain Na,K-ATPase activity at a level necessary to maintain the *trans*-membrane Na/K gradient. A compromised gradient alters membrane potential and affects a number of other transport and co-transport processes. In addition, depletion of cellular

ATP compromises other essential metabolic tasks. As noted above, alteration in energy stores is critical in neurons undergoing hypoxia or other forms of stress, including glutamate-induced excitotoxicity as may occur in glaucoma.

Sources of stress need not be metabolic in origin but may be initiated by other factors, such as mechanical stress. An example is the postulated block in ganglion axonal transport that occurs when the optic nerve turns at right angles as it enters the optic cup and passes through the cribiform plate as the optic nerve head. It is of considerable interest that at this point there is a transition zone for NOS. Figure 12A and B demonstrate a rather sudden loss of diaphorase activity in ganglion neuron axon bundles as these pass through the cribiform plate and acquire myelination. Because staining in this experiment was done on a longitudinal section of optic nerve, loss of diaphorase does not appear to be an artifact of stain penetration. Because this area of the optic nerve head is also a transition zone for blood flow, additional loss of regulation of the sodium pump, if it were to exist in POAG, would be quite significant.

The fact that NO, glutamate, and certain other transmitters and second messengers can alter the activity of Na,K-ATPase implies that dysfunction of this pathway could affect neuronal survival directly or, minimally, alter the pathogenicity of other factors adversely affecting cell viability. Either underactivity or overactivity of the system could be compromising: underactivity by failing to cause a compensatory upregulation of Na,K-ATPase to deal with increased pumping load, and overactivity leading to excessive use of ATP and depriving the cell of its ability to carry out essential metabolic tasks.

ACKNOWLEDGMENTS

We thank Mary McKee and Colm Scanlon for their contributions, respectively, to the histological and biochemical aspects of this work, and C.G. Moore for assistance in reviewing the literature. This work was supported in part by grants from the National Eye Institute and the American Health Assistance Foundation.

REFERENCES

1. Steardo L, Nathanson JA. Brain barrier tissues: end organs for atriopeptins. *Science* 1987;235:470–3.
2. Steardo L, Owen C, Hunnicutt E, Nathanson JA. Atriopeptin receptors in blood-brain and blood-CSF barrier [Abstract]. *Proc Soc Neurosci* 1986;12:125.
3. Sugrue MF, Viader MP. Synthetic atrial natriuretic factors lowers rabbit intraocular pressure. *Eur J Pharmacol* 1986;130:349–50.
4. Nathanson J. Atriopeptin-activated guanylate cyclase in the anterior segment. *Invest Ophthalmol Vis Sci* 1987;28:1357–64.
5. Mittag TW, Tormay A, Ortega M, et al. Atrial natriuretic peptide, guanylate cyclase, and intraocular pressure. *Curr Eye Res* 1987;6:1189–96.
6. Korenfeld MS, Becker B. Atrial natriuretic peptides: effects on IOP, cGMP and aqueous flow. *Invest Ophthalmol Vis Sci* 1989;30:2385–92.
7. Stone RA, Glembotski CC. Immunoactive atrial natriuretic peptide in the rat eye: molecular forms in anterior uvea and retina. *Biochem Biophys Res Commun* 1986;134:1022–8.

8. Stone RA, Laties AM, Hemmings HC, Ouimet CC, Greengard P. DARPP-32 in the ciliary epithelium of the eye: a neurotransmitter-regulated phosphoprotein of brain localizes to secretory cells. *J Histochem Cytochem* 1986;34:1465–8.

9. Snyder GL, Girault J, Chen J, et al. Phosphorylation of DARPP-32 and protein phosphatase inhibitor-1 in rat CP: regulation by factors other than dopamine. *J Neurosci* 1992;12:3071–83.

10. Ghosh S, Freitag AC, Martin-Vasallo P, Coca-Prados M. Cellular distribution and differential expression of the three α subunit isoforms of the Na,K-ATPase in the ocular ciliary epithelium. *J Biol Chem* 1990;265:2935–40.

11. Sweadner K. Isozymes of the Na,K-ATPase. *Biochim Biophys Acta* 1989;988:185–220.

12. Scavone C, Scanlon C, McKee M, Nathanson JA. Atrial natriuretic peptide modulates Na,K-ATPase through a mechanism involving cGMP and PKG. *J Pharmacol Exp Ther* 1995; 272:1036–43.

13. Mittal CK, Murad F. Guanylate cyclase: regulation of cGMP metabolism. In: Nathanson JA, Kebabian JW, eds. *Handbook of experimental pharmacology.* New York: Springer Verlag, 1982;581:225–60.

14. Wizemann A, Wizemann V. Untersuchungen zur ambulanten and perioperativen Augeninnen-drucksenkug mit organischen Nitraten. *Klin Mbl Augenheilk* 1980;177:292–5. (in German).

15. Yamamoto R, Bredt DS, Snyder SH, Stone RA. The localization of NO synthase in the rat eye and related cranial ganglia. *Neuroscience* 1993;54:189–200.

16. McKee M, Scavone C, Nathanson JA. NO, cGMP, and hormone regulation of active sodium transport. *Proc Natl Acad Sci USA* 1994;91:12056–60.

17. Nathanson JA, Scavone C, Scanlon C, McKee M. The cellular Na,K-ATPase as a site of action for carbon monoxide and glutamate. *Neuron* 1995;14:781–94.

18. Moncada S, Palmet MJ, Higgs EA. NO: physiology, pathophysiology, and pharmacology. *Pharmacol Rev* 1991;43:109–42.

19. Moncada S, Higgs EA. The L-arginine-NO pathway. *N Engl J Med* 1993;329:2002–12.

20. Stuehr DJ, Cho HJ, Kwon NS, Weise M, Nathan CF. Purification and characterization of the cytokine-induced macrophage NO synthase. *Proc Natl Acad Sci USA* 1991;88:7773–7.

21. Nathanson JA, Bartels S, Krug J. Ocular actions of natriuretic peptides and guanylate cyclase activators. In: Drance SM, Neufeld S, Van Buskirk E, eds. *Applied pharmacology of the glaucomas.* Baltimore: Williams & Wilkins, 1993:156–74.

22. Nathanson JA, McKee M. Alterations of ocular NO synthase in human glaucoma. *Invest Ophthalmol Vis Sci* 1995;34:1774–83.

23. Goh Y, Hotehama Y, Mishima HK. Characterization of CM relaxation induced by various agents in cats. *Invest Ophthalmol Vis Sci* 1994;35:4268–75.

24. Elias M, Manenti-Santos C, deLima W, Nathanson JA, Scavone C. NO modulates Na pump activity in rat tracheal tissue. Proc XXI Ann Conf Fed Soc Exp Biol, 1996, Caxamblu, Brazil.

25. Ellis D, Scanlon C, McKee M, Moore C, Nathanson JA. A dual role for acetylcholine and NO in regulating the Na,K-ATPase in bovine ciliary muscle [Abstracts]. *Invest Ophthalmol Vis Sci* 1997;38:S490.

26. Nathanson JA, Erickson K. The effects of endothelin, ANF and nitroglycerine on the outflow facility in the primate eye. In: Lutjen-Drecol E, ed. *Basic aspects of glaucoma research.* Meinz: Schattuer, 1993:275–85.

27. Flugel-Koch C, Kaufman P, Lutjen-Drecoll E. Association of a choroidal ganglion cell plexus with the fovea centralis. *Invest Ophthalmol Vis Sci* 1994;36:11988–92.

28. Tamm E, Flugel-Koch C, Mayer B, Lutjen-Drecoll E. Nerve cells in the human CM: ultrastructural and immunocytochemical characterization. *Invest Ophthalmol Vis Sci* 1995;36:414–26.

29. Rohen JW. The evolution of the primate eye in relation to the problem of glaucoma. In: Lutjen-Drecol E, ed. *Basic aspects of glaucoma research.* Stuttgart: Schattauer-Verlag, 1982:3–33.

30. Wiederhold M, Sturn A, Lepple-Wienhues A. Relaxation of trabecular meshwork and CM by release of NO. *Invest Ophthalmol Vis Sci* 1994;35:1515–20.

31. Kaufman PL, Gabelt BT. Cholinergic mechanisms and aqueous humor dynamics. In: Drance S, Neufeld A, Van Buskirk E, eds. *Applied pharmacology of the glaucomas.* Baltimore: Williams & Wilkins, 1992:64–92.

32. Tsou K, Snyder GL, Greengard P. NO/cGMP pathway stimulates phosphorylation of DARPP-32, a dopamine- and cAMP-regulated phosphoprotein, in the substantia nigra. *Proc Natl Acad Sci USA* 1993;90:3462–5.

33. Al-Aswald L, Adorante JS, Erickson KA. Effects of cell volume regulation on outflow facility in calf and human eyes in vitro [Abstract]. *Invest Ophthalmol Vis Sci* 1995;36:S722.

34. O'Donnell ME, Owen NE. Role of cyclic GMP in ANF stimulation of Na,K-Cl-cotransporter in vascular smooth muscle cells. *J Biol Chem* 1986;261:15461–6.
35. Chang A, Polansky J, Crook RB. Natriuretic peptide receptors on human trabecular meshwork cells. *Curr Eye Res* 1996;15:137–43.
36. Asai T, Katsumori N, Mizokami K. Retinal ganglion cell damage in human glaucoma. I. Studies on the somal diameter. *Folia Ophthalmol Jpn* 1987;38:701–7.
37. Glovinsky Y, Quigley HA, Dunkelberger GR. Retinal ganglion cell loss is size-dependent in experimental glaucoma. *Invest Ophthalmol Vis Sci* 1991;32:484–91.
38. National Advisory Eye Council. *Vision research, A national plan: 1994–1998.* Washington, DC: US Public Health Service, 1993;199–241. NIH publication 93-3186.
39. Lipton SA, Choi Y, Pan Z, et al. A redox-based mechanism for the neuroprotective and neurode-structive effects of NO and related nitroso-compounds. *Nature* 1993;364:626–31.
40. Dawson VL, Dawson TM, Bartley DA, Uhl GR, Snyder SH. Mechanism of NO mediated neurotoxicity in primary brain cultures. *J Neurosci* 1993;13:2651–61.
41. Dreyer EB, Zurakowski D, Schumer RA, et al. Elevated glutamate in the vitreous body of humans and monkey with glaucoma. *Arch Ophthalmol* 1996;114:65:643–51.
42. Liu S, Chiou GC, Verma R. Improvement of retinal functions after ischemia with L-arginine and its derivatives. *J Ocular Pharmacol* 1995;11:261–5.
43. Coyle JT, Puttfarcken P. Oxidative stress, glutamate, and neurodegenerative disorders. *Science* 1993;262:689–95.
44. Ames A, Li Y. Energy requirement of glutamatergic pathways in rabbit retina. *J Neurosci* 1992;12:4234–42.

Nitric Oxide and Endothelin in the Pathogenesis of Glaucoma, edited by I. O. Haefliger and J. Flammer. Lippincott–Raven Publishers, Philadelphia © 1998.

17

The Glaucoma Excitotoxicity Theory

Claude Bonne and Agnes Muller

Laboratoire de Physiologie Cellulaire, Université de Montpellier, Montpellier, France

The pathogenic mechanisms responsible for the loss of retinal ganglion cells (RGC) in glaucoma have not yet been elucidated.

RGC damage is commonly attributed to the high intraocular pressure (IOP) recorded in the majority of patients. However, evidence from the study of low-tension glaucoma and ocular hypertension suggests that high IOP is neither necessary nor sufficient to explain glaucomatous neuropathy even if it is a major risk factor.

Other problems, such as blood flow deficiency due to vascular and hemorrheologic dysfunctions, have been evoked and well argued (1). Metabolic abnormalities have also been suggested to be risk factors. For example, a defect in neurotrophic factors could be involved in the neuropathy, because it is known that they can protect RGC against mechanical or ischemic insults (2,3).

Studies in the central nervous system during the past 20 years have shown that both traumatic and ischemic neuronal injury can be mediated by increased extracellular levels of the excitatory neurotransmitter glutamate (GLU) and excessive stimulation of its receptors, an effect that can also be involved in the pathogenesis of degenerative neuropathies (4,5). Today, it appears that these processes may be involved in the apoptotic death of RGC.

This review reports the main data that support the excitotoxicity theory of glaucoma and discusses some potential new therapeutic approaches to this neuropathy.

THE BASES OF THE THEORY

Vitreous GLU Level Is Increased in Glaucoma

The excitotoxicity theory of glaucomatous neuropathy was put forward for the first time at ARVO in 1992 by Dreyer and Lipton (6). In their initial study, they showed a twofold elevation in the level of GLU in the vitreous body of a group of 26 patients with glaucoma plus cataract compared with that in a control population of patients with cataracts only. In a following article published in 1996, these authors, in association with others (7), confirmed and completed their results, showing an even greater increase in GLU level in the vitreous of monkeys made glaucomatous for 4–8 months by argon laser burns of the trabeculum. Moreover, in monkeys with glaucoma, the greatest level of GLU was observed in the posterior vitreous, suggesting that the source of the amino acid was the retina.

Another animal study in the rabbit (8) also confirmed that an increase in vitreous GLU concentration to a level that is potentially toxic to neurons can be induced by chronic elevations in IOP.

The chronicity of the stress appears to be a major factor in the induction of this biochemical abnormality. In fact, experiments performed in the rabbit with an acute and drastic increase in IOP (100 mm Hg) were unable to demonstrate such a specific elevation in the extracellular GLU level (9). It appears important to bear this observation in mind with regard to the specificity of the retina, because in such acute conditions GLU is effectively released in the ischemic areas of the central nervous system (see below).

GLU and Glaucoma Induce RGC Apoptosis

Apoptosis, in contrast to necrosis, is a mode of cell death that is an active process depending on gene expression (10). This programmed cell death, which is not accompanied by inflammatory reaction, is an important physiologic event during development. For example, it is responsible for the selection of one million RGC that constitute the mature optic nerve from the several million cells originally present in the embryonic nerve.

Recent histologic studies of the retina in experimental glaucoma (11) and in glaucoma patients (12,13) have suggested that RGC die by an apoptosis-like mechanism. Among the various effectors capable of inducing apoptosis, GLU is a possible candidate. It has been repeatedly demonstrated that exogenous GLU is able to kill neurons by triggering their apoptosis (14,15).

These recent studies confirmed and specified the data obtained from the pioneer work by Lucas and Newhouse (16), which showed that high doses of GLU subcutaneously administered to young mice provoked degeneration of retinal neurons and of RGC in particular.

GLU Ionotropic Receptor Antagonists Are Retinal Neuroprotective Agents

The initial steps of the GLU neurotoxic mechanism of action are those that mediate its excitatory neurotransmitter function, i.e., binding and activation of its postsynaptic ionotropic membrane receptors. Several types of ionotropic GLU receptors have been characterized (NMDA, AMPA, and kainate) and all these receptors can be implicated in neuron toxicity (17). However, pharmacologic data obtained from cell cultures stressed with GLU and protected by specific antagonists emphasize the predominant role of the NMDA (*N*-methyl-D-aspartate) receptor in GLU-induced RGC damage (18,19). It is also of interest that NMDA receptor antagonists protect RGC from GLU chronical toxicity in vivo (20). Moreover, it has been shown that the larger RGC were the most sensitive to NMDA cytotoxicity (21), a situation that appears similar to glaucoma because larger RGC are primarily affected in this disease.

THE MECHANISM OF GLU ACCUMULATION

GLU is present as a neurotransmitter in a variety of retinal neurons, including bipolar cells. When synaptically released under physiologic conditions, GLU is obviously not toxic because uptake systems efficiently transport extracellular GLU to cells, particularly to Müller cells. It has been shown that a long-term doubling of the extracellular (vitreal) GLU concentration is toxic to mammalian RGC (20), raising the question of the mechanism responsible for its elevation in the vitreous of glaucoma patients.

There are several possible sources for excess GLU. Traumatic or ischemic insult to neurons could damage cell membranes and release intracellular GLU, which could, in turn, lead to additional excitotoxicity. A close possibility is that the initial insult can lead to energy depletion and depolarization of presynaptic neurons, and then to unregulated release of the neurotransmitter. Moreover, under these depolarizing conditions, uptake reverses, releasing nonvesicular GLU into the extracellular space (22). Several mechanisms can be jointly responsible for extracellular GLU accumulation, related either to release of vesicular and nonvesicular amino acids or to inhibition of glial and neuronal reuptake. As far as this latter mechanism is concerned, many secondary metabolic disturbances induced by ischemia can also interfere with this major neuroprotective machinery. In particular, it has been shown that arachidonic acid released from membrane phospholipids is able to block GLU reuptake by interfering with the GLU/Na^+ membrane transporter. In the same way, oxygen-derived free radicals (OFR) and H_2O_2 generated under hypoxia can inhibit this transporter, as demonstrated in cultured cortical astrocytes (23) and Müller cells (unpublished data).

As reported above, the retina appears to be more efficiently protected than the brain from GLU accumulation in extracellular space. No GLU release can be detected by retinal microdialysis in the rabbit under acute ischemia (9), even if some GLU-related dysfunctions can be recorded under these conditions. The unique organization of Müller cells in this neural tissue may be of special importance to protect the retinal neurons from GLU toxicity, and a primary functional defect of these glial cells could hypothetically occur in glaucoma.

THE MECHANISM OF GLU TOXICITY

The Ionotropic NMDA Receptor and the Role of Ca^{2+}

The NMDA receptor is a protein complex that binds GLU and its synthetic analogue NMDA (Fig. 1). This complex is also an ion channel permeant to Na^+, K^+, and Ca^{2+}. By increasing Na^+ and Ca^{2+} conductance, GLU provokes depolarization of the postsynaptic neurons and activates Ca^{2+}-dependent enzymes, leading to information transfer. Under conditions of overstimulation due to an increased GLU level, an overload of Ca^{2+} is produced, which can trigger a series of cytotoxic events. Ca^{2+} overload can result from direct opening of the receptor channel and also of voltage-operated Ca^{2+} channels in neuron membranes (24).

Overload of Ca^{2+} in GLU-hyperactivated neurons stimulates various Ca^{2+}-dependent enzymes, including calpaine, phospholipase A_2, and nitric oxide synthase (NOS). These enzymes contribute to GLU toxicity, as demonstrated by the pharmacologic protection afforded by their inhibitors (25–29).

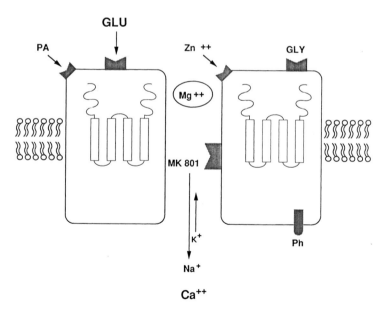

FIG. 1. The NMDA receptor. The neurotransmitter glutamate (GLU), by binding to the receptor, opens a channel permeant to Na^+, K^+, and Ca^{2+}. Mg^{2+} ions that block the channel are mobilized by depolarization initiated by activation of other receptors. The receptor is regulated by a variety of ligands of allosteric binding sites. Glycine (GLY) stimulates the GLU effect. In contrast, polyamines (PA) and Zn^{2+} lower its efficacy. Phosphorylation sites (Ph) located on intracellular domains can be also implicated in the receptor/channel modulation. The drug MK 801 is a noncompetitive antagonist frequently used as a tool to study the involvement of NMDA receptors in excitotoxic processes.

The Role of OFR in Excitatory Amino Acid Toxicity

OFR are reactive derivatives of molecular oxygen produced mainly in biologic tissues by oxidases and oxygenases (Fig. 2). Neurons stressed by excitatory amino acids (EAA) generate OFR through a Ca^{2+}-dependent pathway, as demonstrated by electron spin-resonance spin trapping (30,31). There are several sources of OFR in GLU-activated cells. Calpaine, a proteolytic enzyme activated in EAA-stimulated neurons (25), has been shown to be responsible for conversion of xanthine dehydrogenase to xanthine oxidase, a source of superoxide (O_2^-) production. Phospholipase A_2, which releases arachidonic acid from membranes, allows its oxidative metabolism and the generation of OFR as a byproduct (29). Constitutive neuronal NOS is a Ca^{2+}/calmodulin-dependent enzyme that generates NO from arginine. The role of this messenger is discussed below.

It has been shown that OFR generated in neurons under GLU stimulation were able to induce necrosis or apoptosis, depending on the magnitude of the

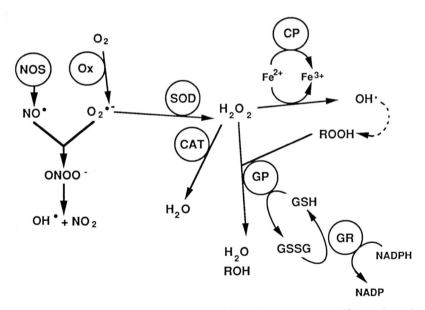

FIG. 2. Enzymatic production and destruction of OFR. Molecular oxygen (O_2) can be reduced by various enzymatic reactions, mainly by oxidases (Ox) and oxygenase cascades. Superoxide radical (O_2^-) can be reduced to hydrogen peroxide (H_2O_2), a reaction that is catalyzed by superoxide dismutases (SOD). H_2O_2 is destroyed by catalase (CAT) and by glutathione peroxidase (GP) in the presence of reduced glutathione (GSH). This enzyme is also able to detoxify lipid peroxides (ROOH). Oxidized GSH (GS SG) is recycled to the reduced form by glutathione reductase (GR) with NADPH as co-factor. When produced in excess, H_2O_2 can be reduced in the presence of ferrous ions (Fe^{2+}) to the hydroxyl radical (OH$^\bullet$), the most reactive OFR. Ceruleoplasmin (CP) contributes to OFR defenses by oxidizing Fe^{2+} to Fe^{3+}. Nitric oxide synthase (NOS), which produces NO$^\bullet$ from arginine, can also contribute to oxidative stress. NO can combine with O_2^- leading to formation of the very reactive entity peroxinitrite anion (ONOO$^-$), which can further decompose into OH$^\bullet$.

stimulus (32). For apoptotic neuronal cell death, a variety of experiments have emphasized the role played by OFR (10). Apoptosis is a complex process that requires gene expression and which is regulated by an equilibrium between proapoptotic and antiapoptotic proteins. In neurons, apoptosis can be induced by suppression of neurotrophic factors or by GLU overstimulation, two stimuli that can be antagonized by antioxidants. It is interesting that one function of neurotrophic factors is to regulate the enzymatic activity of glutathione peroxidase, a central defense against oxidative stress. Moreover, it has been shown that H_2O_2 is a potent inducer of apoptosis and that the most studied antiapoptotic protein, Bcl_2, may act by increasing the defense against OFR (33).

The Double-Edged Role of NO in GLU Toxicity

NO is synthesized by three isoforms of NOS. Neuronal and endothelial isoforms, termed constitutive NOS, are regulated by intracellular Ca^{2+}. In this way, neuronal NOS (NOS-I) is activated in neurons stimulated by GLU, in which NO plays the role of a retrograde neurotransmitter in glutamatergic synapses. In contrast, inducible NOS activity (NOS-II) is independent of Ca^{2+} and the enzyme is expressed in various cells, such as macrophages, neutrophils, microglial cells, and glial cells, in response to inflammatory stimuli such as cytokines. In the retina this isoform, present in retinal pigment epithelium and Müller cells, is induced by ischemia/reperfusion and can be involved in retinal injury. Constitutive neuronal NOS-I, also present in Müller cells, appears to be implicated in EAA-induced neuron damage (26,28–32).

Several mechanisms can be invoked to explain the toxicity of NO. Because of the pleotropic activity of this messenger, these mechanisms are more easily analyzed in neuron cultures, which eliminate interfering vascular effects. First, it has been demonstrated that NO cytotoxicity is not mediated by activation of guanylate cyclase, because guanylate cyclase inhibitors do not affect NMDA neurotoxicity and 8-bromo-cGMP does not induce cell damage (34). Experiments showing that the so-called NO donors sodium nitroprusside (SNP) and SIN-1 kill the neurons do not afford clear demonstration of a direct toxicity of NO, because SNP can have additional activities owing to its ferrocyanide moiety and SIN-1 can also decompose into $O_2^{·-}$. It is now generally believed that NO toxicity is mediated by its reaction product with $O_2^{·-}$, the peroxinitrite anion ($ONOO^-$), a powerful oxidant that further decomposes into $OH^·$ and NO_2 (35).

Both peroxinitrite and $OH^·$ are very toxic agents that can react with DNA, enzymes, and membranes, and kill the cells by necrosis or apoptosis. The neurotoxicity of NO is demonstrated in neuron cultures stressed either with hypoxia or with large concentrations of EAA. Under these conditions, the cells can be protected by NOS inhibition or scavenging of NO.

Although it is well established that NO participates in GLU toxicity, there are also experimental data demonstrating that some effects of this molecule may contribute to protect neurons against GLU insult. The NO neuroprotective effect is believed to involve several pathways that affect GLU receptors. The first mechanism is related to cGMP formation through the stimulation of guanylate cyclase. For example, it has been recently shown that cGMP reduces GLU-induced membrane current in retinal cells (36). A second mechanism, demonstrated in cortical cells in culture, is related to the redox modulation of the GLU (NMDA) receptor. Depending on the ambient redox milieu, NO can be converted into NO^+, which downregulates the NMDA receptor by S-nitrosylation of thiol groups in a modulatory site (35).

CONCLUSION

A growing number of observations support the excitotoxicity theory of glaucoma. However, to reinforce the theory a series of questions must be answered. For example, what is the source of vitreous GLU? What are the respective roles of axonal trauma and ischemia in GLU accumulation? Can the topography of NMDA receptor distribution explain glaucomatous lesions? Is NOS present in vulnerable RGC? Is GLU excitotoxicity a primary or secondary cause of RGC apoptosis?

If the role of GLU excitotoxicity is confirmed in glaucoma, several new therapeutic approaches will be offered. For example, scavenging of OFR with antioxidants and inhibition of Ca^{2+} overload with noncompetitive antagonists of NMDA receptors have already been shown to be neuroprotective in experimental models. Moreover, even if GLU toxicity is only a secondary phenomenon, the way to anti-apoptotic drugs is open.

REFERENCES

1. Drance SM. Glaucoma: changing concept. *Eye* 1992;6:337–45.
2. Siliprandi R, Canella R, Carmignoto G. Nerve growth factor promotes functional recovery of retinal ganglion cells after ischemia. *Invest Ophthalmol Vis Sci* 1993;34:3232–45.
3. Mansour-Robaey S, Clarke DB, Wang YC, Bray GM, Aguayo AJ. Effects of ocular injury and the administration of brain-derived neurotrophic factor (BDNF) on the survival and re-growth of axotomized retinal ganglion cells. *Proc Natl Acad Sci USA* 1994;91:1632–6.
4. Meldrum B, Garthwaite J. Excitatory amino acid neurotoxicity and neurodegenerative disease. *Trends Pharmacol Sci* 1990;11:379–87.
5. Beal MF. Mechanisms of excitotoxicity in neurologic diseases. *FASEB J* 1992;6:3338–44.
6. Dreyer EB, Lipton SA. Excitatory amino acids in glaucoma: a potentially novel etiology of neuronal loss [Abstract]. *Invest Ophthalmol Vis Sci* 1992;33:S2002.
7. Dreyer EB, Zurakowski D, Schumer RA, Podos SM, Lipton SA. Elevated glutamate levels in the vitreous body of humans and monkeys with glaucoma. *Arch Ophthalmol* 1996;114:299–305.
8. Nguyen QD, Kaiser PK, Dreyer EB. The buphthalmic/glaucomatous rabbit eye: amino acid analysis [Abstract]. *Invest Ophthalmol Vis Sci* 1995;36:S4467.
9. Muller A, Villain M, Bonne C. The release of amino acids from ischemic retina. *Exp Eye Res* 1997;64:291–3.
10. Bredesen DE. Neural apoptosis. Review. *Ann Neurol* 1995;38:839–51.
11. Garcia-Valenzuela E, Shareef S, Walsh J, Sharma SC. Programmed cell death of retinal ganglion cells during experimental glaucoma. *Exp Eye Res* 1995;61:33–44.
12. Bonfoco E, Nicotera P, Smith JA, Dreyer EB, Lipton SA. Retinal ganglion cells die by an

apoptotic-like mechanism in human glaucoma [Abstract]. *Invest Ophthalmol Vis Sci* 1995; 36:S4444.

13. Kerrigan LA, Pease ME, Green WR, Quigley HA. Studies of presumed apoptosis in human primary open-angle glaucoma [Abstract]. *Invest Ophthalmol Vis Sci* 1996;37:S3811.

14. Lam TT, Fu J, Li SH, Abler AS, Tso MOM. N-methyl-D-aspartate (NMDA)-induced apoptosis in rat retina [Abstract]. *Invest Ophthalmol Vis Sci* 1995;36:S4301.

15. Dreyer EB, Zhang DX, Lipton SA. Transcriptional or translational inhibition blocks low dose NMDA-mediated cell death. *Neuroreport* 1995;6:942–44.

16. Lucas DR, Newhouse JP. The toxic effects of sodium L-glutamate on the inner-layers of the retina. *Arch Ophthalmol* 1954;58:193–201.

17. Mosinger JL, Price MT, Bai HY, Xiao H, Wozniak DF, Olney JW. Blockade of both NMDA and non-NMDA receptors is required for optimal protection against ischemic neuronal degeneration in the in vivo adult mammalian retina. *Exp Neurol* 1991;113:10–7.

18. Sucher NJ, Aizenman E, Lipton SA. N-methyl-D-aspartate antagonists prevent kainate neurotoxicity in rat retinal ganglion cells in vitro. *J Neurosci* 1991;11:966–71.

19. Kitano S, Morgan J, Caprioli J. Hypoxic and excitotoxic damage to cultured rat retinal ganglion cells. *Exp Eye Res* 1996;63:105–12.

20. Vorwerk CK, Lipton SA, Zurakowski D, Hyman BT, Sabel BA, Dreyer EB. Chronic low-dose glutamate is toxic to retinal ganglion cells—toxicity blocked by memantine. *Invest Ophthalmol Vis Sci* 1996;37:1618–24.

21. Dreyer EB, Pan ZH, Storm S, Lipton SA. Greater sensitivity of larger retinal ganglion cells to NMDA-mediated cell death. *Neuroreport* 1994;5:629–31.

22. Szatkowski M, Attwell D. Triggering and execution of neuronal death in brain ischaemia: two phases of glutamate release by different mechanisms. *Trends Neurosci* 1994;17:359–65.

23. Volterra A, Trotti D, Racagni G. Glutamate uptake is inhibited by arachidonic acid and oxygen radicals via two distinct and additive mechanisms. *Mol Pharmacol* 1994;46:986–92.

24. Sucher NJ, Lei SZ, Lipton SA. Calcium channel antagonists attenuate NMDA receptor-mediated neurotoxicity of retinal ganglion cells in culture. *Brain Res* 1991;551:297–302.

25. Dykens JA, Stern A, Trenkner E. Mechanism of kainate toxicity to cerebellar neurons in vitro is analogous to reperfusion tissue injury. *J Neurochem* 1987;49:1222–8.

26. Dawson VL, Dawson TM, London ED, Bredt DS, Snyder SH. Nitric oxide mediates glutamate neurotoxicity in primary cortical cultures. *Proc Natl Acad Sci USA* 1991;88:6368–71.

27. Pellegrini-Giampietro DE, Cherici G, Alesiani M, Carla V, Moroni F. Excitatory amino acid release and free radical formation may cooperate in the genesis of ischemia-induced neuronal damage. *J Neurosci* 1990;10:1035–41.

28. Cazevieille C, Muller A, Meynier F, Bonne C. Superoxide and nitric oxide cooperation in hypoxia/reoxygenation-induced neuron injury. *Free Rad Biol Med* 1993;14:389–95.

29. Cazevieille C, Muller A, Meynier F, Dutrait N, Bonne C. Protection by prostaglandins from glutamate toxicity in cortical neurons. *Neurochem Int* 1994;4:395–8.

30. Lafon-Cazal M, Pietri S, Culcasi M, Bockaert J. NMDA-dependent superoxide production and neurotoxicity. *Nature* 1993;364:535–7.

31. Dutrait N, Culcasi M, Cazevieille C, et al. Calcium dependent free radical generation in cultured retinal neurons injured by kainate. *Neurosci Lett* 1995;198:13–6.

32. Bonfoco E, Krainc D, Ankarcrona M, Nicotera P, Lipton SA. Apoptosis and necrosis, two distinct events induced, respectively by mild and intense insults with NMDA or nitric oxide/superoxide in cortical cell cultures. *Proc Natl Acad Sci USA* 1995;92:7162–6.

33. Hockenbery DM, Oltvai Z, Yin XM, Milliman C, Korsmeyer SJ. Bcl-2 functions in an antioxidant pathway to prevent apoptosis. *Cell* 1993;75:241–51.

34. Dawson VL, Dawson TM, Bartley DA, Uhl GR, Snyder SH. Mechanism of nitric oxide-mediated neurotoxicity in primary brain cultures. *J Neurosci* 1993;13:2651–61.

35. Lipton SA, Choi YB, Pan ZH, et al. A redox-based mechanism for the neuroprotective and neurodestructive effects of nitric oxide and related nitroso-compounds. *Nature* 1993;364:626–32.

36. McMahon DG, Ponomareva LV. Nitric oxide and cGMP modulate retinal glutamate receptors. *J Neurophysiol* 1996;76:2307–15.

Nitric Oxide and Endothelin in the Pathogenesis of Glaucoma, edited by I. O. Haefliger and J. Flammer. Lippincott–Raven Publishers, Philadelphia © 1998.

18

Mechanisms of Neuronal Apoptosis

Denis Monard

Friedrich Miescher Institut, Basel, Switzerland

Two types of cell death, necrosis and apoptosis, have been defined during development or in pathologic situations. Necrosis is characterized by cell swelling, cell lysis, and spillage of cell content into the extracellular space. It always leads to an inflammatory response. Apoptosis is characterized by cell shrinkage and fragmentation of the nucleus, sometimes associated with degradation of the DNA into oligomers. Apoptosis requires an intrinsic active suicide program that depends on transcription and translation of new genes. There is no leakage of cell content into the extracellular space and therefore no induction of an inflammatory reaction. Nevertheless, the apoptotic cells are rapidly phagocytosed by neighboring cells or macrophages. Necrosis and apoptosis can take place in all organs. This communication focuses on the apoptotic cell death program that takes place in the nervous system.

BIOLOGIC RELEVANCE OF APOPTOSIS IN THE NERVOUS SYSTEM

During development, the neuroblasts migrate to reach the location at which they will further differentiate. At this stage they extend processes called neurites to establish contacts with the cells from which they will receive information, or with the target cells that they will stimulate. The afferent neurites will become the dendrites and the efferent neurite the axon. The phase of neurite outgrowth is influenced by a multiplicity of molecules found or released in the environment by neighboring cells. Among these molecules, trophic factors play a very important role. When an axonal neurite has reached its target, its growth cone establishes contacts that with time differentiate into functional synapses. The target cell also releases trophic factors. Some of them react with specific receptors at the presynaptic terminal of the innervating neuroblast and are taken up to be retrogradely transported along the axon. This phenomenon is crucial to the survival of the innervating neuron. Disruption of the retrograde axonal transport by ligation or by disruption of the cytoskeletal structure of the axon leads to the death of the innervating neuron. It is therefore quite possible that, in glaucoma, the pressure exerted on the optic nerve is one of the causes that leads to the death of the retinal ganglion cells.

The importance of the target for survival of the innervating neuron has been nicely demonstrated in experiments performed by Hamburger (1). Removal of the developing limb of a chick embryo results in a marked decrease in the number of motor neurons, and transplantation of an extra limb bud before the normal period of cell death leads to a marked increase in the number of motor neurons. These phenomena and subsequent experiments have led to the ''neurotrophic hypothesis'' which postulates that (a) certain neuronal populations depend on exogenous neurotrophic factors for normal survival, and (b) the factors are present in insufficient quantities to maintain alive all the neurons generated during development.

What is the relevance of apoptosis in the nervous system? During development an excessive number of neuroblasts are generated. Apoptosis is required to eliminate cells that had only a transient function (e.g., in guiding the migration of freshly born cells or influencing the pathfinding of their neurites) and that are no longer needed. Another important feature is performance of ''size matching,'' i.e., eliminating the excess of neuroblasts that have not been solicited to obtain a functional wiring. In fact, in certain structures of the nervous system, up to 50% of the generated neuroblasts die before embryonic development ends.

IDENTIFICATION OF MOLECULES INVOLVED IN THE APOPTOTIC PATHWAY

Studies in tissue culture and in very simple organisms have provided seminal information about the mechanisms of apoptosis. In tissue culture, the survival of neuronal cells requires the presence of trophic factors, such as, e.g., the neurotrophins. Lack of these specific factors rapidly leads to apoptosis. A series of experiments has demonstrated that apoptosis does not take place when transcription of new mRNAs or translation of new proteins is blocked. These results suggest that cell death is due to an active ''suicide program.'' To understand this program, it became essential to identify the molecules involved.

Studies with the nematode *Caenorhabditis elegans* have provided invaluable information in this search (2). *C. elegans* is a very simple organism in which each one of its 1,090 cells has been identified. The developmental cell lineage leading to this set of cells has also been unraveled, and 131 cells were found to die through apoptosis before the animal reaches maturity. After exposition to mutagenetic agents, many *C. elegans* mutants with a modified cell fate program have been generated. In one of these mutants, the mutations prevented the normal cell death program, thus leading to a viable organism in which an excess of cells was detected. These mutations allowed the identification of two genes, called *ced-3* and *ced-4,* that code for proteins actively involved and required for apoptosis. Another of these mutants showed an opposite phenotype, i.e., many cells normally surviving in the wild type die. This phenomenon leads to a strong reduction in the total number of cells and to a nematode that dies early in development. These results indicated that the gene identified, called *ced-9*, was coding for a protein whose function is to put a brake on the suicide program.

This idea was further sustained by the characterization of another mutant in which the *ced-9* gene was abnormally activated, leading to an organism in which apoptosis did not take place and to an excess of surviving cells, similar to the phenotypes caused by inactivation of the apoptosis-triggering *ced-3* and *ced-4*. In mutants in which both *ced-3* and *ced-9* are inactivated, the normal cell death program does not take place. This supports the idea that these two genes encode proteins that antagonize each other and therefore that they are involved in the same apoptotic pathway.

THE MAMMALIAN HOMOLOG OF *ced-9*

Today's molecular biology methodology allows the sequencing of genes, such as *ced-3*, *ced-4*, and *ced-9*, that have been identified because of the detection of an abnormal phenotype after in vivo mutagenesis. The nucleotide sequence of *ced-9* turned out to be homologous with an oncogene called *bcl-2*, first identified as being overexpressed in certain B-cell lymphomas and thus causing the behavior of their tumor cells. *Bcl-2* expression was shown to prevent lymphocytes from undergoing programmed cell death, including the apoptosis of normal lymphocytes that takes place in these cells after withdrawal of their supply of cytokines. A series of experiments demonstrated that *ced-9* and *bcl-2* are similar in their function as well. First, expression of *bcl-2* in sympathetic neurons prevented their apoptosis on withdrawal of nerve growth factor (NGF), the neutrophin required for their survival. Second, *bcl-2* prevented cell death when inserted into *C. elegans*. In agreement with this survival function, *bcl-2* is expressed in the developing nervous system of embryonic and neonatal mice at the time when the decision between neuronal survival or apoptosis is taking place. Such results were sufficient to motivate many laboratories to search for further homologues of *bcl-2* in mammalian cells.

THE *bcl-2* FAMILY

Again, the power of molecular biology led to the identification of many genes whose function was tested by overexpression in different cellular systems. This approach provided the realization that some of them act, like *bcl-2*, as inhibitors of apoptosis but that others, called *bax* and *bak*, function as promoters of cell death. The genes of the *bcl-2* family are differently organized and are transcribed as different spliced forms of mRNAs. The corresponding proteins (Bcl-2, Bcl-xL, Bak, Baxα, Baxβ, Baxγ) have distinct overall sequences. They do, however, reveal domains of strong homology through which they can interact to form homodimers and heterodimers. It has been proposed that the formation of Bcl-2 homodimers promotes cell survival and that the formation of Bax or Bak homodimers reinforces the apoptosis program. Consequently, because of the possibility of dimer formation, reinforcement of the cell death program would depend on the relative intracellular concentration of both types of proteins. However, the recent discovery of mutant forms of Bcl-xL that fail to interact with Bak or Bax but that nevertheless maintain their cell death-inhibiting function revealed the existence of a Bax/Bak-independent apoptotic pathway. It also supported the idea that the Bax/Bak proteins do not promote apoptosis per se but that, if present in sufficient amounts, they are able to sequester the Bcl-2/Bcl-xL proteins and thus prevent their braking function on different cell death programs (3).

THE MAMMALIAN HOMOLOGUES OF *ced-3*

The *ced-3* and *ced-4* genes identified by the mutations as genes required for somatic cell death during *C. elegans* development have also been sequenced. As in the case of *ced-9*, it was hoped that their sequence could lead to the identification of homologous mammalian genes encoding proteins required for the process of apoptosis.

The first CED-3 mammalian homologue found is a protein called, corresponding to its enzymatic activity, interleukin-1β-converting enzyme, or ICE. ICE belongs to a new family of cysteine proteases that have the unusual property of cleaving peptide bonds after aspartic residues (4–6). Peptide derivatives that can inhibit ICE activity have been generated and were shown to interfere with the cell death program. However, extracts derived from cells undergoing apoptosis were not able to generate interleukin-1β by specific cleavage of its precursor, as would have been expected in the presence of active ICE. Furthermore, mice lacking ICE, although unable to generate active interleukin-1β, did not exhibit general abnormalities in apoptosis. Taken together, these results indicated that steps of proteolytic degradation are required for apoptosis but that ICE is very unlikely to be the specific cysteine protease involved. This situation promoted the search for other proteins with similar properties, and today at least 10 mammalian homologues of CED-3 and ICE have been identified. They have been given very bizarre names, such as Nedd-2/ICH1, Yama/CPP32/apopain, Tx/ICH2/ICE rel-II, ICE rel-III, Mch2, and ICE-LAP3/Mch3/CMH-1. All of these proteins are members of a family of cysteine proteases that share the same active site comprising the five amino acids QACRG. Because of the complexity of their nomenclature, the experts in this field have recently decided to rename them and propose to call them caspase-1 to caspase-10, "c" standing for cysteine, "asp" for aspartate, and "ase" for protease.

WHICH CYSTEINE PROTEASE IS MOST RELEVANT FOR APOPTOSIS OF NEURONAL CELLS?

Obviously, given this multiplicity of cascades identified, it became important to find out which of these cysteine proteases exerts a decisive function in the apoptotic program and whether the same enzyme is involved in each of the different tissues. Such questions cannot properly be answered without the modern mouse technology. This has, in fact, been illustrated by quite a recent publication that described the phenotype in mice lacking caspase-3 (7). These animals were born at a frequency lower than expected by mendelian genetics, indicating that some embryos are not viable. The animals that were born died at 1–3 weeks of age. Their thymocytes were shown to have retained normal susceptibility to the apoptotic stimuli specifically triggering a form of apoptosis detectable in the immune system, thus indicating that caspase-3 is not the key cysteine protease in the death of those cells. On the contrary, analysis of their nervous system demonstrated that the development of their brains was profoundly affected. The decrease in apoptosis caused a variety of hyperplasias and a disorganized cell deployment in many structures of the brain. For example, the reduced apoptosis during development of the retina led to marked enlargement of the optic stalk. The results clearly demonstrated the importance of precise control of apoptosis for proper morphogenic events to take place during brain ontogenesis. The severity of the phenotype caused by the absence of caspase-3 is intriguing, because other cysteine proteases (caspase-6 and caspase-7) are also expressed in the developing brain. This might indicate that cascade-6 and cascade-7 are not involved in the apoptosis of brain cells. The availability of knockout mice lacking either *caspase-6* or *caspase-7* should provide information confirming or discrediting this possibility. Another explanation could be that *caspase-6* or *caspase-7* is involved in the apoptosis that takes place in brain structures distinct from those revealing the *cascade-3* phenotype. Finally, one cannot yet rule out the existence of different pathways involving caspase-6 and/or caspase-7 and converging to the activation of caspase-3. This last hypothesis is certainly in line with the fact that many proteases can activate other proteases by cleaving their precursor polypeptide. In fact, sequential proteolytic activation is required in many complex cellular events.

The fact that the abnormal phenotype was restricted to the nervous system revealed the key importance of caspase-3 in this tissue and also suggested that other members of this family of cysteine proteases may prove to be important in the apoptosis that takes place in other tissues. The results may also imply a redundancy of different apoptotic pathways in some tissues.

PROTEASE INHIBITORS AS INHIBITORS OF APOPTOSIS

Given the importance of cysteine proteases as one of the steps leading to apoptosis, the discovery that certain inhibitors of proteases were indeed able to prevent programmed cell death appears to be a logical consequence. For example, a Baculovirus protein called p35, which is likely to inhibit members of the CED-3/ICE family of cysteine proteases, was shown to antagonize cell death when expressed in mammals, insects, and nematodes. More surprising are the following observations. CrmA, a Cowpox protein of the serpin (serine protease inhibitor) superfamily, was shown to block apoptosis induced by different types of pathways in different types of cells. Similarly, SPI-1, a Poxvirus serpin that has an inhibitor specificity distinct from that of CrmA, was identified as being able to prevent Poxvirus-induced apoptosis. Finally, protease nexin-1, a mammalian serpin, has been reported to antagonize in vivo neuronal apoptosis during development of the chick nervous system or after facial nerve lesioning in newborn rats or mice. It is unlikely that these different serpins act at the same level or that they all directly inhibit members of the cysteine proteases mentioned above. Therefore, to explain their antagonistic effect on apoptosis, it can be postulated that they interfere with the activity of serine proteases whose function is to specifically cleave inactive precursors to generate active cysteine proteases. This mode of activation has, for example, been demonstrated for the cysteine protease stromelysin, which is activated by cleavage of its inactive precursor by a serine protease. Serine proteases and their inhibitors could therefore be members of cascades of proteolytic activation in which different types of proteases are sequentially activating each other. Consequently, it can be predicted that many other proteases and protease inhibitors will eventually be identified as involved in the regulation of apoptosis.

WHAT ARE THE ULTIMATE SUBSTRATES OF THE APOPTOTIC PROTEASES?

The cascades of proteolytic activation are believed to be set up to ensure very efficient degradation of ultimate target proteins, a phenomenon with determining biological consequences. The search for these final protease targets, whose degradation will initiate or reinforce the cell death program, is still in progress. In a first approach, biochemical assays or tissue culture experiments did indeed allow identification of proteins that are potential targets of cysteine proteases, i.e., components of the nucleus, such as the lamins or enzymes involved in the metabolism and/or the repair of RNA or DNA, such as the poly (ADP-ribose) polymerase (PARP), the 70 kDa component of U1 small nuclear ribonucleoprotein or the D4 guanine nucleotide dissociation inhibitor. Other possible targets have been found among the proteins involved in the regulation of gene expression, such as the sterol element binding proteins or the protein kinase Cδ.

The case of the PARP clearly illustrates that a second complementary in vivo approach is required to firmly establish whether the degradation of these potential substrates is really one of the key events in the mechanisms of apoptosis. In tissue culture experiments, PARP was found to be degraded during many, if not all, forms of apoptosis. Because degradation of PARP is assumed to have fatal consequences for the metabolism of nucleic acids, the observation clearly made sense. However, mice lacking PARP have been generated. These animals develop normally, and no significant perturbations of apoptosis have been noted. This appears to rule out a definitive consequence of PARP degradation in the execution phase of apoptosis. It also indicates that similar in vivo experiments will be required to truly establish the biological relevance of the cleavage of the other potential targets.

WHAT IS THE FUNCTION OF *ced-4*?

Ced-4 has also been cloned, and the protein that it codes has been identified at the level of the amino acids sequence. Despite this knowledge, no mammalian homologues have yet been found, and the function of *ced-4* in the mechanisms of apoptosis has remained a mystery for many years. Very recent reports (8– 12) have started to shed light on the role of the CED-4 protein. To bypass the absence of mammalian homologues, the *C. elegans* CED-4 has been expressed in mammalian cells and has been shown to trigger cell death. This CED-4– induced mammalian apoptosis was blocked by overexpression of Bcl-X_L and by caspase inhibitors. These results indicated that the function of CED-4 is under control of the Bcl-2 family and that CED-4 causes cell death through activation of caspases.

Immunoprecipitation experiments with a set of specific antibodies have shown that CED-4 can bind independently and simultaneously to CED-9 and CED-3. Similar experiments have also indicated that such interactions also take place between the mammalian homologues, i.e., between members of the Bcl-2 family and members of the caspase family. Indirect evidence has also indicated that the formation of such high molecular weight complexes can occur in the absence of CED-4, suggesting that an unidentified CED-4 mammalian homologue can promote these protein–protein interactions.

The specific antibodies were also used, together with the powerful confocal microscopy, to localize these different proteins within the cell. This study showed that the induction of high molecular weight complexes led to a redistribution of the antigens, which were no longer able to diffuse in the cytoplasm but formed a granular pattern. Cell fractionation analysis revealed that the proteins were shifted from a cytosolic to a membrane fraction rich in mitochondria after formation of complexes. These results have led to the hypothesis that CED-9/Bcl-2, located at the mitochondrial membrane, binds and modulates CED-4 (or its mammalian homologue), which subsequently binds CED-3/caspase and inactivates it. Inversely, CED-4 binding to CED-3/caspase could lead to caspase activation, but this activation would be prevented if CED-4 is also interacting with CED-9/Bcl-2. Only the caspases with a long prodomain appear to be able to be involved in the formation of these complexes of many proteins. This may mean that CED-4 binds certain proenzymes and therefore modifies their folding to optimally present the critical site that has to be cleaved by a serine protease to generate an active caspase. Such a co-factor function would not be possible if CED-4 is simultaneously bound to CED-9/Bcl-2.

Bcl-2, CYTOCHROME C, AND CASPASE ACTIVATION

Other results published very recently indicated that cytochrome C released from mitochondria can, together with other cytosolic factors, cause caspase activation. This pathway in the execution of cell death is blocked by the inhibitors of caspases which, however, do not affect the release of cytochrome C from mitochondria. Overexpression of Bcl-2 blocks the translocation of cytochrome C from mitochondria to cytosol. This also prevents the activity of this apoptotic pathway.

CONCLUSIONS

Obviously, the knowledge accumulated in recent years indicates that apoptosis is an active cellular process that can be influenced by many metabolic pathways. These apoptotic cascades most probably interact to ensure efficient elimination of cells that become superfluous during development or whose functions are impaired under pathologic conditions. The years to come will certainly enable us to determine which of these cascades are most relevant to apoptosis of the neuronal cells.

REFERENCES

1. Hamburger V. Cell death in the development of the lateral motor column of the chick embryo. *J Comp Neurol* 1975;160:535–46.
2. Ellis HM, Horvitz HR. Genetic control of programed cell death in the nematode *C. elegans*. *Cell* 1986;44:817–29.
3. Chinnaiyan AM, Dixit VM. The cell-death machine. *Curr Biol* 1996;6:555–62.
4. Martinou JC, Sadoul R. ICE-like proteases execute the neuronal death program. *Curr Opin Neurobiol* 1996;6:609–14.
5. Kumar S. ICE-like proteases in apoptosis. *Trends Cell Biol* 1995;20:198–202.
6. Martin SJ, Green DR. Protease activation during apoptosis: death by a thousand cuts? *Cell* 1995;82:349–52.
7. Kuida K, Zheng TS, Na S, et al. Decreased apoptosis in the brain and premature lethality in CCP32-deficient mice. *Nature* 1996;384:368–72.
8. Goldstein P. Controlling cell death. *Science* 1997;275:1081–2.
9. Chinnaiyan AM, O'Roorke K, Lane BR, et al. Interaction of CED-4 with CED-3 and CED-9: a molecular framework for cell death. *Science* 1997;275:1122–6.
10. Wu D, Wallen HD, Nunez G. Interaction and regulation of subcellular localization of CED-4 by CED-9. *Science* 1997;275:1126–9.
11. Yang J, Liu X, Bhalla K, et al. Prevention of apoptosis by Bcl-2: release of cytochrome C from mitochondria blocked. *Science* 1997;275:1129–32.
12. Kluck RM, Bossy-Wetzel E, Green DR, Newmeyer DD. The release of cytochrome c from mitochondria: a primary site for Bcl-2 regulation of apoptosis. *Science* 1997;275:1132–6.

Nitric Oxide and Endothelin in the Pathogenesis of Glaucoma, edited by I. O. Haefliger and J. Flammer. Lippincott–Raven Publishers, Philadelphia © 1998.

19

Delayed Retinal Neuronal Death in Glaucoma

Satoshi Kashii

Department of Ophthalmology and Visual Sciences, Graduate School of Medicine, Kyoto University, Kyoto, Japan

Glaucoma has been studied in terms of glaucomatous optic neuropathy. However, retinal ischemia is already present in glaucoma, especially early in the disease state. To determine the pathogenesis of early stages of glaucoma, it is necessary to elucidate the underlying mechanism of retinal ischemia.

GLAUCOMA AND RETINAL ISCHEMIA

Two separate vascular systems are present in the ocular blood circulation. The retina depends on the retinal vessels and the choroid. The retinal vessels that originate from the central retinal artery are distributed in the inner layers of the retina, extending from the inner aspect of the inner nuclear layer (INL) to the retinal ganglion cell layer (GCL), whereas the outer layers of the retina, from the outer aspect of the inner nuclear layer (INL) to the photoreceptors (R) and retinal pigment epithelium, are nourished by the choroid, which is derived from the posterior ciliary arteries (Fig. 1A). Therefore, central retinal artery occlusion (CRAO) is not an appropriate example for retinal ischemia, because the cherry red spot, a typical feature of CRAO, reflects patent choroidal circulation. Total retinal ischemia develops only when obstruction occurs at the level of the ophthalmic artery and both the ciliary (i.e., choroidal) and the retinal circulations are disrupted at the same time. Although reported in the literature (1), ophthalmic artery occlusion is extremely rare in clinical practice.

Recently, color Doppler analysis of ocular blood flow has demonstrated that blood flow in the central retinal artery as well as posterior ciliary arteries is reduced early in glaucoma before visual field defects can be detected (2). The study was performed by a group at the University of British Columbia, Canada, using a color Doppler imaging technique. It has been reported that patients with primary open-angle glaucoma and normal-tension glaucoma have lower blood

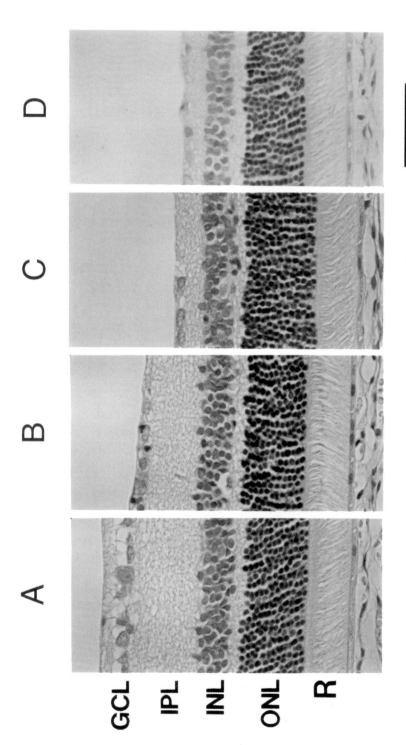

FIG. 1. Photomicrographs of transverse sections of rat retina demonstrating delayed retinal neuronal death after ischemia. Histologic sections were obtained from an untreated eye (**A**) and from eyes at various reperfusion period after 60-min ischemia, i.e., postischemic days 4 (**B**), 7 (**C**), and 14 (**D**). The entire retina was submitted to ischemia, but a selective part of the retina demonstrated marked cell death in a delayed fashion. GCL, retinal ganglion cell layer; IPL, inner plexiform layer; INL, inner nuclear layer; ONL, outer nuclear layer; R, photoreceptors. Bar = 50 μM. Reproduced from ref. 8 with permission from the *J Jpn Ophthalmol Soc.*

flow velocities and higher resistive indices in the central retinal artery, as well as shorter posterior ciliary arteries, than do normal control subjects (3–5). They found that the eyes with normal visual fields and normal appearing optic nerve discs in patients with asymmetric glaucoma had reduced blood flow velocity and higher resistance in both the central retinal artery and short posterior ciliary arteries (2). Their findings imply that all the layers of the retina are subject to ischemia early in the course of glaucomatous disease.

The optic nerve head (ONH) has been extensively studied in terms of the pathogenesis of glaucomatous optic nerve damage, regardless of whether it may be based on the mechanical or the vascular theory, or on a combination of the two. Nasal visual field loss is known to be produced by a compressive lesion at the anterior angle of the optic chiasm, notably with a giant internal carotid artery aneurysm (6). In contrast to glaucomatous optic neuropathy, it has been long known that successful treatment of such internal carotid aneurysms results in marked improvement of vision in some cases of compressive optic neuropathy (7). In contrast, successful surgical decompression of the elevated intraocular pressure (IOP) by any type of glaucoma surgery cannot recover vision once it is lost in a patient with glaucoma. The apparent difference in postoperative visual outcomes strongly indicates the presence of some other mechanisms operating in glaucoma other than axonal damage, which is the primary cause of compressive optic neuropathy. Considering the early presence of retinal ischemia in glaucoma, it is reasaonable to assume that the mechanism responsible for cell death in retinal ischemia must be involved, especially in the early stages of pathogenesis. Focusing on this aspect, this chapter reviews the pathogenesis of glaucoma in terms of cell death, based on our experiments.

DELAYED RETINAL NEURONAL DEATH IN RETINAL ISCHEMIA

To study retinal ischemia, in vivo experiments are necessary. Various methods have been used to study retinal ischemia, including vascular ligation and focal ischemia produced by photothrombosis. We employed a pressure-induced model that has been most widely used. A 27-gauge needle was inserted into the anterior chamber of the rat and connected to a bottle of irrigating solution. Retinal ischemia was induced by elevation of the IOP regulated by the height of the bottle. Figure 1 shows the temporal profile of the histologic changes after retinal ischemia (8). Histologic sections were obtained after various reperfusion periods following 60-min ischemia. The number of retinal ganglion cells (GC) and the thickness of the IPL were more prominently reduced with progressing time after the ischemia. In contrast, the structures of the outer retina were preserved. Although the entire retina was submitted to ischemia, but a selective part of the retina, i.e., the inner part of the retina, demonstrated marked cell death in a delayed fashion. This is the phenomenon known as delayed neuronal death in the central nervous system (9).

RETINAL ISCHEMIA AND GLUTAMATE-INDUCED NEUROTOXICITY

According to our in vivo retina microdialysis study in the cat (8), an increase in the release of glutamate occurs during ischemia, and a much greater increase in the release of glutamate is observed during the reperfusion period (Fig. 2). Serine, a non-neurotransmitter, showed no significant change in concentration. A similar pattern of greater release of glutamate during reperfusion has been reported in the the rabbit retina (10). In contrast, transient cerebral ischemia is reported to produce a spike-like release of glutamate during the period of ischemia (11–13). The apparent difference in the time course of glutamate release may be related to differences in target tissue and experimental conditions.

Glutamate exerts its action through its receptors. Glutamate receptors are subdivided into three classes; N-methyl-D-aspartate (NMDA), non-NMDA (kainate/AMPA), and metabotropic receptors. In our experimental settings, histologic changes after ischemia occurred almost exclusively in the inner part of the retina, where NMDA receptors are distributed (14). Therefore, we studied the effects

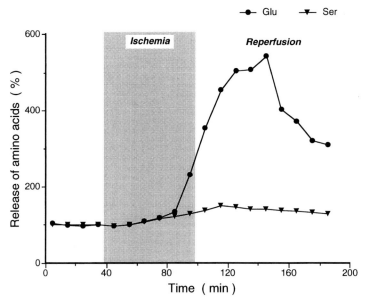

FIG. 2. Time course changes in the microdialysate levels of glutamate (Glu) and serine (Ser) from the cat retina subjected to 60-min ischemia. Microdialysate samples (20 ml) were collected until 90 min after cessation of ischemia at 10-min intervals. Amino acid concentrations in each sample were calculated as percentages of baseline concentrations of samples collected immediately before ischemia. An increase in the release of glutamate occurred during ischemia, and a much greater increase in the release of glutamate was observed during the reperfusion period, whereas serine, a non-neurotransmitter, showed no significant changes in concentration. Reproduced from ref. 8 with permission from the *J Jpn Ophthalmol Soc.*

TABLE 1. *Quantifying analysis of the effects of MK-801 on histologic changes caused by pressure-induced ischemia*[a]

		Postreperfusion day 7 after 60 min ischemia		
	Control (% control)	Nontreatment (% control)	Pretreatment with vehicle (% control)	Pretreatment with MK-801 (3.0 mg/kg) (% control)
Cell number in GCL	104.9 ± 4.3	48.9 ± 4.9	57.0 ± 7.4	91.9 ± 4.0*
Thickness of IPL	100.7 ± 3.6	50.0 ± 8.3	48.3 ± 6.5	85.3 ± 1.2*

[a] Mean ± SE; n = 4–7 animals in each group.
* $p < 0.05$ compared with the group of pretreatment with vehicle (Mann–Whitney's U test).

of MK-801, a selective NMDA receptor antagonist, on the histologic changes after ischemia. In animals pretreated with MK-801, reduction in the number of GC as well as the thickness of the IPL was dose-dependently inhibited (Table 1). In contrast, marked cell death occurred in the inner retina of animals pretreated with vehicle. These findings suggest that NMDA receptors mediate retinal ischemia.

NITRIC OXIDE AND GLUTAMATE-INDUCED NEUROTOXICITY

Our in vitro experiments using cultured retinal neurons revealed that nitric oxide (NO) has dual actions in glutamate neurotoxicity (15). Primary cultures obtained from fetal retinas were used for the experiments. After 7 days of plating, non-neuronal cells were removed by addition of cytosine arabinoside and only those cultures maintained for 10–12 days in vitro were used. Our cultured neurons consisted mainly of amacrine cells (16). The neurotoxic effects of a drug on the retinal cultures were quantitatively assessed using the trypan blue exclusion method (17). Special care was taken to use Mg^{2+}-free medium for making the NMDA solution, and neither glycine nor strychnine was added to the NMDA solution according to findings from our previous study (16). Figure 3 shows typical examples of glutamate neurotoxicity in cultured retinal neurons. Immediately after 10-min exposure to glutamate (1 mM), cell viability did not change. However, further incubation in glutamate-free medium produced significant cell death (Fig. 3B). The delayed response after exposure of cultured retinal neurons to glutamate is compatible with the delayed appearance of the ischemic injury in the inner part of the retina.

NO is synthetized by an enzyme, nitric oxide synthase (NOS). Three types of isoforms are identified. The neuronal type is found in neurons that are primarily amacrine cells in the retina (18,19). Type III is found in the vascular endothelium. Type II is induced by macrophages in response to inflammation. Our previous biochemical study revealed that cultured retinal neurons possess one-third of the activity of adult rat retinal tissue (15). To elucidate how NO is involved in

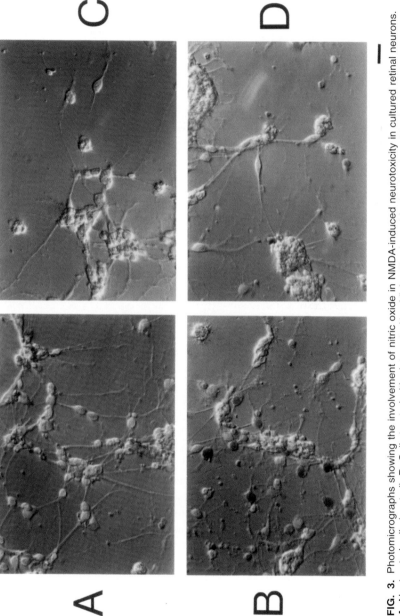

FIG. 3. Photomicrographs showing the involvement of nitric oxide in NMDA-induced neurotoxicity in cultured retinal neurons. **A:** Nontreated cells (control). **B:** Cells treated with glutamate (1 mM) for 10 min and further incubated in glutamate-free medium for 1 h. The cells were stained with trypan blue dye immediately after the 1-h incubation in glutamate-free medium. **C:** Cells treated with glutamate (1 mM) and N^ω-nitro-L-arginine (N-Arg, 300 μM) or (**D**) hemoglobin (Hb, 20 μM) for 10 min and further incubated in glutamate-free medium for 1 h. Simultaneous application of N-Arg or Hb with glutamate inhibited glutamate-induced neurotoxicity. Bar = 50 μm. Reproduced from ref. 8 with permission from the *J Jpn Ophthalmol Soc.*

glutamate-induced neurotoxicity, we first studied the effect of NOS inhibitors on glutamate-induced neurotoxicity. Simultaneous application of N^ω-nitro-L-arginine (N-Arg, 300 μM) with glutamate (1 mM) inhibited glutamate-induced neurotoxicity (Fig. 3C). Second, hemoglobin (Hb, 20 μM), which binds NO and removes it from the medium, reduced the amount of cell death induced by glutamate (Fig. 3D). These results indicate that NO is involved in glutamate-induced neurotoxicity.

Sodium nitroprusside (SNP) and S-nitrosocystein (SNOC) are both NO donors. Immediately after 10-min exposure to SNP (500 μM) or SNOC (500 μM), cell viability did not change. Further incubation in the medium devoid of NO donors for more than 1 h was required to observe significant cell death. Therefore, NO-induced neurotoxicity also takes place in a delayed manner. A radical form of NO readily reacts with superoxide, and peroxynitrite is formed as a result. Superoxide dismutase (SOD), a radical scavenger, removes superoxide. Simultaneous application of SOD with SNP or SNOC inhibited NO-induced neurotoxicity, indicating that NO itself is not toxic but that superoxide is required to see neurotoxicity induced by NO (15). It is peroxynitrite, formed by the reaction of NO with superoxide, that leads to cell death.

When we examined the effects of NO on NMDA-induced neurotoxicity, we encountered an interesting phenomenon. NO donors (SNP or SNOC) at 50 μM had no effects on cell viablity when they were applied alone. However, simultaneous application of these donors at 50 μM with NMDA inhibited NMDA-induced neurotoxicity. The results indicate that NO at low concentrations has a protective effect against NMDA-induced neurotoxicity and that NO at higher concentrations mediates glutamate neurotoxicity (15). According to our previous electrophysiologic study using a patch-clamp technique (20), pretreatment with SNP or SNOC completely abolished the entire cell currents induced by NMDA. The inhibition induced by NO was specific for NMDA receptor, because pretreatment with SNP or SNOC did not affect the response induced by kainate. Therefore, in summary, NO at low concentrations inhibits NMDA receptors and thereby prevents neuronal death, whereas NO at higher concentrations, interacting with the oxygen radical, becomes toxic and mediates glutamate neurotoxicity.

NO AND RETINAL ISCHEMIA

To determine whether NO is involved in retinal ischemia, we studied the effects of N^ω-nitro-L-arginine methyl-ester (L-NAME), a competitive NOS inhibitor, on the histologic changes after retinal ischemia. The specimens were obtained after 7 days of reperfusion following 60-min ischemia. L-NAME (3.0 mg/kg) or nitro-D-arginine-methyl-ester (D-NAME; optical isomer of L-NAME, 3.0 mg/kg) was administered i.v. 30 min before ischemia. Pretreatment with L-NAME restored the number of ganglion cells to 81% of controls and the thickness of the IPL to 85% of controls. In contrast, D-NAME was ineffective in counteracting the ischemic injury to the inner retina. A similar observation was made in the rat using N-Arg, another NOS inhibitor (21). Furthermore, the protective action of L-NAME was also observed when we studied the effects of intravitreous administration of L-NAME (3 pmol to 3 nmol) on the histologic changes after intravitreous injection of NMDA (200 nmol) (22). Therefore, the protective action of L-NAME against retinal ischemia is considered to result from its inhibition of NMDA-induced neurotoxicity.

CONCLUSIONS

Our in vivo study indicates that NO plays a key role in glutamate-induced neurotoxicity and that glutamate neurotoxicity is responsible for the pathogenesis of retinal ischemia. On the other hand, retinal ischemia is present early in the disease process of glaucoma. It has been demonstrated by histopathologic and by psychophysical and electrophysiologic studies that glaucoma in its early stage preferentially damages larger retinal ganglion cells projecting to the magnocellular layers of the dorsal lateral geniculate nucleus (23–28). Recently, Lipton and associates demonstrated that larger retinal ganglion cells are more susceptible to NMDA-mediated neurotoxicity (29), suggesting that glutamate-induced loss seen first in larger retinal ganglion cells by way of NMDA receptors may explain the pattern of loss seen in glaucoma. Therefore, investigations of the role of NO in retinal ischemia will contribute to future understanding of glaucomatous retinal ganglion cell damage and raise the possibility of active intervention in preventing ischemic damage in its early stage.

REFERENCES

1. Brown CG, Magargal LE, Sergott R. Obstruction of the retinal and choroidal circulation. *Ophthalmology* 1986;93:1373–82.
2. Nicolela MT, Drance SM, Rankin SJA, Buckley AR, Walman BE. Color Doppler imaging in patients with asymmetric glaucoma and unilateral visual field loss. *Am J Ophthalmol* 1996;121:502–10.
3. Rojanapongpun P, Drance SM, Morrison BJ. Ophthalmic artery flow velocity in glaucomatous and normal subjects. *Br J Ophthalmol* 1993;77:25–9.
4. Rankin SJA, Walman BE, Buckley AR, Drance SM. Color Doppler imaging and spectral analysis of the optic nerve vasculature in glaucoma. *Am J Ophthalmol* 1995;119:685–93.
5. Harris A, Sergott RC, Spaeth GL, Katz JL, Shoemaker JA, Martin BJ. Color Doppler analysis of ocular vessel blood velocity in normal tension glaucoma. *Am J Ophthalmol* 1994;118:642–9.
6. Farris BK, Smith JL, David NJ. The nasal junction scotoma in giant aneurysms. *Ophthalmology* 1986;93:895–905.
7. Bird AC, Nolan B, Gargano FP, David NJ. Unruptured aneurysm of the supraclinoid carotid artery: a treatable cause of blindness. *Neurology* 1970;20:445–54.
8. Kashii S. The role of nitric oxide in the ischemic retina. *J Jpn Ophthalmol Soc* 1995;99:1361–76.

9. Kirino T. Delayed neuronal death in the gerbil hippocampus following ischemia. *Brain Res* 1982;239:57–69.
10. Louzada JP, Dias JJ, Santos WF, Lachat JJ, Bradford HF, Coutinho NJ. Glutamate release in experimental ischemia of the retina: an approach using microdialysis. *J Neurochem* 1992;59:358–63.
11. Benbeniste H, Drejer J, Shousboe A, Diemer NH. Elevation of the extracellular concentrations of glutamate and aspartate in the rat hippocampus during transient cerebral ischemia monitored by intracerebral microdialysis. *J Neurochem* 1984;43:1369–74.
12. Globus MYM, Busto R, Martinez E, Ginsberg MD. Comparative effect of transient global ischemia on extracellular levels of glutamate, glycine and γ-aminobutyric acid in vulnerable and nonvulnerable brain regions in the rat. *J Neurochem* 1991;57:470–8.
13. Uchiyama TY, Araki H, Tae T, Otomo S. Changes in the extracellular concentrations of amino acids in the rat striatum during transient focal cerebral ischemia. *J Neurochem* 1994;62: 1074–8.
14. Dixon DB, Copenhagen DR. Two types of glutamate receptors differentially excite amacrine cells in the tiger salamander retina. *J Physiol* 1992;49:589–606.
15. Kashii S, Mandai M, Kikuchi M, et al. Dual actions of nitric oxide in *N*-methyl-D-aspartate receptor-mediated neurotoxicity in cultured retinal neurons. *Brain Res* 1996;711:93–101.
16. Kashii S, Takahashi M, Mandai M, et al. Protective action of dopamine against glutamate neurotoxicity in the retina. *Invest Ophthalmol Vis Sci* 1994;35:685–95.
17. Choi DW, Maulucci-Gedde M, Kriegstein AR. Glutamate neurotoxicity in cortical cell culture. *J Neurosci* 1987;7:357–68.
18. Yamamoto R, Bredt DS, Snyder SH, Stone RA. The localization of nitric oxide synthase in the rat eye and related cranial ganglia. *Neuroscience* 1993;54:189–200.
19. Osborne NN, Barnett NL, Herrera AJ. NADPH diaphorase localization and nitric oxide synthetase activity in the retina and anterior uvea of the rabbit eye. *Brain Res* 1993;610:194–8.
20. Ujihara H, Akaike A, Tamura Y, et al. Blockade of retinal NMDA receptors by sodium nitroprusside is probably due to nitric oxide formation. *Jpn J Pharmacol* 1993;61:375–7.
21. Geyer O, Almog J, Lupu-Meiri M, Lazar M, Oron Y. Nitric oxide synthase inhibitors protect rat retina against ischemic injury. *FEBS Lett* 1995;374:399–402.
22. Morizane C, Adachi K, Furutani I, et al. L-NAME protects retinal neurons against NMDA-induced neurotoxicity in vivo. *Eur J Pharmacol* (in press).
23. Arden GB, Jacobson JJ. A simple gating test of contrast sensitivity: preliminary results indicate value in screening for glaucoma. *Invest Ophthalmol Vis Sci* 1978;17:23–32.
24. Quigley HA, Sanchez RM, Dunkelberger GR, L'Hernault NL, Baginski TA. Chronic glaucoma selectively damages large optic nerve fibers. *Invest Ophthalmol Vis Sci* 1987;28:913–20.
25. Quigley HA, Dunkelberger GR, Green WR. Chronic human glaucoma causes selectively greater loss of large optic nerve fibers. *Ophthlamology* 1988;95:357.
26. Chaturvedi N, Hedley-Whyte ET, Dreyer EB. Lateral geniculate nucleus in glaucoma. *Am J Ophthalmol* 1993;116:182–8.
27. Silverman SE, Trick GL, Hart WMJ. Motion perception is abnormal in primary open angle glaucoma and ocular hypertension. *Invest Ophthalmol Vis Sci* 1990;31:722–9.
28. Howe JW, Mitchell KW. Electrophysiologically determined contrast sensitivity in patients with ocular hypertension and chronic glaucoma. *Doc Ophthalmol* 1992;80:31–41.
29. Dreyer EB, Pan Z-H, Storm S, Lipton SA. Greater sensitivity of larger retinal ganglion cells to NMDA-mediated cell death. *NeuroReport* 1994;5:629–31.

Nitric Oxide and Endothelin in the Pathogenesis of
Glaucoma, edited by I. O. Haefliger and J. Flammer.
Lippincott–Raven Publishers, Philadelphia © 1998.

20

Medical Therapy of Glaucoma Patients

Günter K. Krieglstein

Universitäts-Augenklinik, Köln, Germany

Despite the ongoing refinement of our antiglaucomatous microsurgical techniques (1), the majority of our glaucoma patients are still treated medically. In the rank order of glaucoma therapy, medical treatment is usually the option to start with. New developments in this field have essentially broadened our ability to lower the elevated intraocular pressure (IOP). The multiplicity of compounds not only provides many choices but also provides more and more possibilities of combinations. The most difficult part, however, is the question of when to start medication.

WHEN TO START MEDICATION?

Before and during this century the medical therapy of glaucoma has been limited to reduction of IOP. The efficacy of IOP reduction with the long-term goal of preserving visual function is quite debatable in many patients diagnosed with ocular hypertension (2). However, it also appears debatable in a good portion of patients diagnosed with late-stage glaucoma. Therefore, there is good agreement among experts that if there is relevant efficacy of IOP reduction it must appear in "early glaucoma." What is "early glaucoma"?

If there are morphometric findings (3,4) at the optic nerve head or at the retinal nerve fiber layer and if perimetric findings indicative of neuronal damage are present, one can assume early glaucoma with great certainty. Elevated IOP can be self-explanatory as related to the risk for development of glaucomatous damage. We know from different longitudinal population surveys that there is a continuum of IOP and that the risk for development of glaucomatous field loss begins within normal IOP ranges and rises nonlinearly with the increase in IOP. Extensive long-term follow-ups by Armaly et al. (2) revealed that if the relative risk for glaucomatous field loss in IOP below 16 mm Hg is set to be 1.0, it is already 10.5 at IOPs above 24 mm Hg. David et al. followed ocular hypertensive patients for over 12 years, which indicates that the relative risk for glaucomatous field loss is 1 in a pressure range from 20 to 25 and rises to 15 at IOP levels above 30 mm Hg. However, there is enormous interindividual variability in this IOP/field loss risk relationship. Apart from the chances that an individual may develop IOP-independent field loss, other risk factors have to be considered carefully to modify the significance of elevated IOP (5).

The question of when to begin medication can be answered in the following way:

1. If damage is evident.
2. If identifiable risk factors, including IOP, make damage inevitable.
3. If IOP level as the sole risk factor appears to be decisive.

An applicable rule of thumb can be:

1. To begin medication at IOP levels exceeding 26 mm Hg. This, in principle, appears to be justified in view of the safety of drugs we are able to use.
2. To begin medication at IOP levels exceeding 22 mm Hg if there are meaningful risk factors apart from the elevated IOP.
3. To begin medication at any IOP level if glaucomatous damage is identifiable at the time of diagnosis.

PRINCIPAL ASPECTS OF MEDICAL THERAPY

No doubt the art of medical treatment of glaucoma lies in the individualization of concepts and strategies. However, some principal aspects apply to nearly all our patients. Because glaucoma medication is usually designed to be a lifelong therapy, the clinician must consider the costs of medications and the potential side effects compared to the presumed protective properties in the individual patient. Side effects may reduce the patient's quality of life, and primary surgery may be preferable in some cases. We need to keep in mind that multiple medical therapy may have a negative impact on the prognosis of anti-glaucomatous surgery. It is not wise to expect the patient to tolerate side effects when surgery will become necessary in the foreseeable future. If we do not consider these limitations, the patient will respond with poor compliance. It is necessary to respect the patient's specific requirements from the very beginning of medical therapy. A unilateral therapeutic trial may contribute to sorting out the pros and cons of medication in the individual patient.

Compliance (6) decreases with the number of medications. For this reason, substitution should take precedence over the addition of another drug. The drug regimen should be titrated to the simplest form possible, which will be rewarded with good patient compliance.

Defining a successful medical anti-glaucomatous treatment requires a continuing search for side effects associated with a search for lack of compliance. This necessarily includes communication with family members of the patient as well as with the family physician. A written dosage schedule should be provided to the patient, and the patient must be enlightened regarding the drug profile. IOP levels during treatment should be taken at different times of day to evaluate IOP fluctuation under therapy. Discontinuation of medication from time to time may be helpful in deciding on gradual subsensitivity or drug-independent decrease of IOP (i.e., so-called "burned out glaucomas"). As at the beginning of treatment, the patient must be enlightened about the nature of the disease. Alertness to changes in the course of the disease cannot be abandoned.

THE SPECTRUM OF DRUGS

What do we have available to tackle elevated IOP? Miotics have been important allies for over a century (7). Epinephrine has been available for over four decades. Different α_2-agonists and a series of β-blockers (8), recently developed topical CAIs (9), and prostaglandin analogues round up our multifold options to lower IOP medically. Among these medications are different mechanisms of action. Miotics improve the outflow facility in a mechanical way (10), whereas epinephrine compounds improve outflow facility in a nonmechanical way. α_2-Agonists reduce inflow in the same way as β-blockers (11) or topical CAIs. Prostaglandins improve the unconventional uveoscleral outflow routes (12,13). Therefore, many concepts of additivity and drug combinations can be designed.

Among our drug armamentarium are "winners" and "losers." Anticholinesterases, so-called "strong miotics," are definite losers. Epinephrine is slipping more and more into the background (14). Many patients develop follicular conjunctivitis and suffer from a vicious cycle with conjunctival hyperemia from usage of epinephrine over a long period (15). There is more and more doubt as to whether epinephrine constitutes a really effective long-term treatment.

Recent developments in the field of α_2-agonists, such as apraclonidine and brimonidine, offer promise compared to the mother compound, clonidine. However, the test of time is still ahead of us. The new topical CAI dorzolamide frees the glaucoma patient from the annoyances of the peroral CAIs. Dorzolamide offers a maintained IOP reduction of about 18% relatively. It is a good adjunct to other medications. Unfortunately, however, in some patients it causes bitter taste and conjunctival allergy. The prostaglandin analogue latanoprost opens a new horizon of medical glaucoma treatment. In addition to acceptable ocular tolerance, it has high potency with treatment once a day. However, the long-term significance of increased iris pigmentation that occurs in many blue-eyed and hazel-eyed patients has yet to be determined.

WHAT ARE THE PERSPECTIVES?

At this time we do not have a medical glaucoma treatment that does not aim at reduction of IOP. The concept of neuroprotection appears very attractive for the preservation of visual function. Neuroprotection might be mediated by calcium channel blockers, excitory amino acid antagonists, or free radical scavengers, all of which may be effective in reducing ganglion cell death during the disease course. Drugs that specifically improve optic nerve head perfusion would constitute another fascinating concept of glaucoma treatment. Medications to restore original trabecular facility have already been tested in experimental animals. One day a medication such as this may be available for humans as well. Agents to increase mechanical resistance of the optic nerve head represent another concept of neuroprotection. Although still speculative for clinical use, the experimental data are already encouraging. Substances that interfere with signal transduction as related to ganglion cell apoptosis are one more outlook. ''We are not at the beginning of the end but on the end of the beginning,'' as was once stated by Winston Churchill in a different context.

REFERENCES

1. Jacobi PhC, Krieglstein GK. Trabecular aspiration. A new mode to treat pseudoexfoliation glaucoma. *Invest Ophthalmol Vis Sci* 1995;36:2270–6.
2. Armaly MF. Ocular pressure and visual fields: a 10-year follow-up study. *Arch Ophthalmol* 1969;81:25.
3. Bartz-Schmidt KU, Jonescu-Cuypers CP, Thumann G, et al. The normalized rim/disc area ratio line. *Int Ophthalmol* 1996;19:331–5.
4. Bartz-Schmidt KU, Sengersdorf A, Esser P, Walter P, Hilgers RD, Krieglstein GK. The cumulative normalised rim/disc area ratio curve. *Graefes Arch Clin Exp Ophthalmol* 1996;234:227–31.
5. Kaiser HJ, Flammer J. Systemic hypotension: a risk factor for glaucomatous damage. *Ophthalmologica* 1991;203:105.
6. Ashburn FS Jr, Goldberg I, Kass MA. Compliance with ocular therapy. *Surv Ophthalmol* 1980;24:237.
7. Krieglstein GK. Cholinergic drugs in the treatment of chronic open-angle glaucoma. *New Trends Ophthalmol* 1987;2:29.
8. Boger WP. Timolol: short-term 'escape' and long-term 'drift.' *Ann Ophthalmol* 1979;11:1239.
9. Bron A, et al. Multiple-dose efficacy comparison of the two topical carbonic anhydrase inhibitors sezolamide and MK-927. *Arch Ophthalmol* 1991;109:50.
10. Bárány EH. The mode of action of pilocarpine on outflow resistance in the eye of a primate (Cercopithecus ethiops). *Invest Ophthalmol* 1962;1:712.
11. Coakes RL, Brubaker RS. The mechanism of timolol in lowering intraocular pressure. *Arch Ophthalmol* 1978;96:2045.
12. Alm A, Stjernschantz J, and the Scandinavian Latanoprost Study Group. Effects on intraocular pressure and side effects of 0.005% latanoprost once daily, evening or morning: a comparison with timolol [Abstract]. *Ophthalmology* 1994;101(Suppl):80.
13. Bito LZ. Prostaglandins, old concepts and new perspectives. *Arch Ophthalmol* 1987;105:1036.
14. Becker B, Pettit TH, Gay AJ. Topical epinephrine therapy of open-angle glaucoma. *Arch Ophthalmol* 1961;66:219.
15. Krieglstein GK. The uses and side effects of adrenergic drugs in the management of intraocular pressure. In: Drance SM, Neufeld A, eds. *Applied pharmacology in the medical treatment of glaucomas.* New York: Grune & Stratton, 1984.

Nitric Oxide and Endothelin in the Pathogenesis of
Glaucoma, edited by I. O. Haefliger and J. Flammer.
Lippincott–Raven Publishers, Philadelphia © 1998.

21

Glaucoma Surgery for Normal-Tension Glaucoma

Roger A. Hitchings

Moorfields Eye Hospital, London, England

Normal-tension glaucoma (NTG) can be viewed as a subset of primary open-angle glaucoma (POAG) in which the intraocular pressure (IOP) lies within the normal range. Total population surveys have shown a prevalence of this subset in different Caucasian populations of up to 30% (1–3). Because the diagnosis of asymptomatic glaucoma in the United Kingdom is based principally on tonometry, the age at presentation of NTG tends to be approximately 10 years later than for the high-tension variety of POAG and correspondingly more advanced (unpublished data). Although the rates of progression may vary and are often quite slow, most cases do progress, making the condition a significant cause of visual loss and worthy of treatment.

At Moorfields Eye Hospital I have charge of a clinic devoted solely to patients with this condition. We have over 400 patients with the disease, many of whom have been followed for more than 10 years. For that period we have performed visual fields on an average of three times a year, diagnosed progression on the basis of significant negative (linear) regression slopes, and treated primarily by lowering IOP those demonstrated to be deteriorating.

DEFINITION OF NTG

At the NTG Clinic in Moorfields Eye Hospital, a diagnosis of NTG is considered when, in the presence of POAG, there is no history to suggest past episodes of elevated IOP, nor does the mean IOP rise above 21 mm Hg on diurnal curves, with no individual pressure exceeding 24 mm Hg.

ASSOCIATED FEATURES OF NTG

Patients may have one or more of the following characteristics:

1. Vasospasm, with a history of migraine, cold extremities, and Raynaud's phenomenom (4).

2. Systemic hypotension with a low body mass, low systolic and diastolic blood pressure, and nocturnal dips in blood pressure (5).
3. Systemic hypertension with the treatment causing nocturnal dips (5).
4. Asymmetric IOP with the eye having the higher IOP having the worse visual field (6).
5. Unilaterality of disease, the left eye being more severely affected than the right (7).

THERAPEUTIC OPTIONS FOR NTG

Treatment for NTG can be directed toward the lowering of IOP or toward improving optic nerve blood supply by non-pressure-lowering drugs. This chapter reviews recent results of glaucoma surgery for this condition. A comprehensive review has summarized earlier attempts (8). The IOP lowering needed to prevent further progression has been put at 30% (9–11). The recognition that an IOP reduction of less than 25–30% would not be followed by significant changes in visual field decay led the collaborative NTG study to use 30% lowering as the benchmark for successful treatment in its treatment arm (11). Earlier attempts at treatment using both laser and or medical means have not been shown to affect the eyes demonstrating progressive visual loss (8), although the NTG study group reported some successes (11). As a result of these observations and codes of practice The Moorfields Normal Tension Glaucoma Clinic has offered surgery to those patients with progressive disease. This chapter discusses recent results. The success or otherwise of treatment has to be measured against non-IOP parameters. We have used changes in the visual field for this purpose.

ESTIMATING VISUAL FIELD PROGRESSION

Currently available commercial software has relied on methods of detecting global change (global indices) or focal change (by comparing pointwise sensitivity with an earlier determined reference level), or by comparing the shape of cumulative frequency curves of visual function. To assess progression it is necessary to measure both the rate and the location of any change in retinal function. Linear progression best fits the mode of change in untreated NTG (12–14). We have developed a method of measuring linear progression at individual retinal locations (Fig. 1) (15). Progression at any location can be defined as the slope with a statistically significant negative regression slope ($p < 0.001$). Both the rate and the location of the slope can be identified.

This chapter reviews the results of IOP lowering in patients with progressive NTG. We have carried out two studies, a within-patient and a within-eye study.

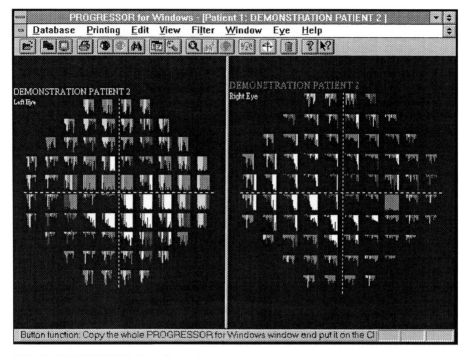

FIG. 1. PROGRESSOR. The illustration of a demonstration patient shows how pointwise retinal sensitivity for right and left eye can be demonstrated in a Windows-based format for management of patients with chronic glaucoma.

THE WITHIN-PATIENT STUDY

Eighteen patients with bilateral progressive NTG were selected for this study. No patient had received anti-glaucoma treatment. The eye with the worse visual field (suggested by a difference in the extent of the visual field defect) was offered fistulizing surgery. A standard Cairns-type guarded sclerostomy without antimetabolites was performed. Sequential threshold perimetry with the Humphrey Perimeter using the 30-2 program was performed every 4 months. The number and rate of decline of retinal locations with statistically significant negative regression slopes ($p < 0.05$) were noted.

After 2 years of follow-up a significant divergence in both the number and the rate of decline of deteriorating locations was found (Fig. 2) (16). This was associated with a significant difference in the IOP levels between the two groups.

The study can be criticized on two grounds, first because in some cases preoperative progression was considered to have occurred on the basis of kinetic perimetry, and second because the worse eye was selected for surgery. Despite these criticisms, the results appear to suggest a relationship between IOP reduction and stability of disease.

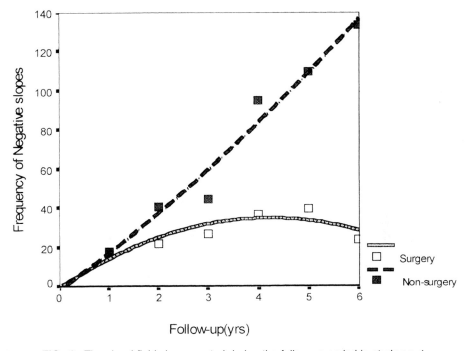

FIG. 2. The visual field change noted during the follow-up period in study no. 1.

THE WITHIN-EYE STUDY

Noting the above criticisms, we repeated the study. We made use of the linear mode of progression seen in the untreated disease. We operated on eyes for which the mean rate of deterioration for those slopes with statistically significant negative regression was known. All eyes had to have four or five fields before surgery. These were compared with the same number of fields after surgery. The change in number of deteriorating slopes and their rate of decline was measured and compared with the pre- and postoperative IOP. We found a significant lowering of IOP as well as a reduction in the number and rate of deterioration (17).

These results also suggested a significant association between IOP change and visual field change as a result of fistulizing surgery. This study could, however, be criticized for the lack of a control group, so that time-related effects were not taken into account. Because of this, we have designed a randomized controlled trial (see below). Not all of our patients subjected to fistulizing surgery maintained a 25% fall in IOP. In embarking on this approach, consideration needs to be given should the necessary IOP lowering not be achieved.

FAILED FISTULIZING SURGERY

Our patients were middle-aged or elderly Caucasians who had not undergone prior medical or surgical treatment. They could be considered free from risk factors for failure of glaucoma surgery. We therefore did not use antiproliferatives for either of these two studies. However, with time a number of patients failed to maintain the 25% IOP decrease. This led to the use of perioperative 5-FU. However, a comparison between eyes receiving perioperative 5-FU with untreated eyes showed no difference between the pre- or postoperative pressures over long-term followup (Fig. 3). As a result it is our current practice to use a low concentration of mitomycin (0.1 mg/ml) perioperatively.

A long term review of the relationship between IOP fall and progressive visual loss has been completed (Fig. 4). This shows, in a small series, that eyes that maintain a 25%+ IOP decrease maintain visual field stability, those whose IOP decrease was c.10% demonstrated visual field loss progression.

MECHANISM OF ACTION OF IOP LOWERING IN NTG

Optic nerve health depends on perfusion. Perfusion pressure is a balance between IOP and intraluminal pressure in the feeder vessels to the optic nerve. Perfusion pressure falls with an increase in the former or a fall in the latter. Lowering IOP, even from within the normal range, appears to have a significant protective effect. This protective effect is also seen in high-tension glaucoma. A 5 mm Hg difference between the medically and surgically treated group in the Moorfields Primary Treatment Trial (18) appears to have been responsible for visual field progression or stability even in high-tension glaucoma. Color Doppler Imaging has demonstrated increased velocity in the ophthalmic artery after glaucoma surgery in high-tension glaucoma, which may be associated with improvements in the appearance of the optic cup. A 5 mm Hg fall in IOP may prevent damage occurring with nocturnal dips in systemic blood pressure in eyes with NTG.

MEDICAL TREATMENT FOR NTG

The studies noted above have suggested that a 25%+ fall in IOP can offer protection against further visual field loss in some patients with NTG. It is the IOP fall, rather than the surgery, which is important. The same IOP decrease obtained by medical means can be expected to achieve the same effect.

CALCIUM-CHANNEL BLOCKERS

Not all patients may be suitable for lowering of the IOP and some may not respond appropriately. For these patients at least, non-pressure–lowering drugs

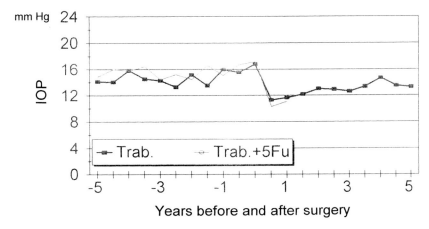

FIG. 3. The change in mean intraocular pressures (IOP) in patients undergoing surgery for normal-tension glaucoma, treated and untreated with perioperative 5-FU.

should be tried. In a prospective study, Kitazawa and associates have shown that the calcium-channel blocker oral brovincamine can exert a beneficial effect on the long-term visual performance of eyes with NTG (19–20). Topical betaxalol has been accepted as a calcium-channel blocker and could be expected to exert a similarly beneficial influence in eyes with NTG. If its effect can be seen to approach that of IOP lowering after fistulizing surgery, but without the risk, then it would become a useful alternative drug.

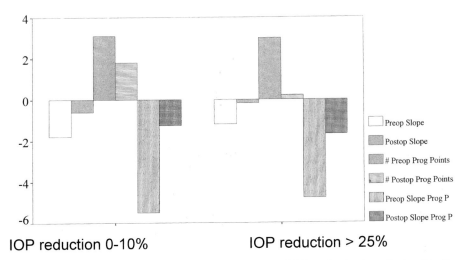

FIG. 4. Visual field progression by intraocular pressure (IOP) reduction in patients with differing mean postoperative pressures in eyes with normal-tension glaucoma.

We have started a randomized prospective study comparing the effect of surgery to topical betaxolol in eyes with progressing NTG. We wish to see if topical betaxolol exerts 80% of the beneficial effect of fistulizing surgery. This prospective study is currently recruiting. The selection criteria include the presence of progressive disease in one or more locations despite normal IOPs. Such eyes will be randomly allocated to either medical or surgical treatment. Surgery will set out to lower IOP by 25%+, and medical treatment (topical betaxolol) will not attempt to affect IOP. The rates of change pre- and post-intervention will be compared.

CONCLUSION

A number of studies from the NTG Clinic at Moorfields Eye Hospital are reviewed. These suggest that significant lowering of IOP has a role to play in the management of progressive NTG. The problems and pitfalls in this therapeutic approach have been identified.

REFERENCES

1. Klein BE, Klein R, Sponsel WE, et al. Prevalence of glaucoma. The Beaver Dam Eye Study. *Ophthalmology* 1992;99:1499–504.
2. Dielemans I, Vingerling JR, Wolfs RCW, Hofman A, Grobbes DE. The prevalence of primary open angle glaucoma in a population based study in The Netherlands. The Rotterdam Study. *Ophthalmology* 1994;101:1851–5.
3. Hollows FC, Graham PA. IOP, glaucoma and glaucoma suspects in a defined population. *Br J Ophthalmol* 1966;50:570–86.
4. Gasser P. Ocular vasospasm: a risk factor in the pathogenesis of low-tension glaucoma. *Intl Ophthalmol* 1989;13:281–90.
5. Hayreh SS, Zimmerman MB, Podhajsky P, Alward WL. Nocturnal arterial hypotension and its role in optic nerve head and ocular ischemic disorders. *Am J Ophthalmol* 1994;117:603–24.
6. Haefliger IO, Hitchings RA. Relationship between asymmetry of visual field defects and intraocular pressure difference in an untreated normal (low) tension glaucoma population. *Acta Ophthalmol* (Copenh) 1990;68:564–7.
7. Poinoossawmy D, Hitchings RA. Frequency of asymmetric visual field defects in normal tension glaucoma and primary open angle glaucoma. [Submitted]
8. Geijssen HC. *Studies on normal pressure glaucoma.* Vol. 1. Amsterdam: Kugler, 1991.
9. Yamamoto T, Ichien M, Suemori Matsushita H, Kitazawa Y. Trabeculectomy for normal-tension glaucoma. *Nippon Ganka Gakkai Zasshi* 1994;98:579–83.
10. Yamazaki Y, Miyamoto S, Hayamizu F, Nakagami T, Koide C. The relationship between visual field defects and clinical factors in normal-tension glaucoma. *Nippon Ganka Gakkai Zasshi* 1995;99:1017–21.
11. Schulzer M. Intraocular pressure reduction in normal-tension glaucoma patients. The Normal Tension Glaucoma Study Group. *Ophthalmology* 1992;99:1468–70.
12. Crabbe D, Fitzke F, McNaught AI, Hitchings RA. Improving the prediction of future visual field status in progressive glaucoma. [Abstract]. *Invest Ophthalmol Vis Sci* 1995;36:S171.
13. McNaught AL, Crabbe DP, Fitzke FW, Hitchings RA. Visual field progression: comparison of Humphrey Statpac2 and pointwise linear regression analysis. *Graefes Arch Clin Exp Ophthalmol* 1996;234:411–8.
14. McNaught AL, Crabbe DP, Fitzke FW, Hitchings RA. Modelling series of visual fields to detect

progression in normal-tension glaucoma. *Graefes Arch Clin Exp Ophthalmol* 1997;233: 750–5.

15. Fitzke FW, Hitchings RA, Poinoosawmy P, McNaught AI. Analysis of visual field progression in glaucoma. *Br J Ophthalmol* 1996;80:40–8.
16. Hitchings RA, Wu J, Poinoosawmy D, McNaught AI. Surgery for normal tension glaucoma. *Br J Ophthalmol* 1995;79:402–6.
17. Bhandari A, Poinoosawmy D, Wu J, Hitchings RA. Surgery slows the rate of visual loss in normal tension glaucoma. *Ophthalmology* 1997;104:1131–7.
18. Migdal C, Gregory W, Hitchings R. Long-term functional outcome after early surgery compared with laser and medicine in open-angle glaucoma. *Ophthalmology* 1994;101:1651–6.
19. Sawada A, Kitazawa Y, Yamamoto T, Okabe I, Ichien K. Prevention of visual field defect progression with brovincamine in eyes with normal-tension glaucoma. *Ophthalmology* 1996;103:283–8.
20. Kitazawa Y, Sawada A, Okabe I, Sato K. Brovincamine fumarate, Ca 2 blocker, favourably influences the prognosis of visual field defects of Normal Tension Glaucoma. *Perimetry Update* 1995;309.

Nitric Oxide and Endothelin in the Pathogenesis of Glaucoma, edited by I. O. Haefliger and J. Flammer. Lippincott–Raven Publishers, Philadelphia © 1998.

22

How Should Glaucoma Patients Be Handled?

Douglas R. Anderson

Department of Ophthalmology, Bascom Palmer Eye Institute, University of Miami School of Medicine, Miami, Florida

On the basis of the scientific information presented here, how, in the end, should we manage our patients with glaucoma?

Science-based management depends on what we understand to be scientifically established facts. Where facts supported by uncontested evidence are lacking, clinicians must still make decisions, and these are based on a working hypothesis of what seems most likely from any incomplete evidence at hand. It is differing ''opinions'' about what is the most likely explanation for all the observations that accounts for different ''opinions'' about management.

INTRAOCULAR PRESSURE IS THE CULPRIT

We probably all accept, almost as a definition of the disease, that in glaucoma an intraocular pressure (IOP) higher than an eye can tolerate results in the type of optic nerve damage and visual dysfunction that we recognize as characteristic of glaucoma. Moreover, we accept that reducing this causal component therapeutically is of benefit.

Of course, there are exceptions. Sometimes the IOP is outside the physiologic or statistically normal range (i.e., the range seen in 95% of people) but has not caused harm to date. We have learned that sometimes such elevated IOP never produces symptomatic harm, so that we may not be aggressive about lowering the IOP—if in our judgment the IOP is not high enough to represent a threat, at least immediately—and especially if available means to lower IOP may be harmful, expensive, or inconvenient. We may also suspect in some cases that the damage observed occurred as an episode when IOP was higher than at present, or when susceptibility was greater than at present (e.g., during a hemodynamic crisis), and that after such an episode is over the expected future course is nonprogressive damage. In such cases treatment is unnecessary. Finally, we sometimes wonder if a particular case is undergoing IOP-independent progressive damage that only *looks* like that produced by excessive IOP, but whose course will be unaffected by lowering the IOP. Indeed, in some of the work presented here, it was noted that some patients continued to experience visual loss after the IOP was lowered, and that their average blood pressure was lower than that in patients whose visual loss halted after IOP was lowered. Of course, there is no way to know if the progression might have been slowed by lowering the IOP and simply not halted completely, so that IOP was indeed still part of the pathogenic equation for damage, but in concept there may be an IOP-independent component of injury in cases that look like glaucoma. Schulzer et al. (1) noted that, in a cluster of cases with clinical evidence of nonvasospastic microvascular disease, the degree of damage appears not to be related to level of IOP.

These exceptions do not change our impression that IOP is nevertheless somehow central to the nature of glaucoma. We note that the classical clinical findings of glaucomatous optic nerve damage result when IOP is raised (in secondary glaucomas and in animals with experimentally induced elevation of IOP), and we listen when experienced clinicians are certain they have seen cases in which progressive visual loss was halted by effective lowering of the IOP, e.g., by surgery. Therefore, without evidence that a particular case represents an exceptional circumstance, we are fairly well agreed that the first line of therapy is to lower the IOP in cases in which the pressure appears to be at an intolerable level.

IOP HAS CO-CONSPIRATORS: IT DOES NOT WORK ALONE

However, we recognize that other factors combine with the level of IOP to cause harm to the optic nerve. Our working hypothesis is that in the absence of these other ''susceptibility factors,'' an eye might tolerate pressures quite a bit higher than the physiologic range. However, in eyes that are made vulnerable by these other factors, IOP-generated forces against the optic disc will produce damage. The IOP may be only slightly above the physiologic (''statistically normal'') range. This is actually a bit of a puzzle, because the physical forces from a pressure of 23 mm Hg (perhaps the average random pressure in eyes with primary chronic open-angle glaucoma) are not greatly increased above those produced by, e.g., 19 mm Hg. Therefore, we now accept that even a ''normal'' IOP of 19 mm Hg may sometimes press on the optic disc tissues sufficiently to produce harm.

The point here, however, is that something that we do not yet fully understand determines what level of IOP will be harmful or how harmful a given level of IOP will be. A more creative statement might be that the level of IOP determines whether or not these other factors will be harmful.

If we wish to alter these susceptibility factors therapeutically, we must consider what these factors might be and formulate a working hypothesis of the pathogenesis of the optic nerve damage in order to interrupt one or another of the steps in the pathogenic pathway. Then we can seek a science-based way to benefit the patient. The purpose of this volume is to display possibly relevant scientific information, with an emphasis on the potential vascular contribution. My task is to discuss whether or not any of this information is ready for clinical application. Therefore, I will formulate in broad terms what currently appear to be the pathogenic mechanisms, explore the existing evidence for the nature of the pathogenic steps or pathway, consider the possible therapeutic measures to change whether or how much the IOP harms the eye, and indicate what further evidence we might like to obtain to eliminate some of the uncertainties.

In considering therapy, we might consider three approaches generally: lowering the IOP, removing the other causal (or, "susceptibility") factors, and interrupting the pathogenic process between the insult and the ultimate damage.

Pathogenesis of Damage

Accepting that the damage of typical cases of glaucoma is dependent on or is affected by the level of IOP, we can look first at the effects of IOP on the eye in the region of the optic disc. It is these effects that combine with or are modified by other contributing susceptibility factors. The level of IOP (a) affects the configuration of and the tissue forces within the lamina cribrosa (and distorts the tissue elements it supports), (b) affects the hydrostatic pressure gradient along the axons as they exit the eye, and (c) affects the transmural pressure difference across blood vessel walls. The pathogenic process probably invokes a harmful consequence of one or more of these physiologic effects.

Lamina Cribrosa Effects

The effect on the lamina cribrosa is a simple elastic change in tissue configuration that results as tissue forces change. We expect connective tissue to undergo elastic conformational changes with body movements and external forces far in excess of that represented by 30 mm Hg without suffering harm. Yet the feature of glaucomatous cupping that makes it different from ischemic optic neuropathy, descending optic atrophy (e.g., from proximal tumor compression), and ascending optic atrophy (from retinal lesions) is that the lamina cribrosa collapses, becomes thin, and bows backward. Does this result from a connective tissue abnormality that makes this specialized tissue disintegrate easily when pressured? And, by chance, does this elastin-containing connective tissue share relevant properties with the ground substance of the juxtacanalicular connective tissue of the trabecular meshwork? Might it be that the same eyes that have abnormal trabecular meshwork and elevated IOP also have weakness of the lamina cribrosa because of a common biochemical abnormality?

In this regard, the recent report (2) defining a genetic defect in families with glaucoma points to a gene relating to a connective tissue component that is seemingly unique to the trabecular meshwork and ciliary body (not found in other connective tissues, which explains why there is not a generalized connective tissue disease associated with it). However, I wonder if the lamina cribrosa has been examined for expression of this gene. It is an old concept that in glaucoma the trabecular meshwork and the optic nerve are each "sclerotic," so that cupping and elevated IOP are simply dual manifestations of a common etiology, without the elevated IOP having caused the cupping. Historically, we finally discarded this concept because cupping develops with secondary elevation of IOP in eyes without constitutionally abnormal trabecular meshwork. Yet in the present day, we might again mull over the observation that the IOP elevation in primary glaucoma is often not so great, and yet the laminar collapse is considerable.

Hydrostatic Pressure Gradient

The hydrostatic pressure gradient along the axon and across the stretched lamina cribrosa is the second natural effect of an IOP that is higher than the pressure in the cerebrospinal fluid compartment. It is the obvious existence of this pressure gradient that made Bárány (3) suggest that an impairment of axoplasmic flow might be pathogenically important in glaucoma. With more knowledge of axoplasmic events, we now recognize that the pressure gradient affects "slow axoplasmic flow" in the reverse condition of elevated intracranial pressure to produce papilledema (4) but that this is a nonlethal effect for the axon. However, bidirectional rapid axonal transport is blocked when IOP is elevated. Such blockage is not necessarily caused by a longitudinal hydrostatic pressure gradient per se but might result from an indentation of the axon if its support structures are severely distorted, and is certainly blocked in any axon segment with inadequate ATP, as would occur in ischemia with reduced supply of glucose and oxygen. Blockage of axonal transport is a lethal injury, equivalent to axonotomy. Without transport of trophic signals from the synapse, the ganglion cell body undergoes apoptosis.

Vascular Effects

We come next to the third effect of IOP, the simple mathematical fact that the transmural pressure difference in intraocular vessels is the intraluminal pressure minus the external tissue pressure, the IOP. As long as the intraluminal pressure exceeds IOP, the vessel diameter is a function of the transmural pressure difference and the tone of the vessel wall. When the intraluminal pressure is lower than IOP, the vessel collapses. This occurs physiologically in veins as they exit from the eye, with the result that, at some point just upstream from the constriction, the venous pressure is just enough higher than IOP to keep the vessel distended. The perfusion pressure relevant for intraocular vessels which, along with resistance in the vascular bed, determines the flow through it, is therefore arterial pressure minus IOP. Elevation of IOP therefore challenges the blood flow by reducing the perfusion pressure.

As has been demonstrated, it appears that the blood flow is not typically reduced when the perfusion pressure is reduced either by elevating the IOP or by lowering the blood pressure. The explanation is that the vascular resistance is adjusted to keep flow constant, a physiologic process known as autoregulation. This term implies that something in the local tissue chemistry reflects whether the tissue is overperfused or underperfused and adjusts the tone in the vascular wall, and thereby its diameter and the resistance to flow through the vessel. Not only the local chemical conditions but also the stretch on the vascular wall and the shear stress of the blood flowing along the endothelium affect individual vessels, including arterioles, capillaries, and veins. Through such a combination of influences, both the volume of blood flow (to supply nutrition such as oxygen and glucose) and the capillary intraluminal pressure (to prevent edema) are controlled. In this volume we have seen that oxygen tension is maintained despite challenge to the circulation, and that when metabolic activity increases during exposure of the retina to flashing light, there is a nitric oxide-mediated increase in blood flow.

The concept that forms the basis of this volume is that somehow in glaucoma the challenge is too great for the regulatory system to handle. In those cases in which the IOP challenge to the circulation is not really so great, we can hypothesize that the regulatory system may be faulty (''dysregulation''), and that circulation is inadequate under a challenge that would have been overcome by a more capable regulatory system. This, we believe, accounts for individual variation in the degree of IOP that is tolerated. Preferential involvement of some parts of the disc may also indicate regional differences of such physiology within the disc(s).

Some of the chapters in this volume deal with pathologic events that might permit ischemia to occur in susceptible individuals. Others deal with the pathophysiologic consequences that are set into motion by the ischemia, leading to neuronal death. Our hope is to understand well enough how the ischemia occurs and the cascade of intracellular consequences, so that we can develop therapy to prevent the ischemia, or to interrupt the agonal cascade of events that results. We should review what we now understand about these things.

Susceptibility to IOP-Induced Ischemia

Our attention has been directed at vascular dysregulation, because ''vasospasm'' sometimes appears to be associated with glaucoma, perhaps especially those in whom the IOP challenge is not so great and whose IOP is at a level we would ordinarily expect to be safe. In addition, we have seen that the diastolic blood pressure tends to be lower in cases with normal-tension glaucoma (NTG) and in cases of ordinary glaucoma that progress despite an IOP that has been lowered.

We have also seen some of the complex interactions and feedback mechanisms that control nutritional perfusion of tissues, some of which involve nitric oxide or endothelin. It is clear that the optic nerve head vessels are affected by nitric oxide, and it can be assumed that these substances are involved in physiologic control of the nourishment of this region. We are left with the impression that when some of these mechanisms are faulty, certain tissues may suffer pathologic effects. Age-related changes in nitric oxide release and in other cardiovascular physiologic mechanisms may, for example, relate to the seemingly greater optic nerve vulnerability with age. We are left to await elucidation of why certain tissues are selectively affected to produce migraine, cold hands, or glaucomatous optic nerve damage.

The reduction in blood pressure during sleep has received attention recently, although it is not clear if the basis for nocturnal hypotension is a reduced cardiac output or a reduced net vascular resistance. Either way, it appears that the physiologic mechanisms of cardiovascular control during sleep may be different from the mechanisms during the awake state. It may not be the hypotension but the change in control mechanisms that make the optic nerve susceptible. We need to better understand how the optic nerve head usually commands its required share of the cardiac output, and exactly how it may not be able to do so during sleeping or awake states. There must be a general mechanism for distributing available cardiac output according to prioritized bodily needs. If there is rationing of a temporarily limited cardiac output, how is it determined if the optic nerve is among the tissues favored?

The implication of the correlation with vasospasm is that when a vessel is spastic, it might may not be able to dilate well enough to meet the challenge presented by the IOP. The vessel can dilate only so much and reduce its resistance to a limited degree, perhaps not enough to meet the challenge. Looked at differently, perhaps the combination of vascular dysregulation and the IOP challenge causes damage that neither would have produced alone. Similarly, a low arteriolar blood pressure reduces the pressure in the reservoir available for use when the IOP challenge is presented. Even with full vasodilation, the minimal resistance that can be achieved may not be sufficient to maintain circulation with the available perfusion pressure. There may be other circumstances that interfere with the ability to regulate blood flow in the optic nerve head. Moreover, even with intact regulatory mechanisms, there may be other causes of ischemia that are moderated by the level of IOP. In any event, we are beginning to accept that somehow there is an IOP-moderated ischemic element to the pathogenic process of glaucomatous cupping, perhaps largely because of the observed association with vasospasm and low blood pressure, although we do not yet know the details as well as we would like.

There are somewhat higher blood levels of endothelin in cases of vasospasm, and levels of vasoconstrictors that by themselves do not cause constriction may make the vessels hyper-reactive to stimuli involved in physiologic control. This sounds like a very logical explanation of vasospasm, e.g., an exaggerated response to cold stimulus. In addition, the aqueous humor has high levels of endothelin in glaucoma, and endothelin may contract trabecular meshwork cells and result in resistance to outflow of aqueous humor. Again, we might raise the question of whether those with mildly elevated IOP also have enhanced susceptibility to damage from pressure, in this case on the basis of a systemic defect that results in generalized excessive production of endothelin. Along the same lines, if there are nerves with nitric oxide synthase in both the trabecular meshwork and the lamina cribrosa, there is a third potential association between characteristics of the trabecular meshwork and the lamina cribrosa, raising again the nagging question of a potential noncausal correlation of IOP elevation and optic disc damage.

We should keep in mind that vasospasm is not evident in all cases of glaucoma and that there may be several ways by which the optic nerve head can become unable to respond to an IOP challenge. In addition, there may be ways for the optic nerve to develop microvascular inadequacy by other mechanisms, perhaps in some cases independent of the level of IOP. In fact, as mentioned earlier, Schulzer et al. (1) found a cluster of patient with glaucoma who had exhibited vasospasm during clinical tests, but another cluster who exhibited clinical abnormalities that might produce nonvasospastic microvascular occlusion or impairment. In these latter cases, strangely, the degree of damage could not be correlated with the level of IOP. These findings warrant confirmation and also exploration of the pathogenic and therapeutic implications of finding distinct groups, not with regard to the cause of elevated IOP, as we presently classify glaucomas, but with regard to the manner by which the optic neuropathy develops. The import is that if different cases have different inciting pathogenic factors, they may differ with respect to vasodirected therapy that might be effective. Antivasospastic drugs may not be the answer for all cases.

Assuming for the moment that the initial insult to the neuron is ischemia, we might review why we consider the optic disc as the site of the insult. From time to time, inner retinal ischemia has been put forth as a potential pathogenic hypothesis, but we always return to the optic nerve head. We note the prominent collapse of the lamina cribrosa, the occurrence of splinter hemorrhages at the disc, and the observed blockage of axonal transport deep in the optic nerve head when IOP is elevated experimentally. No condition of the retina or of the proximal optic nerve that destroys axons results in the kind of excavation of the optic nerve head seen in glaucoma. If a weakness of the lamina cribrosa is not at the center of the pathogenic process, then at least the events that harm the axons must also affect the connective tissue of the lamina cribrosa, which pinpoints the focus of investigation to this region. An unanswered question is how the proposed ischemic events of glaucoma differ from those of anterior ischemic optic neuropathy to account for the different pathologic outcome. Is it the acuteness of onset, severity or chronicity of the hypoperfusion, or that the precise location is slightly different, in one case limited to the pre-laminar optic disc and in the other closer to the lamina cribrosa deep in the optic nerve head? It does appear that in glaucoma the axons are often lost a few at a time, meaning that the insult reaches a lethal threshold of severity and persistence (if these two factors interact) in very small regions at a given time, whereas ischemic optic neuropathy abruptly and severely affects a larger patch of tissue.

Treatment of Postischemic Events

Before looking in more detail at how this ischemic insult occurs and what we might do about it, let us suppose that somehow a small region deep in the optic nerve head one day becomes ischemic. Let us suppose hypothetically that with insufficient glucose and oxygen, ATP formation in a segment of the axon is inadequate to maintain rapid axonal transport or, with a more severe event, cytoplasmic dissolution permits chaotic free radical formation and oxidative stress that might irreparably destroy a small axon segment. If an axon segment does not maintain axonal transport for a certain length of time, a process is triggered to initiate apoptosis of the retinal cell body, because trophic factors fail to arrive at the ganglion cell body in the retina from the axon terminal. (It doesn't matter whether the axonal transport blockage is caused by ischemic or by nonischemic mechanisms.) In this volume it is also noted that oxidative stress itself may initiate apoptosis. However, it is unclear if the oxidative stress must strike the ganglion cell body itself or if oxidative stress to a distant axon segment is sufficient. Some time after axonal transport is blocked, perhaps a few weeks, the affected ganglion cell(s) would disintegrate, releasing glutamate, not specifically because they are glutaminergic cells but because all cells contain a respectable concentration of glutamate that is much higher than that found in the extracellular tissue fluid. When glutamate stimulates NMDA receptors of neighboring cells, calcium influx stimulates a host of calcium-dependent enzymes, resulting in proteolysis, free radical formation, and other nasty events that kill the affected cells, release additional glutamate, and spread the destruction.

One reason for presenting summarily the pathway is to note that the inciting injury hypothesized to be in the optic nerve head may be very localized and minimal, just sufficient to hamper ATP production, but *without* the full-fledged ischemia that changes local axon membrane potential or permeability, causes intracellular or extracellular edema, or causes necrosis of the local axon segment with calcium influx, free radical formation, and dissolution of tissue elements. These intracellular events typify ischemic necrosis, and may be the events that occur in the optic disc in anterior ischemic optic neuropathy or the inner retina with central retinal artery occlusion. If we focus for the moment on just the initial events in the disc, there may be no alteration of membrane potential, so calcium influx through voltage-gated channels would not be expected and neuroprotection would not be provided by agents that block voltage-gated calcium channels. Moreover, it is not certain that there are NMDA receptors on the axons (as opposed to the cell bodies), so even if there is some glutamate release it may not affect the adjacent axons. Apparently astroglia do not have NMDA receptors and would not be injured by any glutamate release in the optic nerve head, although oligodendroglia (absent in this region, however) may undergo glutamate-induced damage not mediated by receptors. The point is that ischemia, perhaps mild but prolonged but in any event very localized to a short segment of axon, may not produce the same result as the more widespread severe ischemia, as suffered in CNS stroke, that affects the neuronal cell bodies. Not all the scientific information on CNS ischemia, specifically stroke, is necessarily pertinent to the kind of ischemia we hypothesize to occur in the glaucomatous optic disc, in which the tissue elements are axons, astroglia, connective tissue sheets of the lamina cribrosa, and microvessels.

If we look at the next pathogenic step, looking at each step for therapeutic opportunities, it is possible that there is no therapeutic means to overcome impaired transport except by providing sources of energy to produce ATP, which means restoring the impaired blood flow. Energy sources or substitutes for ATP might be provided, but how to supply this at the site needed is not obvious. Similarly, one might attempt to provide the ganglion cell with the trophic factors it is not receiving by retrograde axonal transport, but delivery of the trophic factors to the ganglion cells is problematic. One or another of these avenues of treatment may one day be developed but none is available at present.

If we are unable to restore bloodflow and are unable to provide tropic factors exogenously or by restoring axonal transport, we might next think of an antiapoptotic drug. We might ask if the familial tendency for glaucomatous damage might be related to genetic differences in the apoptotic physiology, a concept that might arise from the review of apoptosis presented in this volume. Antiapoptotic drugs may be possible in the future, however, when such drugs were tried experimentally for some neurodegenerative disorders, carcinomas developed, because apoptosis is an important physiologic means by which the body initiates death of deranged cells. We might await a mechanism to deliver such drugs specifically to the retinal ganglion cell.

Finally, following the pathogenic pathway along, protection of retinal ganglion cells from glutamate toxicity is an intriguing idea. However, in models of acute ischemia (stroke), the drug must be administered in advance of or immediately at the time of ischemia. Moreover, sufficient doses of drugs that block NMDA receptors produce psychotic symptoms, and in theory we might have to worry about effects on intraretinal glutamate-mediated neurophysiology. At present it is not practical to consider systemic administration for a chronic condition when one is not sure on which day and at what hour the insult to the neurons will occur, and local delivery is not yet feasible.

BACK TO ISCHEMIA

For present-day clinical practice, therefore, because it is not yet practical to consider treating the postischemic neuronal events we return to the question of treating the vascular insufficiency itself. The other approaches are worthy of continued research so that one day we can have what is presently science fiction, but efforts to manage the hypoperfusion appear to be much more within our reach. It is also, in principle, more attractive to direct the therapy at the inciting cause(s) or as early in the pathogenic pathway as possible. In other words, if IOP and vascular factors are interacting to produce the initial insult, we should attempt to lower the IOP and to correct the vascular abnormalities.

As shown in this volume, we are learning more and more about the vascular events, but perhaps not enough. We have learned enough to be strongly suspicious that the vascular factors are important, enough to have some ideas about how we might improve the situation, but not enough to be absolutely sure of the benefit. Physicians sometimes (often!) must make therapeutic decisions based on incomplete understanding of the disease, because patients are before them today, not a decade from now when they will know more. Physicians must consider what they *believe* (not what they *know*) is best, and because we have different intuitions, backgrounds, and experiences, our ''opinions'' about management are different. But we should always be clear in our own minds about what we know and what we do not know, and therefore we should not fool ourselves about the basis for our choice of a particular approach.

What do we actually know about vasospasm and its treatment in relation to glaucoma? I believe that we use two lines of evidence. First, we recognize a relationship between vasospasm and glaucoma. If we are precise, we do not know whether there is a cause-and-effect relationship or only an association based on some common etiologic abnormality. For example, excessive endothelin production in the anterior chamber may raise the IOP and excessive endothelin in vascular walls of the same patients may produce vasospasm. This is a wildly speculative hypothesis, not one we might consider likely for use in making clinical decisions, but it must be kept as an open possibility by scientists. Equally reasonable, however, is that vasospastic tendency or vasospastic events make the optic nerve susceptible to harm from a certain level of IOP. Therefore, there is a rationale for use of drugs known to relieve vasospasm.

Second, there are reports that when vasospasm is induced, visual sensitivity declines acutely on visual field testing, and that when vasospasm is reduced with carbon dioxide or calcium-channel blockers, the visual sensitivity improves acutely. Here we again must separate our thinking as clinicians from our thinking as scientists. To a clinician, these observations are interesting, maybe even persuasive. As scientists, we might ask if we know the basis for the observed changes in visual function, and whether they are relevant to the process of axon damage chronically. Are the acute visual changes conceivably induced by altered nutrition to the photoreceptors, changes in electrolyte composition and therefore neuronal activity, and do they have little to do with altering bloodflow in the region of the optic disc? As an analogy, we would not fear that pilocarpine would adversely affect the health of the optic nerve chronically because pilocarpine makes the vision dim acutely. We understand very well that the mechanism of dim vision is not a neurotoxic effect. Therefore, to consider the inverse, we cannot conclude unequivocally that a drug that makes vision brighter acutely necessarily has a beneficial effect on the health of the optic nerve in the long term, unless we know the mechanism to be related to a vascular enhancement or protective effect on the axons.

Nevertheless, it may well be our clinical judgment that it is worthwhile somehow to relieve vasospasm, e.g., with calcium channel blockers or with magnesium, in the belief that it augments the regulatory reserve of the optic disc blood flow. However, it may be of benefit mainly in patients who indeed have vasospastic tendencies. Moreover, if the blood pressure is made lower at the same time, the net effect may be harmful. We must ask if there are effects on the cardiac output that either enhance or reduce the circulation available to be distributed to all body tissues. If there is no effect on cardiac output, are some vascular beds more dilated than others and, if so, is the optic nerve head a tissue with increased or with decreased perfusion? This question applies to any vasodilating drug that may have more effect on one vascular bed than on another. If cardiac output is not changed, then a greater proportion of the total cardiac output will be provided to a particular tissue only if that tissue ends up more dilated than are others. Potentially, if spasm of other vascular beds is more effectively relieved than in the optic nerve by a particular drug, then that drug may actually reduce the proportion of blood flow the optic nerve receives. These considerations simply point out that we cannot be absolutely sure from physiologic and pharmacologic experiments that the drug will have the benefit for which we hope. Moreover, some patients may benefit while others may be harmed. Therefore, as clinicians we must keep an open mind, and if we choose to use vasoactive drugs we must be alert to recognize if a particular patient is not benefiting. One day we may hope to have well-controlled clinical observations that will tell us if some or all of such drugs change the rate of nerve damage and visual loss, and if there are certain kinds of patients that benefit while others do not. Until then, clinicians must simply use their intuition about individual patients, and as clinical scientists must be astutely attentive to the course of patients under their care so that their experience adds to the combined knowledge on which we all depend.

Finally, we must be alert to other causes of vascular dysregulation of insufficiency in addition vasospasm. Therapy directed at vasospasm may appear most suitable for those with evidence of vasospasm as a contributory factor, but other vasoactive agents may be more appropriate for nonvasospastic cases. The challenge is to learn more about the pathogenic mechanism, of the several mechanisms if there are several, and to demonstrate effectiveness of various proposed therapies, first on the abnormal physiology and secondly on the ultimate visual and functional outcome.

ACKNOWLEDGMENTS

This work was supported in part by US Public Health Service Research grants R01 EY 9713 and R01 EY 10465, awarded by the National Eye Institute, Bethesda, Maryland, and in part by a departmental research grant from Research to Prevent Blindness, Inc., New York. Dr. Anderson has been given a Senior Scientific Investigators Award by Research to Prevent Blindness, Inc., New York.

REFERENCES

1. Schulzer M, Drance SM, Carter CJ, et al. Biostatistical evidence for two distinct chronic open angle glaucoma populations. *Br J Ophthalmol* 1990;74:196–200.
2. Stone EM, Fingert JH, Alward WLM, et al. Identification of a gene that causes primary open angle glaucoma. *Science* 1997;275:668–70.
3. Bárány E, as cited by Lampert PW, Vogel MH, Zimmerman LE. Pathology of the optic nerve in experimental acute glaucoma: electron microscopic studies. *Invest Ophthalmol* 1968;7:199–213.
4. Radius RL, Anderson DR. Morphology of axonal transport abnormalities in primate eyes. *Br J Ophthalmol* 1981;65:767–77.
5. Pillunat LE, Anderson DR, Knighton RW, Joos KM, Feuer WJ. Autoregulation in human optic nerve head circulation in response to increased intraocular pressure. *Exp Eye Res* 1997;64:737–44.

Subject Index

Subject Index